Small Intestine Disease

Hoon Jai Chun • Sang-Yong Seol
Myung-Gyu Choi • Joo Young Cho
Editors

Small Intestine Disease

A Comprehensive Guide to Diagnosis and Management

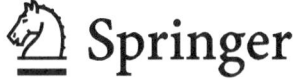

Editors
Hoon Jai Chun
Department of Internal Medicine
Korea University Anam Hospital
Seoul, Korea (Republic of)

Myung-Gyu Choi
Department of Internal Medicine
Seoul St. Mary's Hospital
Seoul, Korea (Republic of)

Sang-Yong Seol
Department of Internal Medicine
Inje University Busan Paik Hospital
Busan, Korea (Republic of)

Joo Young Cho
Department of Internal Medicine
CHA Bundang Medical Center
Seongnam-si, Kyonggi-do
Korea (Republic of)

ISBN 978-981-16-7241-5   ISBN 978-981-16-7239-2   (eBook)
https://doi.org/10.1007/978-981-16-7239-2

This Springer imprint is published by the registered company Springer Nature Singapore Pte Ltd.
The registered company address is: 152 Beach Road, #21-01/04 Gateway East, Singapore 189721, Singapore

I dedicate this work to my talented wife and two children, who have given me an endless supply of love and support, and to Prof. Emeritus Jin Hai Hyun, my wise mentor and friend.

—Hoon Jai Chun

I dedicate my priceless accomplishments to my beloved wife and would also like to express my sincere gratitude to the KSGE (Korean Society of Gastrointestinal Endoscopy) members, who have constantly given me endless support to endure numerous hardships.

—Joo Young Cho

Preface

The small intestine has been uncharted territory for a long time as compared with the stomach and large intestine due to the low incidence of disease and the difficulty of mucosal examination through conventional endoscopy. Since the 2000s, wireless capsule endoscopy and device-assisted endoscopy had been developed and applied to actual clinical practice worldwide. The accumulation of clinical experience of small bowel endoscopy, accompanied with the advent of CT or MR enterography, resulted in great advances in the diagnosis and treatment of small intestine diseases.

This textbook of *Small Intestine Disease—A comprehensive Guide to Diagnosis and Management* will serve as an evidence-based reference in the basic and practical sphere of the small intestine. The comprehensive coverage with well structured five **categories** provides valuable and very informative sources regarding the basics and clinical aspects in the field of small intestine disease. **First**, this book contains the anatomy and physiology of the small intestine, **second**, focuses on the epidemiology, and **third**, describes symptoms and signs of small intestine disease. **Fourth**, summarizes the diagnostic approaches including wireless capsule endoscopy, balloon-assisted endoscopy, radiological images, and so on. **Fifth**, covers various small intestine diseases, including small bowel bleeding and vascular diseases, inflammatory bowel diseases such as Crohn's disease, and tumors. This textbook includes many useful endoscopic or radiological images to share expert's clinical experiences with readers. This textbook has been written by 64 experts with extensive clinical experience in small intestine disease.

We believe that this textbook will be an invaluable guide to gastroenterologists, gastrointestinal surgeons, and primary care physicians searching for a great understanding of the latest diagnostic and therapeutic approaches to small intestine disease. I would like to express my most heartfelt gratitude to all the authors and staff of Springer who have dedicated themselves to the publication of this textbook.

Seoul, South Korea   Hoon Jai Chun

Contents

About the Editors

Hoon Jai Chun is Professor and Chief of the Division of Gastroenterology and Hepatology, Department of Internal Medicine, Korea University College of Medicine, Seoul, Korea. Dr. Chun has established various methods of endoscopic treatment for gastrointestinal diseases and holds numerous patents related to endoscopic diagnostic and therapeutic devices. Furthermore, he has undertaken research studies on the prevention and treatment of functional gastrointestinal disease, *Helicobacter pylori* infection, and gastrointestinal cancer. Dr. Chun has served as Secretary General of the Korean Society of Gastrointestinal Endoscopy and Secretary General of the Korean Society of Gastrointestinal Cancer. Dr. Chun is also a member of many international gastroenterology societies, including the European Society of Gastrointestinal Endoscopy (ESGE) and Japan Gastroenterological Endoscopy Society (JGES), and is a fellow of the American Gastroenterological Association (AGAF). He has published more than 400 full scientific articles in the foremost journals and written numerous book chapters. Dr. Chun has also been an editor and a reviewer of more than 15 prestigious international journals. His contributions to the medical sciences and academic advancement have been recognized with many domestic and international academic awards.

Sang-Yong Seol is Professor of the Division of Gastroenterology, Department of Internal Medicine, Inje University, Busan, Korea. Dr. Seol graduated from Busan National University in 1980. He has served as a leader of Korea ESD study group from 2007 to 2011 and has served as President of KSGE from 2012 to 2013. Now, he works as President of IDEN.

Myung-Gyu Choi graduated from the College of Medicine, the Catholic University of Korea, in 1982, and completed his internship and residency in Internal Medicine at St. Mary's Hospital of the Catholic University of Korea. After obtaining his PhD from the same graduate school in 1993, he served as a visiting scientist at the Mayo Clinic, USA, from 1995 to 1997. He is currently Director of the Gastroenterology Center of Seoul St. Mary's Hospital and Professor in the Department of Internal Medicine at the Catholic University of Korea. Prof. Choi is a pre-eminent leader in gastroenterology, with a particular interest in clinical endoscopy and enteric neuroscience.

He is the past President of the Korean Society of Gastrointestinal Endoscopy from 2013 to 2015 and the Korean Society of Neurogastroenterology and Motility, from 2007 to 2009. He also served as co-president of the OESO 2015. He has served as leader of the Korean Gut Image Study Group during the past decade, which has overseen the National Capsule Endoscopy Registry. He also made important contributions in developing diagnostic and treatment guidelines for gastrointestinal diseases in Korea. Prof. Choi has published more than ten books, including *Clinical Gastrointestinal Endoscopy* (Springer, 1st ed. 2014/2nd ed. 2018) and *Therapeutic Gastrointestinal Endoscopy* (Springer, 1st ed. 2014/2nd ed. 2018). He has also published over 200 original articles in national and international journals.

Joo Young Cho is Professor and Chief of the Division of Gastroenterology, Department of Internal Medicine, Cha Bundang Medical Center, Seongnam, Korea. Dr. Cho first introduced endoscopic submucosal dissection (ESD) and per oral endoscopic myotomy (POEM) in Korea. He was the pioneer of the endoscopic treatments for esophageal and gastric cancer and achalasia patients. He has also developed Hybrid NOTES, a noble technique combining laparoscopic surgery with endoscopy. He has also shown great enthusiasm in sharing information for the development of the Korean medical community. He has always been challenging and innovative in developing safer and more effective endoscopic surgery, winning audiovisual award for 12 years consecutively at the American Society of Gastrointestinal Endoscopy (ASGE). Dr. Cho was able to achieve such accomplishments because of his constant effort to upgrade endoscopic surgery techniques in Korea to the world's highest level. Dr. Cho has been appointed as the next president of the Korean Gastrointestinal Endoscopy Society (KSGE) starting from November 2019.

Contributors

Namyeong Baek Division of Gastroenterology, Department of Internal Medicine, Sungkyunkwan University School of Medicine, Seoul, South Korea

Byoung Wook Bang Inha University College of Medicine, Incheon, South Korea

Jeong-Sik Byeon Department of Gastroenterology, University of Ulsan College of Medicine, Seoul, South Korea

Dong Kyung Chang Division of Gastroenterology, Department of Internal Medicine, Sungkyunkwan University School of Medicine, Seoul, South Korea

Jae Hee Cheon Department of Internal Medicine, Institute of Gastroenterology, Yonsei University College of Medicine, Seoul, South Korea

Dae Young Cheung Department of Internal Medicine, The Catholic University of Korea College of Medicine, Seoul, South Korea

Myung-Gyu Choi College of Medicine, The Catholic University of Korea, Seoul, South Korea

Hoon Jai Chun Department of Internal Medicine, Korea University College of Medicine, Seoul, South Korea

Jaeyoung Chun Gangnam Severance Hospital, Yonsei University College of Medicine, Seoul, South Korea

Jae Hyuk Do Division of Gastroenterology, Department of Internal Medicine, Chung-Ang University College of Medicine, Seoul, South Korea

Chang Soo Eun Department of Gastroenterology, Hanyang University College of Medicine, Seoul, South Korea

In Sub Han Division of Gastroenterology, Department of Internal Medicine, Pusan National University School of Medicine, Pusan National University Hospital, Busan, South Korea

Sung Noh Hong Department of Medicine, Samsung Medical Center, Sungkyunkwan University School of Medicine, Seoul, South Korea

Byung Ik Jang Department of Internal Medicine, Yeungnam University College of Medicine, Daegu, South Korea

Hyun Joo Jang Hallym University of College of Medicine, Division of Gastroenterology, Hwaseong, Korea

Sehyun Jang Korea University Anam Hospital, Seoul, South Korea

Yoon Tae Jeen Division of Gastroenterology and Hepatology, Department of Internal Medicine, Korea University Anam Hospital, Korea University College of Medicine, Seoul, Seongbuk-gu, South Korea

Young Kwan Cho Division of Gastroenterology and Hepatology, Department of Internal Medicine, Gangnam CHA Medical Center, Seoul, South Korea

Sun Hyung Kang Division of Gastroenterology, Department of Internal Medicine, Chungnam National University School of Medicine, Daejeon, South Korea

Bora Keum Korea University Anam Hospital, Seoul, South Korea

Beom-Jin Kim Division of Gastroenterology, Department of Internal Medicine, Chung-Ang University College of Medicine, Seoul, South Korea

Dae Bum Kim Department of Internal Medicine, St. Vincent's Hospital, College of Medicine, The Catholic University of Korea, Seoul, Korea

Duk Hwan Kim Digestive Disease Center, CHA Bundang Hospital, CHA University School of Medicine, Seongnam, South Korea

Eun Ran Kim Division of Gastroenterology, Department of Internal Medicine, Sungkyunkwan University School of Medicine, Samsung Medical Center, Seoul, South Korea

Eun Sun Kim Division of Gastroenterology and Hepatology, Department of Internal Medicine, Korea University Anam Hospital, Institute of Digestive Disease and Nutrition, Korea University College of Medicine, Seoul, South Korea

Hyun Jin Kim Department of Internal Medicine, Gyeongsang National University College of Medicine, Jinju, South Korea

Hyun-Soo Kim Department of Gastroenterology, Chonnam National University Hospital, Chonnam National University Medical School, Gwangju, South Korea

Jae Seung Kim Department of Nuclear Medicine, Asan Medical Center, University of Ulsan College of Medicine, Seoul, South Korea

Ji Hyun Kim Inje University College of Medicine, Busan, South Korea

Jin Su Kim Department of Gastroenterology, The Catholic University of Korea, Seoul, South Korea

Jin-Oh Kim Soonchunhyang University Hospital, Seoul, Korea

Jung Min Kim Department of Internal Medicine and Institute of Gastroenterology, Yonsei University College of Medicine, Seoul, South Korea

Se Hyung Kim Department of Radiology, Seoul National University College of Medicine, Seoul, South Korea

Seong-Eun Kim Department of Internal Medicine, Ewha Womans University College of Medicine, Seoul, South Korea

Seung Han Kim Department of Internal Medicine, Korea University College of Medicine, Seoul, South Korea

Su Hwan Kim Department of Internal Medicine, Seoul National University College of Medicine, Seoul, South Korea

Bong Min Ko Department of Gastroenterology, Soon Chun Hyang College of Medicine, Bucheon, Republic of Korea

Beom Jae Lee Department of Internal Medicine, Korea University College of Medicine, Seoul, South Korea

Bo-In Lee Division of Gastroenterology, Department of Internal Medicine, The Catholic University of Korea, Seoul, South Korea

Hyun Seok Lee Division of Gastroenterology, Department of Internal Medicine, School of Medicine, Kyungpook National University, Kyungpook National University Hospital, Daegu, South Korea

Jun Lee Department of Internal Medicine, College of Medicine, Chosun University, Gwangju, South Korea

Kang-Moon Lee Department of Internal Medicine, St. Vincent's Hospital, College of Medicine, The Catholic University of Korea, Seoul, Korea

Kwang Jae Lee Department of Gastroenterology, Ajou University School of Medicine, Suwon, South Korea

Moon Sung Lee Department of Internal Medicine, Soonchunhyang University College of Medicine, Bucheon, South Korea

Yun Jeong Lim Department of Internal Medicine, Dongguk University Ilsan Hospital, Dongguk University, College of Medicine, Goyang, South Korea

Chang Mo Moon The Department of Internal Medicine, Ewha Womans University College of Medicine, Seoul, South Korea

Jeong Seop Moon Department of Gastroenterology, Inje University Seoul Paik Hospital, Seoul, South Korea

Ji Hyung Nam Dongguk University College of Medicine, Goyang, South Korea

Seung-Joo Nam Department of Internal Medicine, Kangwon National University School of Medicine, Chuncheon, South Korea

Minyoung Oh Department of Nuclear Medicine, Asan Medical Center, University of Ulsan College of Medicine, Seoul, South Korea

Hong Jun Park Department of Internal Medicine, Yonsei University Wonju College of Medicine, Wonju, South Korea

Jae Jun Park Yonsei University, Seoul, South Korea

Junseok Park Soonchunhyang University Hospital, Seoul, Korea

Seun Ja Park Division of Gastroenterology, Department of Internal Medicine, Kosin University Gospel Hospital, Pusan, South Korea

Soo Jung Park Department of Internal Medicine and Institute of Gastroenterology, Yonsei University College of Medicine, Seoul, South Korea

Sung Chul Park Division of Gastroenterology and Hepatology, Department of Internal Medicine, Kangwon National University School of Medicine, Chuncheon, Kangwon-do, South Korea

Yehyun Park Department of Internal Medicine, Institute of Gastroenterology, Yonsei University College of Medicine, Seoul, South Korea

Ki-Nam Shim Department of Internal Medicine, Ewha Womans University College of Medicine, Seoul, Korea

Geun Am Song Division of Gastroenterology, Department of Internal Medicine, Pusan National University School of Medicine, Pusan National University Hospital, Busan, South Korea

Hyun Joo Song Department of Internal Medicine, Jeju National University College of Medicine, Jeju City, Korea

Chung Hyun Tae Department of Internal Medicine, Ewha Womans University College of Medicine, Seoul, Korea

Chang-Hun Yang Dongguk University College of Medicine, Goyang, South Korea

Dong-Hoon Yang University of Ulsan College of Medicine, Seoul, South Korea

Byong Duk Ye Department of Gastroenterology and Inflammatory Bowel Disease Center, Asan Medical Center, University of Ulsan College of Medicine, Seoul, South Korea

Soon Man Yoon Department of Gastroenterology, Chungbuk National University College of Medicine, Cheongju-si, South Korea

Part I

Structure and Function of Small Bowel

Anatomy of the Small Intestine

Chang-Hun Yang and Ji Hyung Nam

Key Points
- The small intestine is divided into the duodenum, jejunum, and ileum.
- The small intestine is served by a complex network of blood vessels, lymphatics, nerves, and muscles for nutrient degradation and absorption.
- The small bowel wall consists of the mucosa, submucosa, muscularis propria, and serosa, with the villi being regarded as the most important anatomical structures as they increase the absorptive area of the small intestine.

Anatomy and Structure of the Wall

Anatomical Division

The small intestine extends from the pylorus to the ileocecal valve and is divided into the duodenum, jejunum, and ileum. Its proximal end is connected to the stomach by the pylorus, whereas its distal end leads to the cecum. The entire length of the small intestine is approximately 6 m in adults, with the duodenal length measuring approximately 30 cm. Excluding the duodenum, the upper 40% of the small intestine is the jeju-

C.-H. Yang · J. H. Nam (✉)
Dongguk University College of Medicine,
Goyang, South Korea

num and the lower 60% is the ileum. The duodenum and jejunum are separated by the duodenojejunal flexure, which is supported by a peritoneal fold known as the ligament of Treitz.

The duodenum surrounds the pancreatic head in a C-shape, and the entire length except for the proximal 2.5 cm is located in the retroperitoneum. Only the ventral portion of the duodenum is covered with the peritoneum, and its dorsal portion is attached to the posterior wall. The duodenum is divided into four parts according to the direction: superior division, descending division, transverse division, and ascending division (Fig. 1). The first portion of the duodenum (i.e., superior division), which is referred to as the duodenal bulb, is enlarged and has no mucosal folds. The second portion (i.e., descending division) has the ampulla of Vater on the medial wall, where the common bile duct and main pancreatic duct open into. The fourth portion (i.e., ascending division) is up to the duodenojejunal angle and is fixed to the abdominal wall.

No obvious anatomical boundary exists between the jejunum and ileum. The jejunum has a slightly larger circumference and thicker wall than the ileum; additionally, the mesenteric fat is much thicker in the ileum than in the jejunum. The small intestinal mucosa is characterized by transverse folds called plicae circularis (valves of Kerckring). These transverse folds are prominent in the distal duodenum and jejunum, but not in the duodenal bulb and distal ileum. Furthermore, the blood supply to the jejunum has only one or

© Springer Nature Singapore Pte Ltd. 2022
H. J. Chun et al. (eds.), *Small Intestine Disease*, https://doi.org/10.1007/978-981-16-7239-2_1

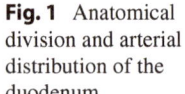

Fig. 1 Anatomical division and arterial distribution of the duodenum

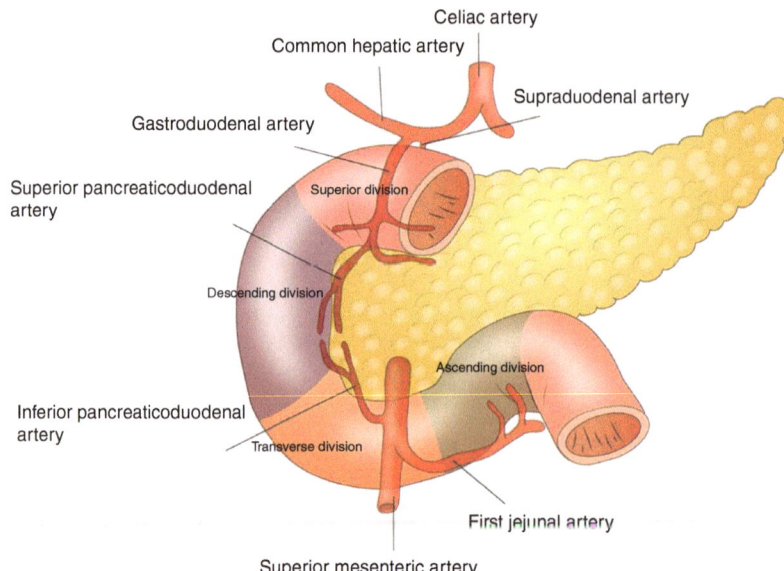

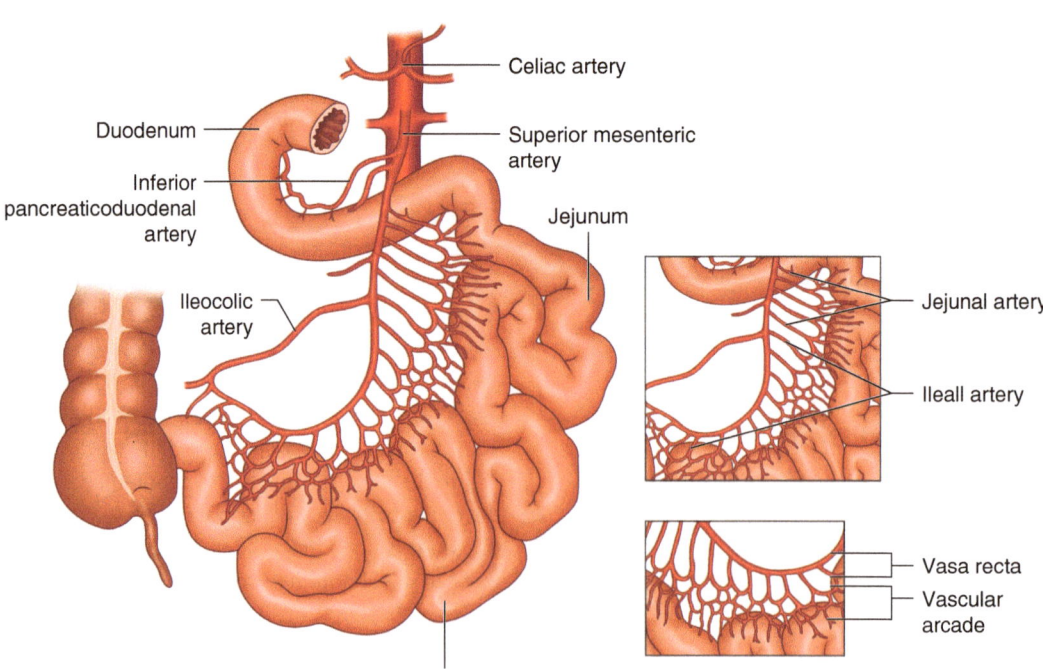

Fig. 2 Arterial distribution of the jejunum and ileum

two vascular arcades with long straight vasa recta, whereas the blood supply to the ileum comprises four to five arcades with shorter vasa recta (Fig. 2). The jejunum is located on the left side of the upper abdomen near the pancreas, spleen, left kidney, and adrenal gland; in contrast, the ileum is mainly located on the right side of the lower abdomen and pelvis.

Structure of the Small Bowel Wall

The small bowel wall consists of the following four layers: mucosa, submucosa, muscularis propria, and serosa, in this order from the lumen (Fig. 3). The main function of the mucosal layer, which comprises three layers—namely, epithelial layer, lamina propria, and muscularis mucosae—is digestion and absorption. Villi are structures in which the epithelial cells surround the lamina propria, and the absorptive enterocytes represent the main cell type of the villous epithelium. The villi protruding into the lumen are considered the most critical anatomical structures for maximal absorptive surface area. The villi are tallest in the distal duodenum and jejunum, gradually shorten toward the distal portion, and disappear from the terminal ileum. Located between the villi and at the base are the crypts of Lieberkühn, which open to the lumen. The villus-to-crypt length ratio is approximately 3:1 to 5:1. The main function of the crypt epithelium is cell renewal, proliferation, and secretion. Progenitor cells at the base of the crypts differentiate into various cells: absorptive cells, enteroendocrine cells, Paneth cells, goblet cells, tuft cells, cup cells, and M cells. Most of these cells migrate vertically to form the villi and crypt surfaces, whereas the Paneth cells are located at the base of the crypts and control normal intestinal flora. The lamina propria is a connective tissue layer with blood vessels, lymphatics, fibroblasts, and smooth cells and is responsible for immunological function. The immune cells in the lamina propria include plasma cells, lymphocytes, mast cells, eosinophils, and macrophages. The muscularis mucosae is a thin layer of muscle that supports the mucosal layer.

The submucosa is a connective tissue layer composed of fibroblasts and mast cells and contains dense blood vessels, nerves, and lymphatic tissues. Meissner's plexus, located at the base of the submucosal layer, controls intestinal peristalsis.

The muscularis propria is divided into outer longitudinal layers and inner circular layers. The outer longitudinal layers shorten and lengthen in the longitudinal direction, whereas the inner circular layers contract and relax in the direction of the lumen, thereby moving the intestinal contents

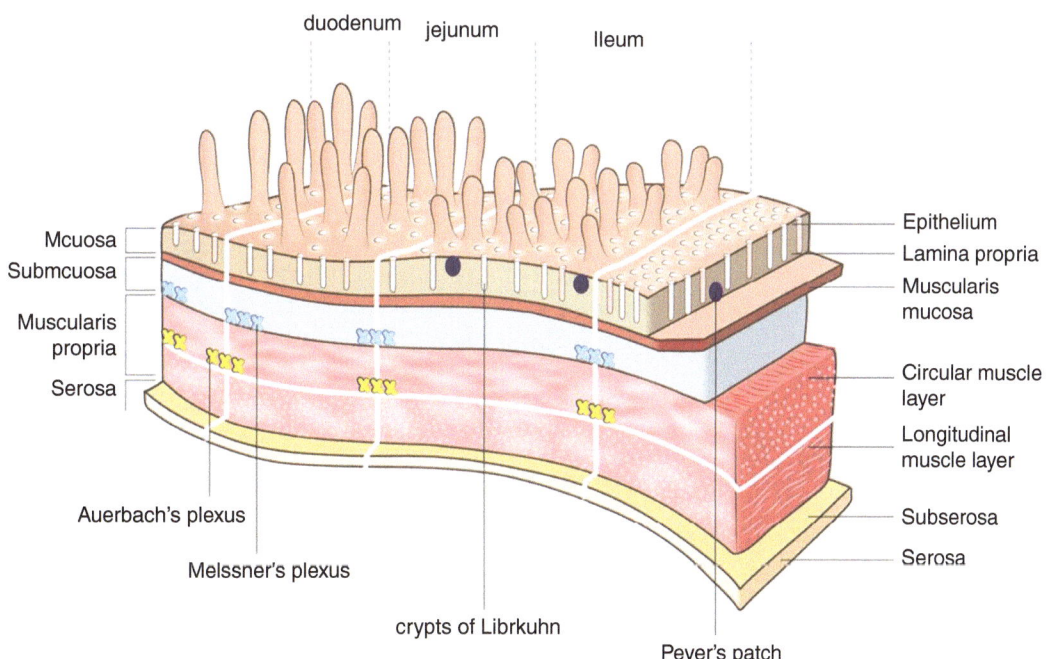

Fig. 3 Structure of the small bowel wall

to the distal portion. Auerbach's plexus, located between the two muscle layers, is associated with Meissner's plexus, which is involved in the movement of muscle layers.

The serosa, the outermost surface of the small intestine, is a structure in which the subserosal layer of loose connective tissues is surrounded by a serosal layer of mesothelial cells and epithelial cells. The serosa consists of the visceral peritoneum, which encircles the entire jejunum and ileum, and anterior surface of the duodenum.

Vascular and Nerve System

Blood Vessels and Lymphatics

The small intestine is served by rich vascular and lymphatic supplies through the mesentery. The mesenteric root passes obliquely and inferiorly from the left of the second lumbar vertebra to the right sacroiliac joint. Despite being only 15–20 cm in length, the mesentery supplies blood to the entire small intestine. Arterial supply to the small intestine is provided by the celiac trunk and superior mesenteric artery (Figs. 1 and 2). The superior mesenteric artery is the second branch of the abdominal aorta, which serves the ascending and transverse colon as well as the small intestine except for the duodenum. The superior pancreaticoduodenal artery originating from the gastroduodenal artery (a branch of the celiac

trunk) and the inferior pancreaticoduodenal artery (the first branch of the superior mesenteric artery) supply blood to the duodenum. The jejunum and ileum have collateral blood supplies from the vascular arcade of the mesentery; however, obstruction of the superior mesenteric artery itself or its main branch can lead to small bowel necrosis. The venous system flows into the superior mesenteric vein and meets with the splenic vein to form the portal vein. Small intestinal lymphatics are characterized by Peyer's patches, which are prominent in the ileum. Lymphatic drainage proceeds from the villus lacteals to the lymph nodes adjacent to the superior mesenteric vessels, and the lymph ultimately flows through the cisterna chyli and thoracic duct to the confluence of the left internal jugular and subclavian veins.

Nervous System

The innervation of the small intestine is provided by the parasympathetic and sympathetic nerves of the autonomic nervous system. The parasympathetic fibers come from the vagus nerve and regulate intestinal secretion and motility. The sympathetic nerves are derived from the splanchnic nerve and are involved in blood vessel motility, pain sensation, and intestinal secretion and motility.

Physiological Function of the Small Intestine

Seun Ja Park

Key Points
- Most of the nutrient absorption in the gastrointestinal tract occurs in the small intestine.
- The intestinal mucosa utilizes the shape of its villi for maximum absorption.
- The physiology of the small intestine involves motion, secretion, digestion, and absorption, interaction between neurons, hormones, and enzymes.

Most of the nutrient absorption in the gastrointestinal tract takes place in the small intestine. The small intestine mucosa utilizes the shape of its villi for maximum absorption. Additionally, the interaction between neurons, hormones, and enzymes assists in nutrient absorption through processes such as gradual movement of the content, secretion effects via serous fluid, and chemical digestion of carbohydrate, protein, and fat. In this chapter, the function of the small intestine is divided into movement, absorption, and secretion of the small intestine [1].

Movement of the Small Intestine

The movement provided by the small intestine is divided into mixing contraction and propulsive contraction. However, all movements of the small intestine induce both mixing and propulsion [1, 2].

When food is consumed, the food is mixed with gastric juice, bile, and pancreatic juice, and the digested material naturally moves with propulsive contraction. During fasting, the periodic intestinal motility called the migrating motor complex functions to discharge the undigested remnant. This intestinal contraction lasts for an average of 4 minutes and occurs every 60–90 min. Irregular mixed contractions with relatively low amplitude occur in the small intestine, except in the ileum. In the distal ileum, strong contractions occur intermittently, pushing out the large fragments. Several centimeters of the direct superior portion of the ileocecal valve are made up of an annular muscle layer, which is called the ileocecal sphincter. This sphincter slows the release of the contents into the cecum, allowing the distal ileum to function as a reservoir. This allows time to reabsorb water, electrolytes, and nutrients. The movement of the small intestine ends in the ileocecal valve, which prevents the reflux of colonic material from the large intestine. The function of the small intestine is to control the rate of nutrient uptake.

S. J. Park (✉)
Division of Gastroenterology, Department of Internal Medicine, Kosin University Gospel Hospital, Pusan, South Korea

© Springer Nature Singapore Pte Ltd. 2022
H. J. Chun et al. (eds.), *Small Intestine Disease*, https://doi.org/10.1007/978-981-16-7239-2_2

Absorption of Small Intestine (Fig. 1)

In the small intestine, hundreds of grams of car-bohydrate, approximately 100 grams of fat, approximately 50–100 grams of amino acid, approximately 50–100 grams of ion, and 7–8 L of water is absorbed. Approximately 1 L of the unabsorbed contents moves to the large intestine. However, it is known that the absorption capacity of the normal small intestine is much larger than this.

Nutrient Absorption

Fat Absorption

Fat is digested and absorbed differently than other nutrients through an intestinal digestion process, mucosal absorption process, and post-absorption transport process. If any of these processes is dis-rupted, steatorrhea occurs. The digestion process can be divided into the processes of lipolysis and micelle formation. Fat is broken down into fatty acid, monoglyceride, and glycerol by lipase and colipase in the stomach, duodenum, and proximal jejunum. The degraded material reaches the sur-face of chorionic epithelial cells in the form of an aqueous mixed micelle. The process of mucosal absorption is mainly performed by passive diffu-sion. For absorption after migration, the degraded material should be in chylomicron form. This 'transport' function by micelle is essential for fat absorption. Approximately 97% of fat is absorbed when there are enough micelles; however, with-out enough micelles, only approximately 40–50% of fat is absorbed. Chylomicrons are absorbed into the lymphatic system, and not into the portal vein.

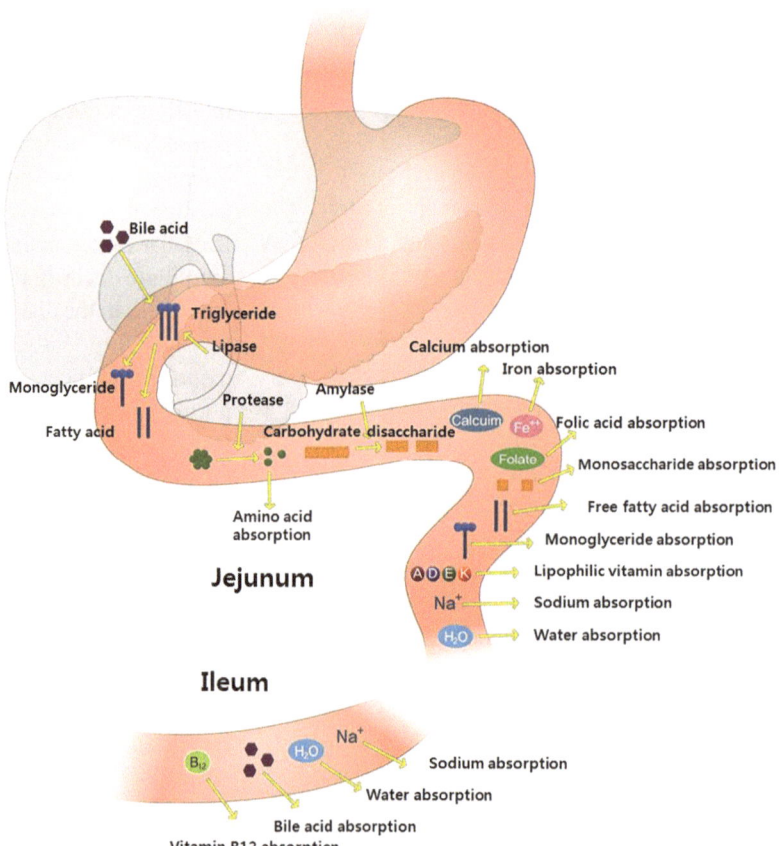

Fig. 1 Absorption of small intestine

Direct Absorption of Fatty Acids through the Portal Vein

In general, lipid digestion products are absorbed through lymphatic circulation after conversion into triglycerides in epithelial cells. Small amounts of fatty acids are absorbed directly into the portal vein via capillaries. The reason for this phenomenon is that, unlike long-chain fatty acids, short-chain fatty acids are relatively water-soluble, and thus, are not converted into triglycerides through the endoplasmic reticulum. Therefore, short-chain fatty acids pass through the epithelial cells and are absorbed directly into the capillaries of the intestinal villi [1, 3].

Monosaccharides: The Primary Absorption Form of Carbohydrates

Dietary carbohydrates are present in the form of starch, disaccharides, and glucose. Carbohydrates are also absorbed in the form of monosaccharides, but only in the small intestine. The most common form of monosaccharide is glucose, which accounts for approximately 80% of the total calories produced by carbohydrates. The remaining 20% are fructose, which is the degraded product of galactose (a component of milk) and sugar. All monosaccharides are absorbed through an active movement process. Lactose is a disaccharide present in milk; it is degraded into glucose and galactose by lactase. In most people, lactase activity is maintained lifelong, but when lactase activity is reduced or deficient, people can exhibit symptoms of lactose intolerance.

Glucose Absorption

Without the transfer of sodium through the serous membranes, glucose cannot be absorbed. This is because when sodium moves, glucose is co-transported and moves together with sodium. When sodium moves into the intercellular space through the basal membrane of the epithelial cells, energy is released to move glucose through the cell membrane.

Galactose Absorption

Galactose is absorbed similarly to glucose. However, fructose is not absorbed through the sodium co-transport process but is instead absorbed through the epithelial cells by facilitated diffusion. Most of the fructose is converted to glucose by phosphorylation and passing through the cell membrane, and then absorbed into the blood. Since fructose is not co-transported with sodium, the rate of transportation is only half that of glucose or galactose.

Proteins Absorbed in Dipeptides, Tripeptides, and Amino Acid Form

Most dietary protein is in the form of a polypeptide. Thus, for absorption, it must be broken down into amino acids, dipeptides, and tripeptides,in the stomach and small intestine. This is accomplished by pepsinogen, trypsinogen, and proteinase. Protein degradation products are also absorbed through the same reaction as that of sodium co-transportation that occurs in glucose absorption. When peptides or amino acids bind to specific transport proteins and sodium, they are absorbed into the epithelial cells through microvilli [1, 4].

Absorption of Water by Osmosis

Water is absorbed through the intestinal wall by diffusion through osmosis. Accordingly, when the chyme is appropriately diluted, water is absorbed into the blood vessels of villi by osmosis. Conversely, water can also move from the plasma to the chyme, which is different from the way it is absorbed. This phenomenon occurs when the hyper-osmotic fluid passes from the stomach to the duodenum. In this case, the water in the plasma moves to the chyme within a few minutes, and the chyme becomes isosmotic.

Ion Absorption

Bicarbonate Absorption In the Duodenum and Jejunum

Since a large amount of bicarbonate is secreted through the pancreatic and bile juice, it is reabsorbed in the upper part of the small intestine. The exchanged hydrogen ions released into the digestive tract when sodium ions are absorbed bind to bicarbonate ions to form carbonic acid (H_2CO_3), which then dissociates into water and carbon dioxide. A mixture of water and the chyme remains in the bowels, but carbon dioxide is rapidly absorbed into the blood and excreted through the lungs.

Absorption at Ileum

The proximal small intestine absorbs most of the nutrients and minerals, while the ileum absorbs vitamin B12 and bile.

Active Transport of Sodium

On average, we consume 5–8 g of sodium per day, and approximately 20–30 g of sodium is secreted from the intestines. To prevent loss of sodium in the feces, the intestinal tract absorbs approximately 25–35 g of sodium, which is approximately 1/seventh of the total body sodium. When the loss of sodium is very high due to severe diarrhea, the amount of sodium in our body can be lowered to a life-threatening amount within a few hours. However, since most sodium is rapidly absorbed in the intestines, the final fecal loss of sodium is only approximately 0.5%. The absorption of sodium in the small intestine is primarily through electrical means, and absorption occurs in the apical membrane. Active transport proteins present in apical membranes allow the absorption of sodium to be coupled to monosaccharides. Therefore, sodium is also important for absorbing glucose and amino acids. Some sodium is absorbed together with chloride ions. Since sodium ions are cations and chloride ions are anions, they are "attracted" by electrical forces [5].

Active Absorption of Calcium, Iron, Potassium, Magnesium, and Phosphorus

Absorption of calcium ions is regulated by vitamin D and parathyroid hormone secreted from the parathyroid glands. They are absorbed in the duodenum only as much as is necessary for our body. Iron ions are also actively absorbed in the small intestine. Many small ions, including potassium, magnesium, and phosphorus, are also actively absorbed through the intestinal mucosa.

Secretory Function of Small Intestine

Mucus Secretion

The wider distribution of the mixed glands is called the Brunner gland, which is located between the duodenal bulb and papilla of Vater. This gland secretes a large amount of alkaline mucus to prevent digestion of the duodenal wall due to the high concentration of acidic gastric juice released from the stomach. In addition, mucus contains a large amount of bicarbonate ions that combine with the bicarbonate ions of the pancreatic juice and liver bile to neutralize the stomach's hydrochloric acid entering the duodenum [5, 6].

Secretion of Bile Acid

Generally, approximately 500 mg of bile acid is produced in the liver and secreted into the duodenum in the form of bile. Secreted bile acid helps in the digestion and absorption of fat in the proximal small intestine.

Gastrointestinal Secretion

The small depressions over the entire surface of the small intestine are called the crypts of Lieberkuhn, which are located between the villi. The surface of both the crypts and villi are covered with goblet cells and enterocytes. Goblet cells secrete mucus to lubricate and protect the surface of the gut. The enterocytes secrete large amounts of water and electrolytes in the crypts. They allow water and electrolytes to be reabsorbed along with the digestive end products on the entire surface of the adjacent villi. Approximately 1800 mL per day intestinal secretions is performed by enterocytes.

Digestive Enzyme

The enterocytes of the mucous membranes covering the villi help absorption of certain food through digestive enzymes. [1] Peptidase breaks down small peptides into amino acids [2]. The four enzymes, sucrase, maltase, isomaltase, and lactase, break down disaccharides into monosaccharides [3]. A small amount of intestinal lipase converts triglycerides to glycerols and fatty acids [1].

References

1. Hall JE. Textbook of Medical Physiology. 12th ed. Philadelphia, PA: Elsevier; 2011.
2. Grundy D, Al-Chaer ED, Aziz Q, et al. Fundamentals of neurogastroenterology: basic science. Gastroenterology. 2006;130:1391–411.
3. Black DD. Development and physiological regulation of intestinal lipid absorption. I. Development of intestinal lipid absorption: cellular events in chylomicron assembly and secretion. Am J Physiol Gastrointest Liver Physiol. 2007;293:G519–24.
4. Broer S. Amino acid transport across mammalian intestinal and renal epithelia. Physiol Rev. 2008;88:249–86.
5. Barrett KE. New ways of thinking about (and teaching about) intestinal epithelial function. Adv Physiol Educ. 2008;32:25–34.
6. Allen A, Flemstrom G. Gastroduodenal mucus bicarbonate barrier: protection against acid and pepsin. Am J Physiol Cell Physiol. 2005;288:C1–19.

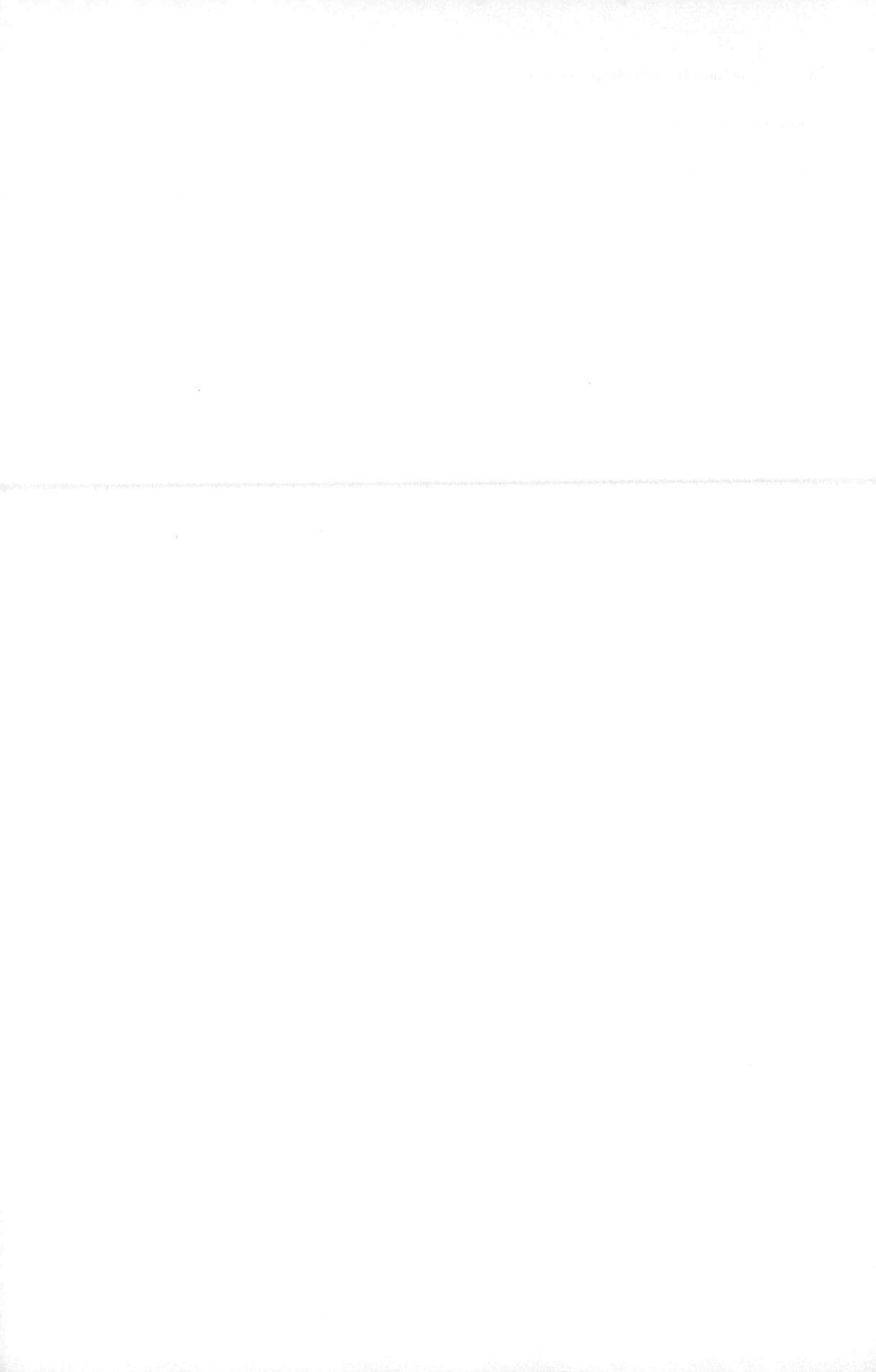

Part II

Epidemiology of Small Bowel Diseases

Small-bowel Bleeding

Seung-Joo Nam

Key Points

- The common and representative diseases that can cause small-bowel bleeding include angiodysplasia, small-bowel ulcer/inflammation, and small-bowel neoplasia.
- The cause of small-bowel bleeding varies with age.
- For overt obscure gastrointestinal bleeding, it is desirable to perform a small-bowel endoscopy (capsule endoscopy or deep enteroscopy) as soon as possible for an accurate diagnosis.

Small-bowel bleeding is an uncommon disease that accounts for 5–10% of all gastrointestinal bleeding cases [1]. With the development of capsule endoscopy and deep enteroscopy, most of the cases (~75%) of obscure gastrointestinal bleeding in the past have been identified as small-bowel bleeding [1]. The purpose of this chapter is to discuss the distribution and frequency of lesions causing small-bowel bleeding and the diagnostic yield of small-bowel evaluation according to clinical presentations.

S.-J. Nam (✉)
Department of Internal Medicine, Kangwon National University School of Medicine,
Chuncheon, South Korea

Causes and Prevalence of Small-bowel Bleeding

There are various lesions that can cause bleeding in the small intestine. Typically, they include (i) vascular lesions such as angiodysplasia and Dieulafoy's lesion; (ii) neoplastic lesions such as lymphoma, adenocarcinoma, neuroendocrine tumor, and leiomyoma; and (iii) inflammatory lesions such as ulcers, vasculitis, Crohn's disease, and non-steroidal anti-inflammatory drug (NSAID) enteritis. In addition to these representative conditions, there are various lesions that can cause small-bowel bleeding, such as diverticulum, infection, and amyloidosis.

Vascular lesion (angiodysplasia) is the most common cause of small-bowel bleeding diagnosed by capsule endoscopy or deep enteroscopy, followed by inflammatory lesions and neoplastic lesions [1]. However, the causes of small-bowel bleeding are different according to the patients' age. Crohn's disease and Meckel's diverticulum are frequent causes of small-bowel bleeding in patients aged 40 years or younger. Vascular lesions, including angioectasia or erosions/ulcers associated with NSAID use, are common in those older than 40 years [1]. Dieulafoy's lesions can occur at any age; however, the mean age of presentation is known to be the fifth decade of life [2]. Small-bowel neoplasms are usually diagnosed in patients in their 40s and 60s, on average, although the mean age differs according to the histologic diagnosis [3]. The causes of small-bowel bleeding are summarized in Table 1.

© Springer Nature Singapore Pte Ltd. 2022
H. J. Chun et al. (eds.), *Small Intestine Disease*, https://doi.org/10.1007/978-981-16-7239-2_3

Table 1 Causes of small-bowel bleeding [1]

Common causes		Uncommon causes
Patients aged <40 years	Patients aged >40 years	
• Inflammatory bowel disease. • Neoplasia. • Dieulafoy's lesion. • Meckel's diverticulum. • Polyposis syndromes.	• Angioectasia. • NSAID ulcer. • Neoplasia. • Dieulafoy's lesion.	• Vasculitis (e.g., Henoch-Schönlein purpura). • Small-bowel varices/portal hypertensive enteropathy. • Amyloidosis. • Radiation enteritis. • Mesenteric ischemia. • Endometriosis. • Intestinal infestation by worms. • Aorto-enteric fistula. • Hemobilia. • Inherited polyposis syndromes. • Osler-Weber-Rendu syndrome. • Kaposi's sarcoma with AIDS. • Plummer-Vinson syndrome. • Ehlers-Danlos syndrome. • Malignant atrophic papulosis. • Blue rubber bleb nevus syndrome. • Pseudoxanthoma elasticum.

NSAID non-steroidal anti-inflammatory drug, *AIDS* acquired immunodeficiency syndrome
Modified from Gerson et al. [1]

Table 2 Causes of small-bowel bleeding by age according to the Korean Capsule Endoscopy Nationwide Database Registry (modified from Song et al.) [4]

	< 30 years	30–39 years	40–49 years	50–59 years	60–69 years	70–79 years	≥ 80 years
Angiodysplasia	14.2%	7.2%	13.5%	15.6%	19.7%	20.8%	34.2%
Other vascular diseases	2.2%	2.6%	3.5%	1.3%	1.5%	2.2%	2.7%
Crohn's disease	12.0%	9.7%	1.7%	1.9%	1.2%	0.3%	0%
NSAID enteropathy	3.8%	3.6%	6.6%	7.5%	9.6%	9.4%	8.7%
Small-bowel ulcer	6.6%	3.6%	12.2%	11.1%	10.8%	14.7%	11.4%
Other inflammatory diseases	4.9%	10.8%	3.8%	8.9%	7.6%	5.5%	1.3%
Small-bowel neoplasia	2.2%	5.1%	4.2%	6.2%	4.2%	3.6%	4.0%
Diverticular disease	6.0%	1.5%	0%	1.1%	0.5%	0.3%	0.7%
Disease outside the small bowel	6.6%	8.7%	5.9%	9.4%	7.9%	6.4%	9.4%
Other disease	0.5%	0.5%	0.3%	0.8%	1.5%	0.6%	1.3%
Obscure gastrointestinal bleeding	41.0%	46.7%	48.3%	36.1%	35.5%	36.3%	26.2%
Total	100%	100%	100%	100%	100%	100%	100%

NSAID non-steroidal anti-inflammatory drug

Table 2 shows the causes of small-bowel bleeding for each age group identified by the Korean Capsule Endoscopy Nationwide Database Registry [4].

Epidemiological differences in small-bowel bleeding according to race or ethnicity have not been extensively studied; however, vascular lesions are more common in Western countries, and inflammatory lesions are more common in Eastern countries [5]. Recently, capsule endoscopy registry data analyzed in Korea over 10 years showed similar tendencies, with a prevalence of 28.5% for inflammatory lesions, 15.3% for vascular lesions, and 9.5% for tumors [6].

Diagnostic Yield According to Clinical Manifestations of Small-bowel Bleeding

According to clinical manifestation, gastrointestinal bleeding is divided into "overt," which accompanies gross bleeding such as hematochezia, melena, and hematemesis, and "occult," which may accompany iron deficiency anemia and/or a positive fecal occult blood test but without gross bleeding recognized by the patient or a doctor. The diagnostic yields of small-bowel bleeding differ according to these manifestations.

Capsule endoscopy or deep enteroscopy shows higher diagnostic yield in patients with overt small-bowel bleeding than in those with occult bleeding [1]. In addition, in patients with overt bleeding, the diagnostic yield decreases continuously as the interval between the time of bleeding and the test becomes longer. In a study of capsule endoscopy in patients with obscure gastrointestinal bleeding, the diagnostic yield decreased as follows: 92% when overt bleeding persisted, 67% after 10–14 days, and 33% after 3–4 weeks [7]. In this study, the diagnostic yield of occult bleeding was 44%. A study with double-balloon enteroscopy also showed similar results [8]. Therefore, the European Society of Gastrointestinal Endoscopy and the Japanese Gastroenterological Endoscopy Society recommend capsule endoscopy to be performed within 14 days in patients with overt obscure gastrointestinal bleeding [9, 10]. However, as some studies have shown that capsule endoscopy performed within 2 or 3 days in patients with overt obscure gastrointestinal bleeding can significantly increase the diagnostic yield, it is desirable to proceed with capsule endoscopy or deep enteroscopy as soon as possible after the onset of overt obscure bleeding. The capsule endoscopy guideline developed by the Korean

Society of Gastrointestinal Endoscopy also recommends performing capsule endoscopy as soon as possible from the time of bleeding onset [11].

Remark

Small-bowel bleeding has various causes; it has a different distribution according to the patients' age. With this knowledge in mind, detailed history taking on patients' past history, family history, and medications can help in the diagnosis and management.

In addition, for an accurate diagnosis, it is desirable to perform small bowel evaluation as soon as possible in patients with overt obscure gastrointestinal bleeding.

References

1. Gerson LB, Fidler JL, Cave DR, Leighton JA. ACG clinical guideline: diagnosis and management of small bowel bleeding. Am J Gastroenterol. 2015;110:1265–87. quiz 1288
2. Jeon HK, Kim GH. Endoscopic management of Dieulafoy's lesion. Clin Endosc. 2015;48:112–20.
3. Cangemi DJ, Patel MK, Gomez V, Cangemi JR, Stark ME, Lukens FJ. Small bowel tumors discovered during double-balloon enteroscopy: analysis of a large prospectively collected single-center database. J Clin Gastroenterol. 2013;47:769–72.
4. Song JH, Hong SN, Chang DK, et al. The etiology of potential small-bowel bleeding depending on patient's age and gender. United European Gastroenterol J. 2018;6:1169–78.
5. Xin L, Liao Z, Jiang YP, Li ZS. Indications, detectability, positive findings, total enteroscopy, and complications of diagnostic double-balloon endoscopy: a systematic review of data over the first decade of use. Gastrointest Endosc. 2011;74:563–70.
6. Lim YJ, Lee OY, Jeen YT, et al. Indications for detection, completion, and retention rates of small bowel capsule endoscopy based on the 10-year data from the Korean capsule endoscopy registry. Clin Endosc. 2015;48:399–404.
7. Pennazio M, Santucci R, Rondonotti E, et al. Outcome of patients with obscure gastrointestinal bleeding after capsule endoscopy: report of 100 consecutive cases. Gastroenterology. 2004;126:643–53.

8. Shinozaki S, Yamamoto H, Yano T, et al. Longterm outcome of patients with obscure gastrointestinal bleeding investigated by double-balloon endoscopy. Clin Gastroenterol Hepatol. 2010;8:151–8.

9. Pennazio M, Spada C, Eliakim R, et al. Small-bowel capsule endoscopy and device-assisted enteroscopy for diagnosis and treatment of small-bowel disorders: European Society of Gastrointestinal Endoscopy (ESGE) clinical guideline. Endoscopy. 2015;47:352–76.

10. Yamamoto H, Ogata H, Matsumoto T, et al. Clinical practice guideline for enteroscopy. Dig Endosc. 2017;29:519–46.

11. Shim KN, Moon JS, Chang DK, et al. Guideline for capsule endoscopy: obscure gastrointestinal bleeding. Clin Endosc. 2013;46:45–53.

Inflammatory Diseases of Small Bowel

Geun Am Song and In Sub Han

Key Point

- Inflammatory diseases of the small bowel can develop from infectious causes, including bacteria, virus, fungus, and protozoa, and from non-infectious causes, such as radiation, drugs, autoimmune disease, ischemia, and trauma.

Causes of Inflammatory Diseases of the Small Bowel

Table 1 shows the causes of inflammation in the small bowel.

Infectious Diseases

Most cases of infectious enteritis occur as acute events and are commonly caused by ingestion of foods or drinks contaminated by pathogenic microbes. The symptoms of enteritis may include diarrhea, abdominal pain, nausea and vomiting, and fever. Acute infectious enteritis is mainly caused by viruses and bacteria. The involved viruses are typically norovirus and rotavirus. The disease spreads from person to person, through stool or vomit, and can occur in a large scale through the ingestion of contaminated food or

Table 1 Classification of inflammatory diseases of the small bowel [1]

Infectious diseases	Non-infectious diseases
Bacterial	Radiation enteritis
Salmonella, Shigella	Induced by drugs or
Toxigenic	chemicals
Escherichia coli	NSAID, Potassium
Campylobacter	Cytotoxic chemical
Yersinia, Gonorrhea	agent
Clostridium difficile	Ischemic enteritis
Chlamydia	Eosinophilic enteritis
trachomatis	Inflammatory bowel
Parasitic	disease
Amebiasis,	Crohn's disease
Hookworm	Behcet's disease
Isospora, Trichuris	Ulcerative colitis
trichiura	(backwash ileitis)
Strongyloides	Cryptogenic multifocal
Viral	ulcerous stenosing
Cytomegalovirus	enteritis
Herpes simplex	Amyloidosis
Human	Meckel's diverticulum
immunodeficiency	Small-intestinal bacterial
virus	overgrowth
Fungal	Henoch-Schönlein
Histoplasmosis	purpura
Candida, Aspergillus	Nonspecific multiple
	ulcers of the small bowel
	Autoimmune disease
	Trauma or Surgery

NSAID non-steroidal anti-inflammatory drug

G. A. Song (✉) · I. S. Han
Division of Gastroenterology, Department of Internal Medicine, Pusan National University School of Medicine, Pusan National University Hospital, Busan, South Korea
e-mail: gasong@pusan.ac.kr

© Springer Nature Singapore Pte Ltd. 2022
H. J. Chun et al. (eds.), *Small Intestine Disease*, https://doi.org/10.1007/978-981-16-7239-2_4

water. It can occur at any time of the year, although it appears in high numbers in spring and winter. Of the causative viruses, rotavirus is more common in infants and young children, whereas norovirus is more common in adolescents and adults. Meanwhile, the causative organisms of bacterial enteritis include *Salmonella*, which causes typhoid fever; *Shigella*, which causes bacterial dysentery; *Vibrio*, which causes cholera; *Escherichia coli*, which causes hemorrhagic enteritis; *Campylobacter;* and *Yersinia*. Patients with an impaired immune status may have different severity and chronicity. If salmonellosis, listeriosis, cryptosporidiosis, or cytomegalovirus are identified in patients with enteritis, their immune status should be checked, such as acquired immune deficiency syndrome [1, 2].

Noninfectious Diseases

Radiation Enteritis

Radiation injuries in the small bowel can be subdivided into acute and chronic forms. Acute radiation enteritis usually presents with abdominal pain, bloating, loss of appetite, nausea, diarrhea, and fecal urgency during or after radiotherapy. Almost all patients undergoing pelvic or abdominal radiation therapy experience some gastrointestinal (GI) symptoms. Patients usually notice these symptoms at 2 weeks after treatment initiation, and the symptoms characteristically peak by the fourth to fifth week. The disease is usually self-limiting and often resolves within 3 months; however, appropriate conservative treatment may occasionally be needed. Chronic radiation enteritis typically develops between 18 months and 6 years after a complete course of radiotherapy, but has been reported to occur even up to 30 years later. Chronic radiation enteritis presents with post-prandial pain, acute or intermittent small-intestinal obstruction, nausea, anorexia, weight loss, bloating, diarrhea, steatorrhea, and malabsorption. These can arise from damage to the small bowel itself, associated phenomena such as bile salt malabsorption, bacterial overgrowth, or lactose intolerance. About 90% of patients undergoing pelvic radiotherapy will develop a change in bowel habits [3].

Drug-induced Enteropathy

Drug-induced enteropathy can be caused by using non-steroidal anti-inflammatory drugs (NSAIDs) and chemotherapeutic agents. It has been known that lower GI tract complications occur in about one-third of patients taking NSAIDs. Post-hoc analysis of a large-scale clinical outcome trial showed that lower GI events accounted for 40% of all serious GI events in patients taking NSAIDs. In one study, small-intestinal mucosal breaks were induced in 55% of healthy volunteers who took naproxen for 2 weeks. In another study, 2-week ingestion of slow-release diclofenac resulted in macroscopic injury to the small bowel in 68–75% of healthy volunteers. Further, the mucosal injury occurred in 71% of patients over 3 months of long-term use [4]. Meanwhile, cytotoxic chemotherapy causes mucosal cell damage, such as mucositis in the oral cavity and GI tract. The most common site of GI tract mucositis is the small bowel, and the major symptom is diarrhea. Irinotecan, methotrexate, and 5-fluorouracil are typical cytotoxic chemotherapeutic agents causing enteropathy [5].

Ischemic Enteritis

Ischemic enteritis occurs due to hypoperfusion of mesenteric vessels without major vessel occlusion. Ischemic enteritis is classified into two types: stenotic and transient. In clinical practice, the transient type is usually misdiagnosed because it resolves in a few days. Therefore, most cases of ischemic enteritis are classified as the stenotic type. Although it is difficult to estimate the real incidence of ischemic enteritis, one study reported that only 11 cases (0.1%) of ischemic stenosis of the small bowel were detected among 9536 patients undergoing surgical resection of the small bowel. An analysis study suggested that ischemic enteritis seems to be more common in patients with underlying diseases, such as hypertension, ischemic heart disease, arrhythmias, cerebral infarction, or diabetes, as well as in elderly people with thrombosis and in male patients [6].

Eosinophilic Enteritis

Eosinophilic enteritis is a rare primary eosinophilic GI disorder of unknown etiology, characterized by the presence of intense eosinophilic infiltration on histopathology of the intestinal mucosa. The prevalence is estimated to be 1 per 100,000 population. Eosinophilic enteritis can affect all age groups, with a peak incidence between the third and fourth decades, and has a male predominance. Patients with eosinophilic enteritis have a personal or family history of atrophy or allergy in 25–75% of the cases. In addition, eosinophilic enteritis is believed to be associated with allergy because of the detection of increased serum IgE levels in patients [7].

Inflammatory Bowel Disease

Inflammatory bowel disease, represented by ulcerative colitis and Crohn's disease, is common in Western countries but rare in Korea and other Asian countries. However, the annual incidence has been steadily increasing since the first domestic case reported in the 1960s. In 2001–2005, the incidence of ulcerative colitis and Crohn's disease was 3.08 and 1.34 per 100,000 population, respectively, much higher than the corresponding incidence of 0.34 and 0.05 in 1986–1990 [8]. The increase in the incidence of inflammatory bowel disease in Korea is considered to be related to changes in intestinal bacterial flora associated with Westernized dietary habits, decreased breastfeeding, early infectious diseases and related immune tolerance, and air pollution. Abdominal tuberculosis is divided into tuberculous peritonitis, mesenteric tuberculous lymphadenitis, and intestinal tuberculosis. Intestinal tuberculosis can involve all parts of the GI tract, from the mouth to the anus. In Korea, the prevalence of intestinal tuberculosis has been reported to be approximately in 4.8% in patients with tuberculosis. However, approximately 50% of patients with active pulmonary tuberculosis were suspected to have intestinal involvement on colonoscopy; thus, intestinal tuberculosis is relatively common in Korea, where the prevalence of pulmonary tuberculosis is high. In patients with Bechet's disease, GI tract symptoms are reported in up to 60%. However, the incidence of Behcet's enteritis is reported to be low and to vary widely across different regions. Behcet's enteritis is more common in patients between the second and third decades of life. In East Asia, including Korea, Behcet's enteritis accounts for 10–30% of patients with Behcet's disease. In Korea, Behcet's enteritis frequently occurs in men, although Behcet's disease is more common in women [9].

Cryptogenic Multifocal Ulcerous Stenosing Enteritis (CMUSE)

CMUSE is characterized by multiple unexplained ulcerations and strictures without systemic inflammation of the small bowel in middle-aged or young patients. CMUSE is a rare disease, and its clinical characteristics have not yet been completely evaluated. CMUSE can be subdivided into two categories: MUSE-I (idiopathic MUSE) and MUSE-V (vasculitis-related MUSE). CMUSE has been known to occur in the jejunum or in the proximal ileum. In a domestic study, 15% of patients had extraintestinal symptoms, such as genital ulcers, weight loss, and subclavian vein thrombosis, and female patients had a longer relapse-free survival time than male patients [10].

Amyloidosis

Amyloidosis is a rare disease with a prevalence of 0.5–1.3 per 100,000 population. Of the cases, 1–8% can be confirmed with GI endoscopic biopsy. Amyloidosis is characterized by the deposition of amyloid in the intercellular space and vascular wall. Amyloid deposition leads to dysfunction of the affected organ and causes variable clinical symptoms depending on the involved organ. The most common site of amyloid deposition is the small bowel [11]. The involved site of the GI tract differs depending on the subtype of amyloid. Sixty percent of patients with secondary amyloidosis have GI tract involvement; however, primary amyloidosis rarely involves the GI tract.

Meckel's Diverticulum

Meckel's diverticulum is one of the most common congenital GI tract abnormalities, with a prevalence of approximately 2%. Most patients are asymptomatic. About 2–4% of patients with Meckel's diverticulum may develop asymptomatic bleeding, intussusception, and pain in the right lower abdomen before 2 years of age [2].

Small-intestinal Bacterial Overgrowth (SIBO)

SIBO is characterized by nutrient malabsorption associated with an excessive number of bacteria in the proximal small bowel. The prevalence is not known but is reported to be approximately 2.5–22%. However, the actual prevalence is estimated higher because of either asymptomatic or nonspecific symptoms in SIBO. Depending on the underlying disease, the prevalence can vary, ranging from 30% to 85% in patients with irritable bowel syndrome and 50% in patients with celiac disease. It has been reported that SIBO is common in the elderly and in patients with chronic pancreatitis, chronic renal failure, and

hepatic cirrhosis. Further, 17% of obese individuals without symptoms are reported to be affected. In most cases of SIBO, it does not occur with only one type of organism, but is cause by an increase in the amount of bacteria present in the colon or in the small bowel itself [12].

References

1. Kasper F, Hauser SL, et al. Harrison's principles of internal medicine. 19th ed. New York: McGraw-Hill; 2015.
2. Morpeth SC, Thielman NM. Diarrhea in patients with AIDS. Curr Treat Options Gastroenterol. 2006;9:23–37.
3. Stacey R, Green JT. Radiation-induced small bowel disease: latest developments and clinical guidance. Ther Adv Chronic Dis. 2014;5:15–29.
4. Lim YJ, Yang CH. Non-steroidal anti-inflammatory drug-induced enteropathy. Clin Endosc. 2012;45:138–44.
5. Park Y, Kim YH. Chemotherapy related oral and gastrointestinal mucositis. J Korean Med Assoc. 2009;52:89–906.
6. Koshikawa Y, Nakase H, Matsuura M, et al. Ischemic enteritis with intestinal stenosis. Intest Res. 2016;14:89–95.
7. Pineton de Chambrun G, Desreumaux P, Cortot A. Eosinophilic enteritis. Dig Dis. 2015;33:183–9.
8. Yang SK, Yun S, Kim JH, et al. Epidemiology of inflammatory bowel disease in the Songpa-Kangdong district, Seoul, Korea, 1986-2005; a KASID study. Inflamm Bowel Dis. 2008;14:542–9.
9. Yang SK. Intestinal Behcet's disease. Intest Res. 2005;3:1–10.
10. Chung SH, Park SU, Cheon JH, et al. Clinical characteristics and treatment outcomes of cryptogenic multifocal ulcerous stenosing enteritis in Korea. Dig Dis Sci. 2015;60:2740–5.
11. Ebert EC, Nagar M. Gastrointestinal manifestations of amyloidosis. Am J Gastroenterol. 2008;103:776–87.
12. Se K. Small intestinal bacterial overgrowth. Intest Res. 2010;8:106–16.

Small Bowel Tumors

Su Hwan Kim

Key Points
1. Small bowel malignancies are rare, and their symptoms are nonspecific, which can delay diagnosis.
2. Small bowel adenocarcinoma and neuroendocrine tumors account for a large portion of small bowel malignancies. Their incidences are steadily increasing.
3. Crohn's disease, celiac disease, and inherited syndromes such as familial adenomatous polyposis, Peutz–Jeghers syndrome, and Lynch syndrome are identified as risk factors for small bowel cancer development.

Introduction

Although the small bowel occupies 75% of the length and 90% of the total mucosal surface of the digestive tract, small bowel tumors are rare and account for about 3% of all gastrointestinal neoplasms [1]. Most symptoms of small bowel tumors are vague and nonspecific. Endoscopic access to the small bowel is more difficult than to the stomach or colon. Coupled with the vague clinical presentation, this can delay diagnosis and make the prognosis of the small bowel tumors unfavorable [2].

Epidemiology

Previously, upper gastrointestinal endoscopy, barium imaging, and computed tomography were of limited value in diagnosing small bowel tumors. However, the recent development of video capsule endoscopy and deep enteroscopy has led to increased detection of these tumors. Video capsule endoscopy, in particular, is an effective diagnostic tool and retrospective studies identified small bowel tumors in 4.3–8.9% of patients who underwent this procedure [3, 4]. More than 40 different histologic types of small bowel tumors have been identified. Common benign small bowel tumors include adenomas, hamartomas, lipomas, inflammatory polyps, and angiomas. The most predominant small bowel malignancies are adenocarcinomas, neuroendocrine tumors, lymphomas, and gastrointestinal stromal tumors [5, 6]. Small bowel malignancies showed an incidence ratio of 2 to 2.5, when US and Asian populations were compared. A higher incidence was observed in the African-American US population compared with the Caucasian population. A high incidence was also reported among the Maori of New Zealand and Hawaiians [1].

S. H. Kim (✉)
Department of Internal Medicine, Seoul National University College of Medicine, Seoul, South Korea

© Springer Nature Singapore Pte Ltd. 2022
H. J. Chun et al. (eds.), *Small Intestine Disease*, https://doi.org/10.1007/978-981-16-7239-2_5

According to the Korea National Cancer Incidence Database, among the newly developed 214,701 cancers in 2015, small bowel cancers occupied 0.4% (848 cases). Crude incidence of small bowel cancer was 1.7 per 100,000 individuals, and the male to female ratio was 1.4:1. Small bowel cancers developed most frequently (25.6%) among septuagenarians [7].

Small bowel adenocarcinoma accounts for around 40% of all small bowel malignancies. Duodenal tumors account for 50% of small bowel adenocarcinomas while the tumors of the jejunum and ileum represent 30% and 20%, respectively [8]. Over a 20 year period (from 1992 to 2013), the incidence of small bowel cancers increased in the US from 1.5 to 2.2 cases per 100,000 individuals; over the past 10 years, the incidence has risen by an average of 2.4% per year. Similar time-trend figures were reported in studies from the UK, Sweden, France, and Denmark [1]. To date, the reasons for this increase remain unexplained, although improvements in tumor detection resulting from advances in the endoscopic and radiographic techniques may be partly responsible [2].

There has been a marked increase in the incidence of small bowel neuroendocrine tumors. The small bowel, particularly the ileum, is the most common site where neuroendocrine tumors develop. The reported prevalence was 0.32–1.12 per 100,000 individuals per year. The incidence of small bowel neuroendocrine tumors has increased by 460% over the last 30 years [9]. Small bowel neuroendocrine tumors recently outnumbered small bowel adenocarcinomas in the USA [8].

Small bowel lymphomas account for around 20% of all small bowel malignancies and involve the ileum, jejunum, and duodenum, in decreasing order of frequency. The risk of small bowel lymphoma increases for patients with celiac disease, inflammatory bowel diseases, and immunosuppression.

Common origins of metastatic small bowel cancers are skin melanoma, colorectal cancer, prostate cancer, lung cancer, and breast cancer [10].

Risk Factors

Certain inherited syndromes such as familial adenomatous polyposis, Peutz–Jeghers syndrome, Lynch syndrome, and Cowden's syndrome are associated with an increased risk of small bowel adenocarcinoma. Recognizing these inherited syndromes is important. If an underlying germline mutation can be identified in a patient, all relatives at risk can be gene tested and offered appropriate cancer screening, including screening for small bowel adenocarcinoma [2]. In patients with familial adenomatous polyposis, duodenal adenocarcinoma is the second most common cause of cancer-related death. In familial adenomatous polyposis patients who underwent total colectomy, the main cause of cancer-related death is small bowel adenocarcinoma. Intensive screening is required because duodenal adenomas are present in 80% of familial adenomatous polyposis cases and these develop into adenocarcinoma in 4% of cases. Familial adenomatous polyposis is present in less than 5% of patients with small bowel adenocarcinoma. In patients with familial adenomatous polyposis, small bowel adenocarcinoma developed mainly in the duodenum (71%) and jejunum (29%) [5].

The lifetime cumulative risk of small bowel adenocarcinoma is around 1% in patients with Lynch syndrome. However, DNA mismatch repair phenotyping is recommended for patients with small bowel adenocarcinoma, because such a test can reveal Lynch syndrome [5]. The relative risk of small bowel adenocarcinoma for patients with Lynch syndrome is more than 100, compared with the general population [11]. Patients with Lynch syndrome are also at increased risk of urothelial, gastric, endometrial, ovarian, and biliary tract cancers [2, 6]. In a study employing video capsule endoscopy, 1.5% of asymptomatic mutation carriers of Lynch syndrome were diagnosed with a small bowel tumor, with all tumors located in the duodenum and within the reach of conventional upper gastrointestinal endoscopy [10].

Peutz–Jeghers syndrome is a disorder that predisposes patients to hamartomatous gastrointestinal tract polyposis. The relative risk of small bowel adenocarcinoma for patients with Peutz–Jeghers syndrome was 520, compared with the general population [6]. The estimated cumulative risk of small bowel adenocarcinoma was 13%, and the lifetime cumulative risk for all cancers was 93% at 64 years of age [5]. In patients with Peutz–Jeghers syndrome, increased risk of cancer was identified in the small bowel, breast, ovary, pancreas, stomach, esophagus, and colon [10].

Patients with sporadic colorectal cancer have an increased risk of developing small bowel adenocarcinoma, while those with small bowel adenocarcinoma are at increased risk of colorectal cancer. This correlation suggests shared risk factors [11].

Multiple endocrine neoplasia type 1, von Hippel Lindau disease, and neurofibromatosis type 1 carry increased risk of neuroendocrine tumors [11].

Compared with the general population, the relative risk of small bowel adenocarcinoma was 34 for patients with Crohn's disease affecting the small bowel. The risk of small bowel adenocarcinoma was also correlated with the duration and location of the inflammatory damage. The cumulative risk of small bowel adenocarcinoma was around 0.2% after 10 years and 2.2% after 25 years of Crohn's disease. Small bowel adenocarcinoma in patients with Crohn's disease most frequently developed in the ileum and appeared in younger patients [6].

Celiac disease increased the relative risk of small bowel adenocarcinoma from 10 to 60 compared with the general population. Celiac disease was associated with small bowel adenocarcinoma in 2% of cases, and the main location was the jejunum [5, 11].

Environmental factors including smoking and consumption of alcohol, red meat, and sugar have been reported to increase the risk of small bowel adenocarcinoma, whereas the consumption of fiber, fruits, and vegetables decreased the risk [5]. However, studies on the predisposing factors are limited due to the rarity of the disease.

Conclusion

Small bowel tumors are rare, and the clinical manifestations tend to be nonspecific, resulting in delayed diagnosis. Recent advances in imaging and endoscopic techniques have improved the detection of small bowel tumors. Better understanding of the risk factors, together with heightened vigilance, will provide earlier diagnosis and more appropriate treatment of small bowel tumors.

References

1. Rondonotti E, Koulaouzidis A, Yung DE, Reddy SN, Georgiou J, Pennazio M. Neoplastic diseases of the small bowel. Gastrointest Endosc Clin N Am. 2017;27:93–112.
2. Pourmand K, Itzkowitz SH. Small bowel neoplasms and polyps. Curr Gastroenterol Rep. 2016;18:23.
3. Islam RS, Leighton JA, Pasha SF. Evaluation and management of small-bowel tumors in the era of deep enteroscopy. Gastrointest Endosc. 2014;79:732–40.
4. Shim KN, Jeon SR, Jang HJ, et al. Quality indicators for small bowel capsule endoscopy. Clin Endosc. 2017;50:148–60.
5. Aparicio T, Zaanan A, Mary F, Afchain P, Manfredi S, Evans TR. Small bowel adenocarcinoma. Gastroenterol Clin N Am. 2016;45:447–57.
6. Aparicio T, Zaanan A, Svrcek M, et al. Small bowel adenocarcinoma: epidemiology, risk factors, diagnosis and treatment. Dig Liver Dis. 2014;46:97–104.
7. Jung KW, Won YJ, Kong HJ, Lee ES. Cancer statistics in Korea: incidence, mortality, survival, and prevalence in 2015. Cancer Res Treat. 2018;50:303–16.
8. Locher C, Batumona B, Afchain P, et al. Small bowel adenocarcinoma: French intergroup clinical practice guidelines for diagnosis, treatments and follow-up (SNFGE, FFCD, GERCOR, UNICANCER, SFCD, SFED, SFRO). Dig Liver Dis. 2018;50:15–9.
9. Rossi RE, Conte D, Elli L, Branchi F, Massironi S. Endoscopic techniques to detect small-bowel neuroendocrine tumors: a literature review. United European Gastroenterol J. 2017;5:5–12.
10. Cheung DY, Kim JS, Shim KN, Choi MG. The usefulness of capsule endoscopy for small bowel tumors. Clin Endosc. 2016;49:21–5.
11. Reynolds I, Healy P, McNamara DA. Malignant tumours of the small intestine. Surgeon. 2014;12:263–70.

Other Small-bowel Disorders

Eun Sun Kim

Key Points
- Meckel's diverticulum is the most common congenital gastrointestinal disease, with a 2% prevalence rate and a male-to-female ratio of 2:1.
- Gastrointestinal amyloidosis is present in 3% of all patients with amyloidosis, involving one or more of the following four symptoms: bleeding (25–45%), malabsorption syndrome, protein-losing enteropathy, and chronic gastrointestinal motility disorder.
- Gastrointestinal involvement is common in systemic lupus erythematosus and may occur in 40% of the life span of a patient with lupus (prevalence rate, 40%) in contrast to vasculitis, adverse effects of lupus medication, and infection.
- There are few cases of celiac disease in Korea; however, in the USA, 13,415 screening tests showed prevalence ratios of 1:22 if the disease runs in the immediate family, 1:39 in second-degree relatives, 1:56 in patients with a symptom, and 1:133 in patients with no symptoms and in those with no risk factors.

In this chapter, we investigate the epidemics of different small-bowel disorders excluding inflammatory/neoplastic disorders.

Meckel's Diverticulum

Meckel's diverticulum is the most common congenital abnormality of the gastrointestinal (GI) tract. Because of the formation of an imperfect obstruction in the vitelline duct, Meckel's diverticulum is formed in the small bowel. Most cases of Meckel's diverticulum are painless; however, the disease may also be accompanied by abdominal pain, small-bowel bleeding, or occlusion. Meckel's diverticulum is usually located on the opposite side of the mesentery of the mid or distal ileum.

The prevalence rate of Meckel's diverticulum was reported to be 3% in a study of 7927 people. Moreover, in a systematic review of seven studies involving 31,499 autopsies, a prevalence rate of 1.2% was reported. Generally, Meckel's diverticulum has a prevalence rate of about 2%, a 2:1 male-to-female ratio, a location about 60 cm

E. S. Kim (✉)
Division of Gastroenterology and Hepatology, Department of Internal Medicine, Korea University Anam Hospital, Institute of Digestive Disease and Nutrition, Korea University College of Medicine, Seoul, South Korea

(2 ft) from the ileocecal valve, and a size about 5 cm (2 in), and these characteristics are referred to as "the rule of twos." Of patients with Meckel's diverticulum, 2–4% develop complications, which usually occur at an age of <2 years. The mucous membrane of Meckel's diverticulum, composed of either ectopic mucous membrane of the stomach, pancreas, and large intestine or normal mucous membrane, may show bleeding.

By the age of 80 years, 6.4% of patients with Meckel's diverticulum are known to have undergone a surgery for its complications, and among elderly patients, 4.2% are suggested to develop a symptom during 15 years.

The risk factors associated with Meckel 's diverticulum in 1476 patients followed up for 50 years were age < 50 years (odds ratio [OR] 3.5, 95% confidence interval [CI] 2.6–4.8); male sex (OR 1.8, 95% CI 1.3–2.4); > 2 cm diverticulum (OR 2.2, 95% CI 1.1–4.4); and presence of a site with abnormal histology (OR 13.9, 95% CI 9.9–19.6), which is a risk factor for accompanying symptoms.

Amyloidosis

Amyloidosis is a general term used to describe a phenomenon in which fibril that consists of light-chain subunits of 5–25 kDa, a component of serum, accumulates in extracellular tissue. Fibril appears green and birefringent in Congo red staining, and light green and fluorescent in thioflavin T staining. Amyloidosis is usually classified into two types: AL and AA. AL amyloidosis is a plasma cell disorder in which a protein from a fraction of low molecular immunoglobulin accumulates. AA amyloidosis is due to the production of amyloid A, an acute-phase reactant, caused by constantly recurring inflammation (e.g., chronic degenerative arthritis, rheumatoid arthritis, ankylosing spondylitis, and inflammatory bowel disorder). The other types of amyloidosis include dialysis-related amyloidosis, organ-specific amyloidosis, age-related systemic amyloidosis, and genetic amyloidosis.

GI amyloidosis occurs in 3% of all patients with amyloidosis. Further, 80% of patients with GI amyloidosis have accompanying systemic involvement, whereas 20% show plasma cell abnormality with no organ involvement. Of the amyloidosis cases involving the digestive system, 60% are AA amyloidosis. AL amyloidosis is rare. Amyloid build up in liver tissue appears in 90% of patients with AL amyloidosis and in 60% of patients with AA amyloidosis. Senile amyloidosis can appear in 10–36% of patients aged >80 years. Especially, senile amyloidosis is found in the heart, GI tract, and 41–44% of serous membrane veins of the large intestine.

GI amyloidosis occurs in the serous membrane or neuromuscular layer. GI amyloidosis is accompanied by one or more of the following four symptoms: bleeding (25–45%), absorption disorder, protein-losing enteropathy, and chronic GI motility disorder. The sites of amyloid build-up are the second portion of the duodenum (100%), the stomach and large intestine (90%), and the esophagus (70%). The build-up of amyloid in the neuromuscular layer can cause GI retention, abnormalities in the intrinsic nervous system, and pseudo-obstruction. Especially, when a large extent of the natural muscular layer of the small bowel is involved, it is related to AL amyloidosis or dialysis-related amyloidosis. On the other hand, amyloid build-up in AA amyloidosis usually occurs in the myenteric plexus instead of the muscular layer.

Small-bowel Involvement of Connective Tissue Disorders

Systemic lupus erythematosus (SLE) is a typical connective tissue disorder that can involve the skin, joints, kidneys, lungs, nervous system, serous membrane, and GI tract. GI tract involvement of SLE is common, which may occur in 40% of the lifetime of patients with lupus, in contrast to vasculitis, adverse effects of lupus medication, and infection. Esophageal invasion occurs in 20–70%; however, its pathophysiology is unclear. Esophageal motility disorder caused by lupus is related to Raynaud disease or anti-ribonucleoprotein antibody. Inflammatory reaction of the esophageal muscle and ischemia and vasculitis of Auerbach's plexus may be related to this disorder. Stomach involvement in lupus often causes bleeding, obstruction, and perforation.

When the small bowel is involved, pseudo-obstruction and protein-losing bowel disease may occur. The mechanism of pseudo-obstruction due to lupus remains unknown but is assumed to be related to the infiltration of immune complexes in the small-bowel muscular layer, or to chronic ischemia and hypomotility caused by angiitis.

Protein-losing bowel disease is rarely reported and can be suspected in patients with no albuminuria accompanying systemic edema and decrease in serum albumin level. Half of the patients have accompanying severe diarrhea and, usually, severe lupus symptoms or multiple organ involvement.

Celiac Disease

Celiac disease is also known as gluten-sensitive small-bowel disease or non-tropical sprue. First described by Samuel Gee in 1888, celiac disease is considered similar to the chronic absorption disorder described by Aretaeus of Cappadocia, Turkey, in 2 B.C. Dicke, a Dutch pediatrician, explained the cause of celiac disease as being recurrent diarrhea due to ingestion of bread and grain. A correlation was discovered while observing the improvement in symptoms after the elimination of bread in the diet, as the result of the shortage of grains during World War II. In 1954, the first description of proximal small-bowel lesions caused by celiac disease was reported, which included the basic findings of mucosal inflammation, proliferation of crypts, and atrophy of the villus.

The prevalence of celiac disease was reported to be high in the Western region, with a ratio of 1:152 in the MONICA project, 1:256 in Sweden, 1:99 in Finland, and 1:96 in Italy.

A total of 13,415 screening tests performed in the USA showed a prevalence ratio of 1:22 if there was an immediate family history, 1:39 if there was a history of the disease in second-degree relatives, 1:56 if a patient had a symptom, and 1:133 if a patient had no symptoms or no risk factors.

Punjabi-Gujarati reported that in immigrants from India to the UK, a 2.7 times increased prevalence rate of celiac disease was observed owing to the change to a high-gluten diet, regardless of the different ethnicity.

Primary Lymphangiectasia

Primary lymphangiectasia is an ectasia of the overall or focal small intestinal lymph duct, which can also be related to lymph duct disorder or deformation in other regions. Lymph duct expansion can appear in the mucosal, submucosal, and subserosal layers. In patients with accompanying lymph duct obstruction, congenital lymphangiectasia, and loss of lymphocyte in the intestines, severe lymphocytopenia may occur, which interferes with cellular immunity.

Small-intestinal lymphangiectasia usually occurs in children and young adults, with the average age of onset being 11 years. Although it sporadically occurs, in seems to have a familial tendency in some patients. Further, if CD55 deficiency occurs in bilateral alleles, problems arise in the process of forming a complement, which leads to the onset of hyperactivation of CHAPLE (complement, angiopathic thrombosis, protein-losing enteropathy) syndrome.

The occurrence of secondary lymphangiectasia is related to heart problems or retroperitoneal lymph node enlargement (associated with anti-cancer treatment or infection).

Symptoms and Signs of Suspected Small Bowel Disease

Seung Han Kim

Key Points

1. **Patients with suspected small bowel disease**: Obscure gastrointestinal bleeding, unexplained abdominal pain, weight loss, chronic diarrhea.
2. **Symptoms and signs to check**: Bleeding episodes, abdominal pain, weight loss, diarrhea, nausea, vomiting.
3. **Required physical examination**: General condition, height and weight, body temperature, blood pressure, abdominal mass and tenderness, skin and perianal lesions, joints.

Measuring approximately 6 m in length, the small bowel is a complex organ located between the stomach and colon and is divided into the duodenum, jejunum, and ileum [1]. The small bowel is associated with a wide variety of diseases. However, small bowel diseases often have ambiguous symptoms and are difficult to diagnose owing to poor anatomical accessibility. Therefore, diagnosis and treatment of small bowel diseases are often delayed.

Recent technological advances in endoscopic and medical imaging have facilitated systematic approaches to small bowel diseases. Hence, an understanding of the signs and symptoms of small bowel diseases, along with their prompt and accurate identification, will lead to an improvement in the prognosis of patients with small bowel diseases consequent to their treatment within an appropriate time frame.

Small Bowel Bleeding

Small bowel bleeding is relatively rare, accounting for 5–10% of patients with gastrointestinal bleeding. Most patients who have gastrointestinal bleeding without an apparent bleeding source after upper and lower gastrointestinal endoscopy and radiologic evaluation of the small intestine likely have small bowel bleeding.

When small bowel bleeding is suspected, patient interviews for detailed medical history and physical examination are important to determine the cause of the patient's symptoms. To diagnose small bowel bleeding, particular attention should be paid to the presence of hemorrhagic disease or comorbid condition, current medications (e.g., antithrombotic agents), and surgical history.

The clinical manifestations of small bowel bleeding are related to the amount, rate, and timing of bleeding and accompanying disease. Repeated hematemesis and hematochezia usually signify hemorrhage from the gastrointestinal tract above and below the ligament of Treitz,

S. H. Kim (✉)
Department of Internal Medicine, Korea University College of Medicine, Seoul, South Korea

© Springer Nature Singapore Pte Ltd. 2022
H. J. Chun et al. (eds.), *Small Intestine Disease*, https://doi.org/10.1007/978-981-16-7239-2_7

respectively. However, aspects may vary depending on the amount of bleeding.

Assessing the patient's general condition and measuring weight, height, body temperature, and blood pressure are important to evaluate patient status. Tachycardia or hypotension can serve as a clue as to the amount of bleeding. Additionally, perforation should be suspected when bleeding is accompanied by abdominal pain, particularly in the presence of rebound tenderness or abdominal stiffness. If acute abdominal symptoms are present, perforation must be confirmed and excluded prior to endoscopy. Characteristic skin signs on physical examination can help differentiate gastrointestinal complications of systemic diseases (e.g., hereditary hemorrhagic telangiectasia, amyloidosis) [2].

Inflammatory Diseases of the Small Bowel

Inflammatory diseases of the small bowel are common and may appear in various forms depending on the cause. In several cases, they are mostly expressed as mucosal ulcers and occasionally appear as a change in the mucosal surface layer. Therefore, the patient may present with different symptoms, including abdominal pain, diarrhea, bleeding, anemia, weight loss, absorption disorder and small bowel obstruction [3].

Inflammatory diseases of the small bowel include Crohn's disease and nonsteroidal anti-inflammatory drug (NSAID)-induced enteropathy (see Part II). Small bowel involvement occurs in approximately 66% of patients diagnosed with Crohn's disease; in particular, small bowel Crohn's disease involves the terminal ileum in approximately 90% of patients [4] and young patients with Crohn's disease often only have small bowel involvement. There exists no standard for diagnostic methods, and diagnosis cannot be confirmed by any one symptom or sign. Crohn's disease may be suspected if its main

symptoms (i.e., abdominal pain, diarrhea, and weight loss) persist for more than a few weeks. Young patients with these symptoms should be carefully observed, as Crohn's disease is common among young individuals in their mid-teens and late twenties.

NSAIDs can affect the entire gastrointestinal tract and, when taken, causes intestinal mucosal damage in 55–75% of patients [5]. NSAID-induced enteropathy can result in various abdominal symptoms, including epigastric pain, nausea, indigestion, constipation, and abdominal distension.

Upon collecting data on medical history, the patient must be asked about the onset of symptoms, occurrence of nocturnal symptoms, recent travel history, food intolerance, contact with patients with colitis, medication history (antibiotics, NSAIDs, etc.), smoking history, family history, extraintestinal symptoms (mouth, skin, eyes, joints, etc.), and perianal lesions (perianal abscess, fistula, fissure, etc.).

Physical examination should be performed to check for general condition, blood pressure, pulse rate, body temperature, weight and body mass index, abdominal findings (abdominal mass, distension, tenderness, etc.), and perianal lesions.

Small Bowel Tumors

Malignant small bowel tumors include adenocarcinomas, neuroendocrine tumors, lymphomas, and sarcomas, whereas benign small bowel tumors include adenomas, leiomyomas, fibromas, and lipomas. Small bowel tumors are relatively rare, accounting for only 3–6% of all gastrointestinal tumors and 1–3% of all malignant gastrointestinal tumors. The clinical features of small bowel tumors are usually nonspecific and ambiguous, making diagnosis difficult, which in turn leads to a delay in appropriate treatment.

Obscure gastrointestinal bleeding (OGIB) is the most common clinical manifestation of small bowel tumors. Most small bowel tumors are found during the examination for OGIB or anemia. Partial or complete small bowel obstruction due to a small bowel tumor may result in abdominal pain, nausea or vomiting, and perforation [6]. Furthermore, small bowel obstruction caused by a small bowel tumor is accompanied by repetitive convulsive abdominal pain after meals and is often misdiagnosed as a nonspecific symptom, resulting in delayed diagnosis. Small bowel tumors are responsible for 2% of unexplained abdominal pain [7]. Moreover, weight loss occurs in approximately 30–50% of patients with small bowel tumors; thus, a detailed examination for diagnosis should be conducted in patients aged >50 years if an unexplained weight loss occurs.

Jaundice may occur when a small bowel tumor develops around the ampulla of Vater. If the small bowel tumor progresses and spreads to the retroperitoneal cavity, symptoms may develop with low back pain. Carcinoid syndrome with symptoms such as wheezing, flushing, and watery diarrhea may develop during the progression of small bowel neuroendocrine tumors.

Patients with a family history of hereditary diseases, such as familial adenomatous polyposis, Lynch syndrome, celiac disease, and Peutz–Jeghers syndrome, are at increased risk for small bowel adenocarcinoma; therefore, collecting data on family history from patients is crucial for diagnosis. Celiac disease is also associated with small intestinal T-cell lymphoma, and patients with a history of Crohn's disease or colorectal cancer are more likely to develop small bowel tumors.

Conclusion

The clinical manifestations of small bowel diseases are mostly ambiguous and nonspecific, thereby resulting in delayed diagnosis. Recent technological advances such as capsule endoscopy, enteroscopy, computed tomography enterography, and magnetic resonance enterography have facilitated access to the small bowel and enabled systematic approaches to patients with small bowel disease. Therefore, gastroenterologists should pay attention to small bowel diseases and attempt to improve the prognosis through prompt and appropriate examination and accurate diagnosis in patients with suspected small bowel disease.

References

1. Tortora G. Principles of anatomy & physiology. 15th ed. Danvers, MA: Wiley; 2016.
2. Braverman IM. Skin signs of gastrointestinal disease. Gastroenterology. 2003;124:1595–614.
3. Leighton JA, Pasha SF. Inflammatory disorders of the small bowel. Gastrointest Endosc Clin N Am. 2017;27:63–77.
4. Kim JH, Moon W. Optimal diagnostic approaches for patients with suspected small bowel disease. Clin Endosc. 2016;49:364–9.
5. Lim YJ, Yang CH. Non-steroidal anti-inflammatory drug-induced enteropathy. Clin Endosc. 2012;45:138–44.
6. Cheung DY, Choi MG. Current advance in small bowel tumors. Clin Endosc. 2011;44:13–21.
7. Shim KN, Kim YS, Kim KJ, et al. Abdominal pain accompanied by weight loss may increase the diagnostic yield of capsule endoscopy: a Korean multicenter study. Scand J Gastroenterol. 2006;41:983–8.

Part III

Radiologic and Imaging Studies to Evaluate Small Intestinal Disorders

Radiologic Imaging for Small-Bowel Evaluation

Se Hyung Kim

Key Points
- Modified small-bowel series are commonly used to overcome the limitations, such as collapse and overlap of small-bowel loops, of conventional small-bowel series.
- Barium enteroclysis can be helpful in diagnosing intermittent small-bowel obstructions or fistulas.
- Computed tomography (CT) enterography is the primary imaging method for evaluating small-bowel diseases because it is easy to perform, uses less radiation dose, and increases patients' compliance in contrast to CT enteroclysis.
- CT enterography is the primary imaging modality for the diagnosis of Crohn's disease, especially in an emergency setting or as a first-line diagnostic tool.
- Magnetic resonance enterography can be useful as a follow-up imaging modality for young patients with Crohn's disease because it has no radiation hazard.

Introduction

The small bowel is a challenging organ for both clinicians and radiologists because of the rarity of small-bowel diseases, less availability of endoscopy for the evaluation of this organ, and low diagnostic yield of conventional barium studies. Although large advancements in endoscopic technology have made conventional barium studies and fluoroscopy less important, the relevance of radiologic examinations can still be emphasized because the small bowel is the most difficult organ to reach with endoscopy. Therefore, this chapter will discuss the indications, advantages, and disadvantages of several radiologic modalities that can be used for small-bowel diseases.

Barium Examination

There are two types of barium studies for small-bowel evaluation: small-bowel follow-through and barium enteroclysis. Small-bowel follow-through has several advantages, such as the lack of need for intubation and sedation, less patient discomfort, and less radiation exposure for both patients and radiologists. However, the long examination time and inadequate bowel distention can be potential disadvantages. On the other hand, with barium enteroclysis, the small bowel can be adequately distended with a maximum double-contrast effect, thus allowing the small

S. H. Kim (✉)
Department of Radiology, Seoul National University College of Medicine, Seoul, South Korea

© Springer Nature Singapore Pte Ltd. 2022
H. J. Chun et al. (eds.), *Small Intestine Disease*, https://doi.org/10.1007/978-981-16-7239-2_8

bowel to be adequately imaged during fluoroscopic examination. However, patients frequently feel discomfort during both intubation and examination. In addition, the higher radiation exposure for both patients and radiologists can be another obstacle to the application of barium enteroclysis [1].

Small-Bowel Follow-through

For conventional small-bowel series, low-density barium solution (40–60% weight/volume [w/v]) is usually used. Initially, 500 mL barium solution is orally ingested. When the stomach becomes empty, 120–150 mL barium solution is repeatedly ingested until the terminal ileum is sufficiently filled with the solution. Through fluoroscopic examination, the bowel path, contour abnormality, filling defect, bowel motility, distensibility, and pliability should be assessed. For spot imaging, overhead projection images should be obtained with the patient in a prone position because this position can improve the image quality owing to a compression effect (Fig. 1). The use of a compression device can sometimes be helpful to detect the presence of bowel adhesion through bowel separation.

After fluoroscopic examination, double-contrast small-bowel follow-through can be performed using per-oral methylcellulose or effervescent agents, which can improve small-bowel distensibility and translucency, resulting in increased sensitivity or specificity for the diagnosis of small-bowel diseases. Double-contrast small-bowel follow-through can also be modified. For modified small-bowel series, 22.5% w/v barium solution mixed with methylcellulose is first used, followed by effervescent agents. In addition, 40% w/v barium solution mixed with methylcellulose is first ingested, and 600 mL of 0.5% methylcellulose can be ingested to maximize the double-contrast effect [2] (Fig. 2).

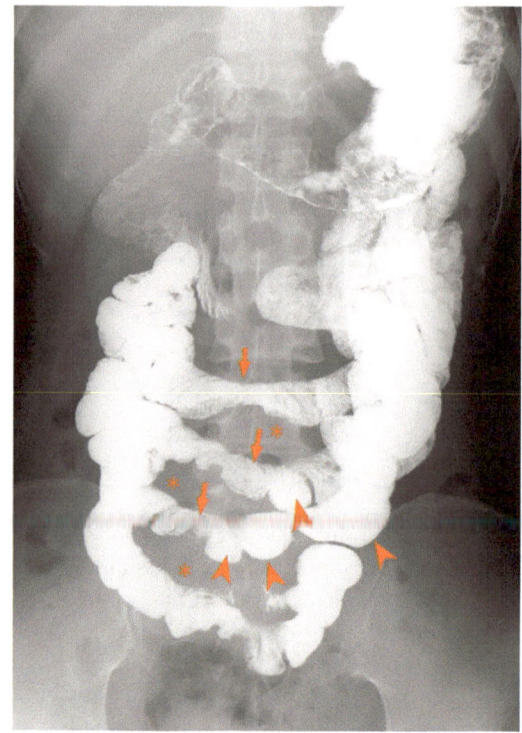

Fig. 1 Overhead image from small-bowel follow-through examination in a 27-year-old woman with Crohn's disease. The small-bowel loops are sufficiently filled with barium solution. Multiple longitudinal ulcerations (arrows) at the mesenteric side of the bowel loops and pseudosacculation (arrowheads) at the anti-mesenteric side are noted. Bowel loops are separated because of thickening of the bowel wall and fibrofatty proliferation (*)

Barium Enteroclysis

For barium enteroclysis, a 12- or 14-F enteroclysis catheter should be inserted through the patients' mouth or nose after spraying with topical anesthetic agents. To prevent reflux of the contrast agent, ballooning should be performed after the catheter is inserted to the proximal jejunum just distal to the ligament of Treitz. For contrast injection, an electronic pump system equipped with a plastic bag and a 50 mL syringe is usually used. Barium enteroclysis can be per-

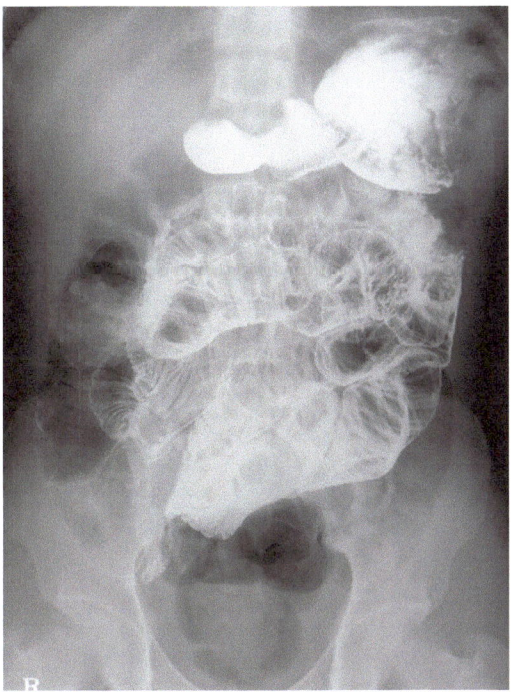

Fig. 2 Modified small-bowel series. The patient first took 40% w/v barium solution mixed with methylcellulose. Thereafter, 600 mL of 0.5% methylcellulose was additionally ingested. The bowel loops are sufficiently distended with better translucency. Therefore, well-distended bowel loops are visible like in barium enteroclysis

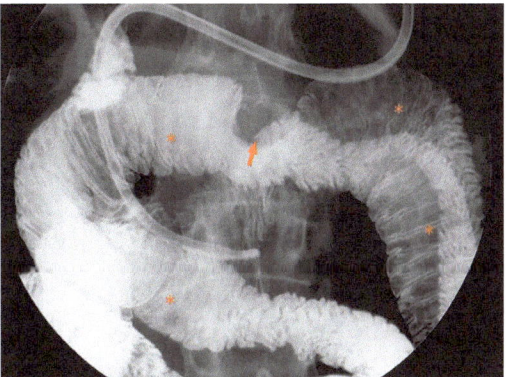

Fig. 3 Barium enteroclysis in a 56-year-old man. There is an eccentric nodule (arrow) at the proximal jejunum. A subepithelial tumor is suspected because of the smooth surface and the obtuse angle between the lesion and the adjacent jejunum. An inserted enteroclysis catheter and well-distended jejunal loops (*) with good translucency can be seen

formed through a single-contrast technique using barium solution alone, a double-contrast technique using both barium solution and methylcellulose, or a biphasic technique in which the single- and double-contrast techniques are used in combination [1]. The biggest advantage of barium enteroclysis is well-distended small-bowel loops with improved translucency, leading to a high diagnostic accuracy (Fig. 3). Because a large amount of contrast agent can be rapidly injected through the catheter and electronic pump system, the examination time can be shortened with less flocculation of contrast agents. Furthermore, because the injection speed can be adjusted, maximum small-bowel distension can be maintained during an entire examination. Barium enteroclysis is especially helpful for patients with suspected malabsorption, partial and intermittent small-bowel obstruction, fistula, or occult gastrointestinal bleeding, which could

not be detected with a conventional barium study [3]. Although barium enteroclysis provides higher diagnostic yield, its result highly depends on the radiologist's experience or expertise.

Computed Tomography (CT) Enterography and CT Enteroclysis

CT enterography and CT enteroclysis are different from general abdominal CT in that CT examinations are performed after the small bowel is fully distended through per-oral (CT enterography) or per-catheter (CT enteroclysis) contrast injection [4, 5]. Furthermore, intramural and extraluminal diseases can also be diagnosed using CT enterography and CT enteroclysis (Figs. 4 and 5), which is not possible with conventional barium studies or enteroscopy. CT enterography is usually preferred over CT enteroclysis because it has better patient compliance, causes less patient discomfort, and requires less radiation dose.

Adequate bowel distension is essential for obtaining high-quality CT enterography images. As oral contrast agents, methylcellulose, polyethylene glycol solution, 3% sorbitol, or mannitol can be used. On the other hand, water is not usually recommended because it does not provide

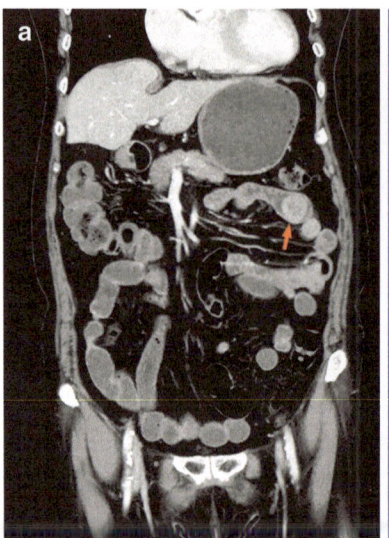 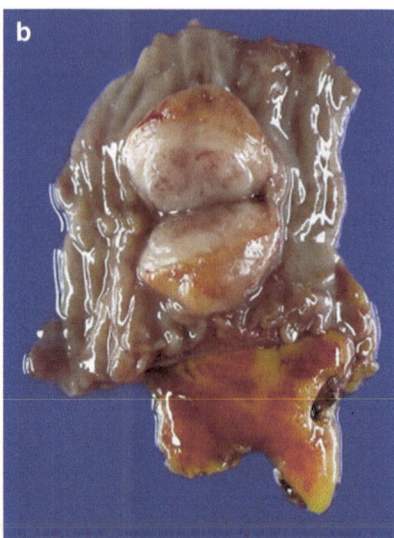

Fig. 4 (**a**) Computed tomography (CT) enterography of the patient in Fig. 3. A 2.3-cm well-demarcated and highly enhancing mass (arrow) is seen at the proximal jejunum. (**b**) Photograph of a gross specimen obtained after small-bowel resection, showing a small subepithelial lesion. The pathologic diagnosis is gastrointestinal stromal tumor. CT enterography reveals the presence and the internal characteristics of the lesion, which is an advantage over a barium study

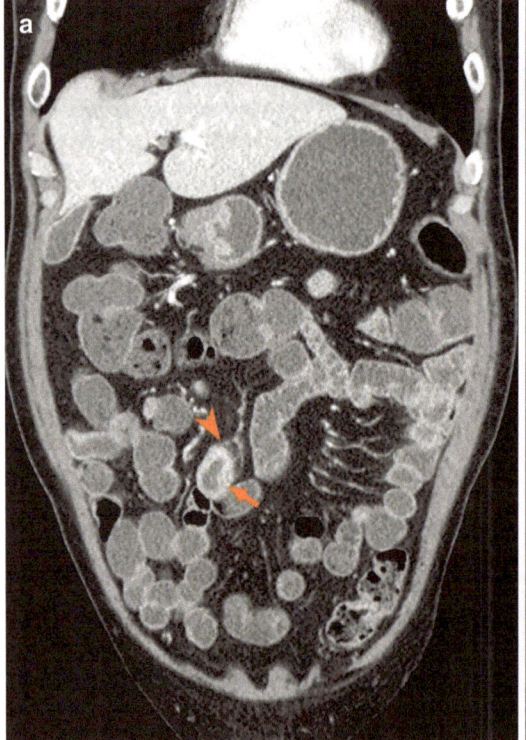
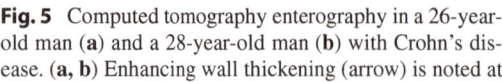
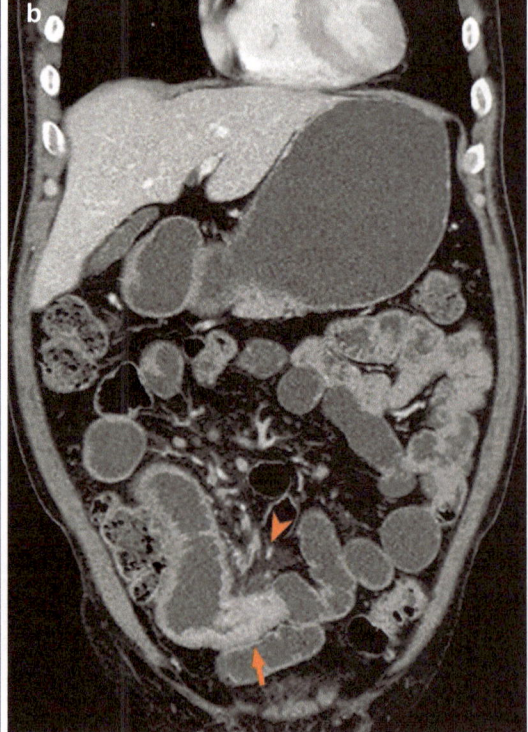

Fig. 5 Computed tomography enterography in a 26-year-old man (**a**) and a 28-year-old man (**b**) with Crohn's disease. (**a, b**) Enhancing wall thickening (arrow) is noted at the distal ileum. Mural stratification is seen at the thickened bowel and perienteric fat stranding (arrowhead) is also noted, suggesting an active inflammation

sufficient bowel distension owing to rapid water absorption through the bowel walls [6]. For CT enterography, patients are asked to drink 150–170 mL of contrast agent repeatedly with 5-min intervals over 60 min (for a total of 1350–1800 mL). For CT enteroclysis, a 12- or 14-F enteroclysis catheter is inserted through the patient's mouth or nose to the proximal jejunum under fluoroscopic guidance. After ballooning of the catheter to prevent reflux of the contrast agent, 1500–2000 mL of the contrast agent is then injected using an electronic motorized pump at an injection rate of 75–200 mL/min [5, 7].

CT scanning can be modified according to the indications. For example, single-phase CT scanning (either enteric or portal phase) is usually performed for the follow-up of patients with Crohn's disease [8], whereas triple-phase CT scanning should be performed when small-bowel tumor or obscured gastrointestinal bleeding is suspected [9].

CT enterography has both advantages and disadvantages compared with magnetic resonance (MR) enterography. CT enterography is easy to perform, inexpensive, less prone to respiratory or peristaltic motion artifacts owing to the short examination time, and provides excellent temporal and spatial resolution; however, it has the unavoidable disadvantage of radiation exposure [9]. Considering that inflammatory bowel disease occurs in young or adolescent patients and shows a waxing-and-waning disease course, radiation hazard can be a problem for those patients, especially when CT enterography is routinely used as a follow-up imaging tool. Fortunately, radiation exposure can be minimized with low-dose CT enterography using an iterative reconstruction technique. Recent studies reported that low-dose CT enterography can reduce the radiation exposure while maintaining the diagnostic accuracy for patients with inflammatory bowel disease [10].

The CT enterography findings of active Crohn's disease include wall thickening >3 mm, strong bowel wall enhancement compared with that of the adjacent normal bowel, mural stratification, comb sign, and fibrofatty proliferation around the involved bowel [11] (Fig. 5). Among

these, the degree of enhancement is known to be correlated with the disease activity of Crohn's disease. In addition, mural stratification is a strong indicator of active bowel inflammation versus homogeneous wall enhancement [12]. When patients with Crohn's disease are admitted to the hospital with a symptom of bowel obstruction, an exact differentiation between medical obstruction by active inflammation and surgical obstruction by chronic fibrosis is important because these conditions require different management plans. Although radiologic differentiation between the two disease conditions is difficult, mural stratification at the transition point with perienteric fat stranding may suggest an inflammatory narrowing, whereas homogeneous wall enhancement with thickening may indicate a fibrotic narrowing [11]. Increased intraluminal pressure caused by bowel obstruction may result in various fistulas at the involved bowels, such as enteroenteric, enterocolic, or enterocutaneous fistula (Fig. 6).

MR Enterography

In the past, MR imaging (MRI) was used in limited cases for gastrointestinal tract imaging mainly because of the long acquisition time. However, with the marked developments in MR technology, such as high-field-strength MR scan-

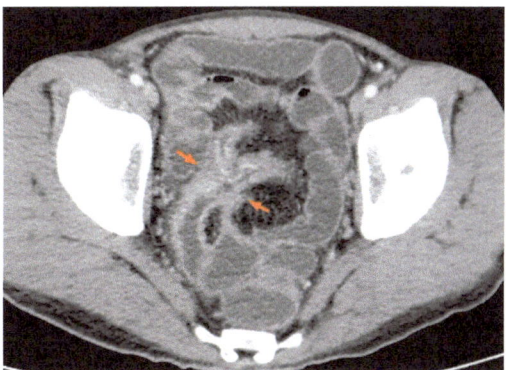

Fig. 6 Computed tomography enterography in an 18-year-old man with Crohn's disease. Thickened and enhancing ileal loops are clearly seen, and there is an enteroenteric fistula (arrows) between the two loops of the involved bowel

ners, multichannel phased array coil, and rapid MR sequences, high-quality MR images can be obtained even for movable organs such as the small bowel [13, 14].

Like in CT enterography, adequate bowel distension is essential to obtain high-quality MR enterography images. The oral contrast agents used for MR enterography can be divided into three types according to the signal intensity on T1- and T2-weighted images: positive, negative, or biphasic [15]. Positive contrast agents (e.g., pineapple juice or blueberry juice) show higher signal intensity than water on both T1- and T2-weighted images, whereas negative contrast agents (e.g., superparamagnetic iron oxide) show lower signal intensity on both T1- and T2-weighted images. Biphasic contrast agents (e.g., methylcellulose, polyethylene glycol solution, 3% sorbitol, and mannitol), which are the most commonly used, show low and high signal intensity on T1- and T2-weighted images, respectively, like water [14, 15]. The contrast administration technique for MR enterography is similar to that for CT enterography.

Because of the relatively long acquisition time, the intravenous use of anti-peristaltic agents is commonly recommended unless there are contraindications. Usually, one-half ampoule of Buscopan® is injected before MR examination and before intravenous contrast injection [16]. First, motion-free sequences, such as single-shot fast spin-echo T2 sequences (i.e., HASTE—half-Fourier single-shot turbo spin-echo), are obtained to identify mural edema or extramural fluid collection or abscess. Thereafter, balanced steady-state free precession sequences, such as true fast imaging with steady-state precession (FISP), are scanned to assess mesenteric findings, including comb sign, fistula, and fibrofatty proliferation. Finally, multiphasic dynamic contrast-enhanced sequences are obtained using a fast three-dimensional spoiled gradient echo T1 fat-saturation sequence to determine the presence or degree of bowel wall enhancement [17] (Fig. 7). Recently, because there have been several reports

showing the usefulness of diffusion-weighted MR sequences for the evaluation of disease activity in Crohn's disease, diffusion-weighted images can be taken before obtaining contrast-enhanced T1 sequences [18].

Compared with CT enterography, the lack of radiation exposure is the biggest advantage of MR enterography. Therefore, bowel movability can be assessed using MR enterography through cine images. Other advantages include better soft tissue contrast, acquisition of functional information through diffusion-weighted or perfusion imaging, and fewer adverse effects of intravenous contrast agents [4]. However, MR enterography also has several limitations, including lower spatial and temporal resolution, longer acquisition time, being prone to artifacts from bowel movement or intraluminal air, high cost, and less availability [9].

Despite such limitations, the American College of Radiology strongly recommends the use of MR enterography for young and adolescent patients with Crohn's disease, especially for follow-up examination and for evaluating perianal diseases [19].

Angiography

Angiography is useful to detect active bleeding (rate: > 0.5 mL/min) or vascular disorders and can be used for the diagnosis of occult gastrointestinal bleeding [20]. Because the angiographic accuracy for gastrointestinal bleeding is strongly related to the speed of bleeding, the diagnostic accuracy rate is 61–72% for the detection of the cause and location of active bleeding, whereas it is <20% when the bleeding speed is slow or when bleeding has stopped [21]. For angiodysplasia, the typical angiographic findings are slowly filling of venous structures at the bowel wall or the presence of vascular bundles and early opacified venous structures [20] (Fig. 8). Angiography can be performed therapeutically as well as diagnostically. The commonly used embolic materials are glue, gelatin sponge, and coil.

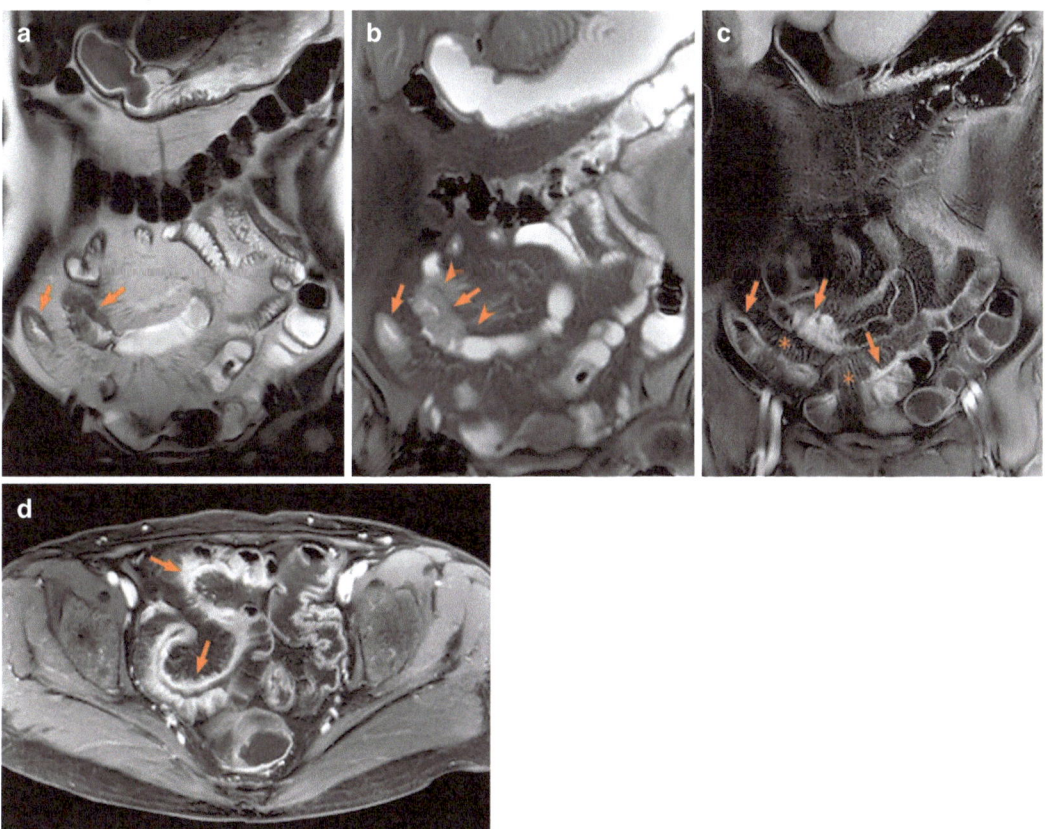

Fig. 7 Magnetic resonance enterography in a 47-year-old woman with Crohn's disease. (**a**) On a HASTE (half-Fourier single-shot turbo spin-echo) sequence image, multifocal wall thickenings (arrows) are seen at the distal ileum. The thickened bowel loops show higher signal intensity than the adjacent muscle, suggesting an active inflammation. (**b**) On a true FISP (fast imaging with steady-state precession) image, dirty fat infiltration (arrowheads) is noted around the thickened bowel (arrows), indicating active inflammation and edema. (**c, d**) Contrast-enhanced coronal (**c**) and axial (**d**) images show a strong enhancement at the involved bowels (arrows) and engorged vasa recta, so-called comb sign (➜), also suggesting active inflammation

Conclusion

By virtue of the rapid advancements in endoscopy, CT, and MRI technology, the use and importance of conventional barium study, which used to be the primary diagnostic tool for small-bowel disease, has been rapidly decreasing. At present, there is a paradigm shift in the diagnosis of small-bowel diseases owing to marked improvements in the diagnostic accuracy of CT or MR enterography. Considering that CT and MR enterography have their own advantages and disadvantages, proper selection should be cautiously made depending on the clinical situation of the patient and the availability of the scanner.

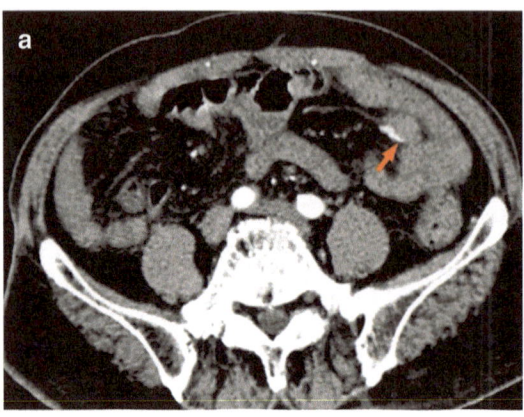
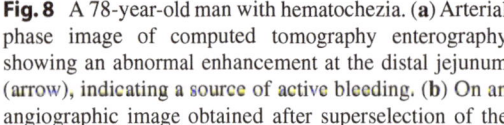
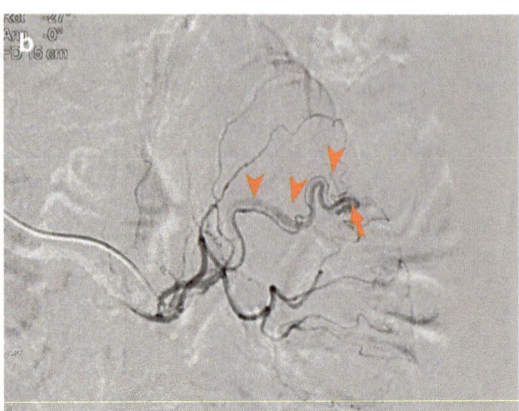

Fig. 8 A 78-year-old man with hematochezia. (**a**) Arterial phase image of computed tomography enterography showing an abnormal enhancement at the distal jejunum (arrow), indicating a source of active bleeding. (**b**) On an angiographic image obtained after superselection of the jejunal branch from the superior mesenteric artery, a small abnormal vascular bundle (arrow) and early draining vein (arrowheads) are seen. Therefore, angiodysplasia can be diagnosed. After embolization using glue, hematochezia was stopped

References

1. Park BJ. Characteristics and selection for small bowel imaging. J 49th Cong Korean Soc Gastrointest Endosc. 2013;2013:356–8.
2. Ha HK, Shin JH, Rha SE, et al. Modified small-bowel follow-through: use of methylcellulose to improve bowel transradiance and prepare barium suspension. Radiology. 1999;211:197–201.
3. Maglinte DD, Chernish SM, DeWeese R, Kelvin FM, Brunelle RL. Acquired jejunoileal diverticular disease: subject review. Radiology. 1986;158:577–80.
4. Raptopoulos V, Schwartz RK, McNicholas MM, Movson J, Pearlman J, Joffe N. Multiplanar helical CT enterography in patients with Crohn's disease. AJR Am J Roentgenol. 1997;169:1545–50.
5. Maglinte DD, Sandrasegaran K, Lappas JC. CT enteroclysis: techniques and applications. Radiol Clin N Am. 2007a;45:289–301.
6. Lee SM, Kim SH, Ahn SJ, Kang HJ, Han JK. Virtual monoenergetic dual-layer, dual-energy CT enterography: optimization of keV settings and its added value for Crohn's disease. Eur Radiol. 2018;28(6):2525–34. https://doi.org/10.1007/s00330-017-5215-z. [Epub ahead of print]
7. Maglinte DD, Sandrasegaran K, Lappas JC, Chiorean M. CT Enteroclysis Radiol. 2007b;245:661–71.
8. Vandenbroucke F, Mortele KJ, Tatli S, et al. Noninvasive multidetector computed tomography enterography in patients with small-bowel Crohn's disease: is a 40-second delay better than 70 seconds? Acta Radiol. 2007;48:1052–60.
9. Hammer MR, Podberesky DJ, Dillman JR. Multidetector computed tomographic and magnetic resonance enterography in children: state of the art. Radiol Clin N Am. 2013;51:615–36.
10. Kaza RK, Platt JF, Al-Hawary MM, Wasnik A, Liu PS, Pandya A. CT enterography at 80 kVp with adaptive statistical iterative reconstruction versus at 120 kVp with standard reconstruction: image quality, diagnostic adequacy, and dose reduction. AJR Am J Roentgenol. 2012;198:1084–92.
11. Hara AK, Swartz PG. CT enterography of Crohn's disease. Abdom Imaging. 2009;34:289–95.
12. Bodily KD, Fletcher JG, Solem CA, et al. Crohn disease: mural attenuation and thickness at contrast-enhanced CT Enterography--correlation with endoscopic and histologic findings of inflammation. Radiology. 2006;238:505–16.
13. Siddiki HA, Fidler JL, Fletcher JG, et al. Prospective comparison of state-of-the-art MR enterography and CT enterography in small-bowel Crohn's disease. AJR Am J Roentgenol. 2009;193:113–21.
14. Ippolito D, Invernizzi F, Galimberti S, Panelli MR, Sironi S. MR enterography with polyethylene glycol as oral contrast medium in the follow-up of patients with Crohn disease: comparison with CT enterography. Abdom Imaging. 2010;35:563–70.
15. Fidler JL, Guimaraes L, Einstein DM. MR imaging of the small bowel. Radiographics. 2009;29:1811–25.
16. Kim SH. Computed tomography enterography and magnetic resonance enterography in the diagnosis of Crohn's disease. Intest Res. 2015;13:27–38.
17. Gee MS, Harisinghani MG. MRI in patients with inflammatory bowel disease. J Magn Reson Imaging. 2011;33:527–34.

18. Kim JS, Jang HY, Park SH, et al. MR Enterography assessment of bowel inflammation severity in Crohn disease using the MR index of activity score: modifying roles of DWI and effects of contrast phases. AJR Am J Roentgenol. 2017;208:1022–9.

19. Expert Panel on Gastrointestinal Imaging. ACR appropriateness criteria on Crohn disease. Am Coll Radiol. 2011;7:1–17.

20. Gunjan D, Sharma V, Rana SS, Bhasin DK. Small bowel bleeding: a comprehensive review. Gastroenterol Rep. 2014;2:262–75.

21. Zuckerman GR, Prakash C, Askin MP, Lewis BS. AGA technical review on the evaluation and management of occult and obscure gastrointestinal bleeding. Gastroenterology. 2000;118:201–21.

Nuclear Medicine Imaging

Jae Seung Kim and Minyoung Oh

Key Points
- When active gastrointestinal bleeding is suspected, a gastrointestinal bleeding scan is helpful to identify and localize the culprit vessel before an endoscopy or angiography.
- ^{99m}Tc-technetium pertechnetate (^{99m}TcO$_4$-), which is taken up by mucin-producing cells of normal or ectopic gastric mucosa and secreted into the gastrointestinal lumen, makes gastric mucosa scanning (scintigraphy for Meckel's diverticulum) possible for detecting ectopic gastric mucosa in a Meckel's diverticulum.
- ^{18}F-fluorodeoxyglucose positron emission tomography (PET) is a useful tool for staging, restaging, and monitoring of cancers in the small intestine, including adenocarcinoma, lymphoma, gastrointestinal stromal tumor, and metastatic small-intestinal tumor. The use of somatostatin receptor imaging, including ^{68}Ga-DOTA-TOC PET, for the assessment of neuroendocrine tumor is increasing because of its high diagnostic accuracy.

J. S. Kim (✉) · M. Oh
Department of Nuclear Medicine, Asan Medical Center, University of Ulsan College of Medicine, Seoul, South Korea
e-mail: jaeskim@amc.seoul.kr; my@amc.seoul.kr

Introduction

Nuclear medicine imaging is a useful diagnostic method for assessing patients with small-bowel disease because it can non-invasively evaluate the physiological and biological changes in the human body. It has been actively used for the evaluation of bleeding and oncologic diseases of the small bowel.

Nuclear Medicine Imaging for Bleeding in the Small Bowel

Gastrointestinal (GI) Bleeding Scan

Introduction
Localization of the bleeding site is important for effective therapy of acute GI bleeding. Upper intestinal bleeding is often diagnosed using gastroscopy and angiography. However, when active and recurrent lower intestinal bleeding is suspected, a GI bleeding scan is helpful for identifying and localizing the culprit vessel before an angiography or endoscopy.

Depending on the radiopharmaceuticals, GI bleeding scans are classified as described below.

^{99m}Tc-sulfur Colloid
Intravenously injected ^{99m}Tc-sulfur colloid is rapidly (within 15 min) extracted from the blood by reticuloendothelial cells of the liver, spleen, and bone marrow. With active bleeding, part of the

© Springer Nature Singapore Pte Ltd. 2022
H. J. Chun et al. (eds.), *Small Intestine Disease*, https://doi.org/10.1007/978-981-16-7239-2_9

injected ^{99m}Tc-sulfur colloid extravasates from the bleeding site into the GI tract lumen, whereas the remaining ^{99m}Tc-sulfur colloid is extracted into the reticuloendothelial system. Persistent extravasation and simultaneous clearance from the blood pool result in a high target-to-background ratio, permitting visualization of the bleeding focus. It is possible to make a diagnosis if dynamic imaging after IV ^{99m}Tc-sulfur colloid injection showed tracer movement into the GI tract. It is sometimes difficult to diagnose bleeding in the splenic flexure or hepatic flexure of the colon owing to high uptake in the spleen or liver. In this case, additional image acquisition in the lateral view would be helpful. It is only possible to diagnose bleeding if it is active at the time of examination with ^{99m}Tc-sulfur colloid, similar to that in angiography. If the result is negative but active bleeding is highly suspected, repeated examination may be necessary.

^{99m}Tc Red Blood Cell (^{99m}Tc-RBC)

Labeling of ^{99m}Tc-RBC

Currently, direct labeling of ^{99m}Tc to RBCs is the most widely used radiopharmaceutical method for a GI bleeding scan. The major advantages of this method over ^{99m}Tc-sulfur colloid are that it is possible to acquire images for a longer period of time, usually up to 24 h, and it is affected only by the half-life of ^{99m}Tc and the stability of ^{99m}Tc-RBCs. This makes it possible to detect intermittent bleeding [1]. The minimal rate of bleeding that can be detected with this method is 0.04 mL/min in animals and 0.1 mL/min in humans [2, 3]. However, it shows a relatively low target-to-background ratio owing to the persistent existence of ^{99m}Tc-RBCs in the blood pool. To achieve a high target-to-background ratio and optimal image quality, the labeling efficiency of ^{99m}Tc-RBCs should be sufficiently high. Unlabeled free pertechnetate could be absorbed into salivary glands and gastric mucosa and secreted into the GI tract lumen, consequently affecting the interpretation of the results of a GI bleeding scan. To increase the labeling efficiency, various techniques of labeling, including in vivo, modified

in vivo, and in vitro methods, have been developed. The in vitro labeling method is widely used because of its high labeling efficiency of >97% with convenient preparation. The lowered labeling efficiency can be explained by the following causes: anticancer drugs, including doxorubicin, heparin (which can form a complex with ^{99m}Tc), methyldopa (which lowers the reducing power by oxidizing tin ion), hydralazine, quinidine (which can promote antibodies to RBCs), and recent history of blood transfusion [4].

Method of Examination

Dynamic images are usually acquired in the supine position from immediately after injection of the radiopharmaceutical to 60–90 min, as active bleeding moves through the GI tract. If bleeding is not detected in the first phase of dynamic imaging, delayed imaging could be achieved usually 2–4 h and up to 24 h after injection. When the bleeding focus is equivocal on dynamic images, single photon emission tomography (SPECT) would be helpful.

Interpretation

Most of the injected radiopharmaceutical is rapidly redistributed to the heart, liver, spleen, and great vessels, while some amount is excreted through the urinary system. A tracer that accumulates and moves over time outside of the organs mentioned above is diagnostic. In the case of bleeding in the large intestine, the tracer moves by making a "rectangle" along the ascending-transverse-descending colon. In the case of small-intestinal bleeding, the tracer starts at the center and moves fast to the outer aspect of the abdomen, with a curved shape (Fig. 1). Localized accumulation of the tracer without movement indicates a solid organ, including an accessory spleen, an ectopic kidney, or a hemangioma. Free pertechnetate moving along the GI tract could be a source of a false-positive finding. In such a case, additional image acquisition in the thyroid and salivary glands could be helpful for the differentiation. Excretion of the tracer through the urinary system could be differentiated through the acquisition of lateral images.

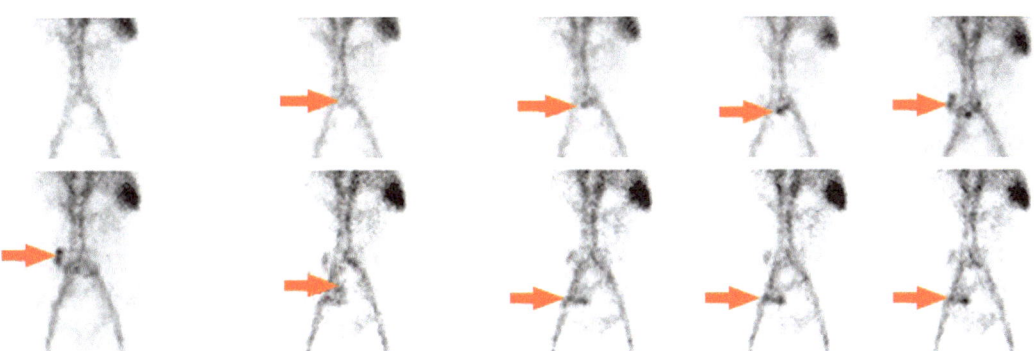

Fig. 1 A ^{99m}Tc red blood cell gastrointestinal bleeding scan showing small-intestinal bleeding that started at the center and moved to the outer aspect of the abdominal cavity

Gastric Mucosa Scan (Scintigraphy for Meckel's Diverticulum)

Introduction

Meckel's diverticulum is a vestigial organ of the omphalomesenteric duct that is present in about 1–3% of the population. It is usually located in the antimesenteric border of the distal ileum within 80–100 cm proximal to the ileocecal valve. Approximately 57% of Meckel's diverticulum contains ectopic gastric mucosa, which secretes gastric acid that leads to ulcer development on Meckel's diverticulum and the adjacent ileum. The most common symptom of Meckel's diverticulum is lower GI tract bleeding with abdominal pain. ^{99m}Tc-pertechnetate is taken up by mucin-producing normal cells of normal or ectopic gastric mucosa and secreted into the GI lumen. This makes gastric mucosa scan (scintigraphy for Meckel's diverticulum) possible for detecting ectopic gastric mucosa in a Meckel's diverticulum. Although the reports vary, overall, a gastric mucosa scan has 85% sensitivity, 95% specificity, and 90% accuracy, if adequately performed [5].

Method

Pretreatment

Fasting before the examination increases the sensitivity of the method by decreasing the silhouette of the stomach. It is recommended to avoid medications or examinations that could affect the GI tract, for 2–3 days before the examination. To increase the sensitivity of the examination, the following medications can be administrated, as recommended by the Society of Nuclear Medicine and Molecular Imaging and European Association of Nuclear Medicine practice guidelines [6]:

- Histamine H2 blocker: By suppressing the secretion of gastric acid from parietal cells, histamine H2 blocker blocks the excretion of ^{99m}Tc-pertechnetate, thereby increasing the sensitivity of Meckel's diverticulum scintigraphy.
- Glucagon: Glucagon causes GI tract muscle relaxation, which leads to some inhibition of intestinal peristalsis, thereby inhibiting the migration of secreted ^{99m}Tc-pertechnetate. However, glucagon must not be administrated to patients with diabetes mellitus.

Method of Examination

Images of the abdominopelvic cavity, including the stomach and urinary bladder, are obtained in the supine position. For infants, chest images should be acquired to exclude possible bronchopulmonary foregut malformation with the ectopic gastric mucosa. Anterior-view images are usually acquired until 30 min after the injection of ^{99m}Tc-pertechnetate. If the initial images are negative, additional images could be acquired up to 60 min after the injection. Images taken after 60 min could show interference from moving ^{99m}Tc-pertechnetate that originated from the stomach. Additional lateral imaging could be helpful for the differentiation of Meckel's diverticulum from uptakes in the kidney. Post-voiding images could be helpful to detect Meckel's diverticulum obscured by the urinary bladder. When there is a high suspicion of Meckel's diverticulum despite the negative results of the standard examination, SPECT would exclude activities from artifacts and the urinary bladder and could be helpful for planning a surgery.

Clinical Application and Interpretation

The goal of a Meckel's scan is to identify the site of ectopic gastric mucosa inside Meckel's diverticulum as a cause of GI tract bleeding. Bleeding caused by Meckel's diverticulum is usually found in children. If there is an active bleeding, performing GI bleeding scan is recommended instead of scintigraphy for Meckel's diverticulum, regardless of age.

^{99m}Tc-pertechnetate used in Meckel's scan is taken up both in normal and ectopic gastric mucosa. Uptake in normal gastric mucosa

appears in the early phase and is maximized 10–15 min after injection. Ectopic gastric mucosa may be suspected when the appearance of focal uptake has a similar pattern to that of the normal gastric mucosa in the right lower abdomen (Fig. 2); however, it may also appear in other locations in the abdominal cavity.

Because of the excretion of radiopharmaceuticals, tracer activity might appear in the small intestine, kidneys, urethra, and bladder. Focal activities could also be seen in cases of hydronephrosis, ectopic kidneys, vesicoureteral reflux, and bladder diverticulum. These activities usually appear later than activities in the normal gastric mucosa.

A false-positive scan could result from duplication cysts containing ectopic gastric mucosa, enteritis, small-bowel obstruction, intussusception, peptic ulcer, angioma, or arteriovenous malformation. A false-negative scan could result if small-bowel series using barium or perchlorate is performed before the examination.

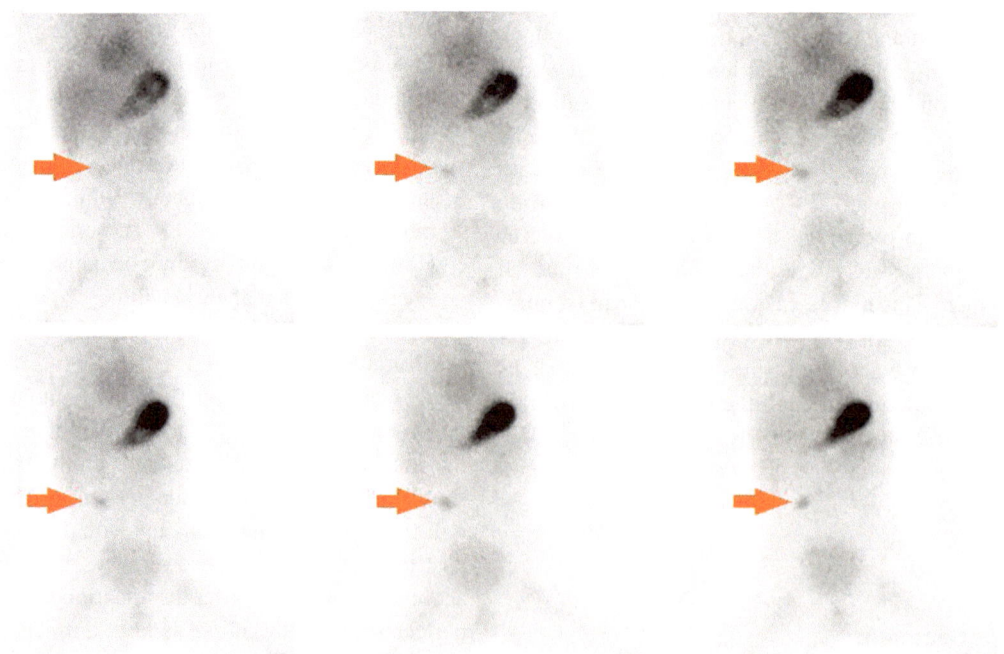

Fig. 2 A positive gastric mucosa scan (scintigraphy for Meckel's diverticulum). There is abnormal accumulation of the tracer in the right lower abdomen (→). Increased accumulation is observed over time, similar to that in the normal gastric mucosa of the stomach

Nuclear Medicine Imaging in Oncology

^{18}F-fluorodeoxyglucose Positron Emission Tomography (^{18}F-FDG PET)

Adenocarcinoma

^{18}F-FDG is a glucose analog labeled with ^{18}F, a radioisotope commonly used in PET scans. It undergoes phosphorylation after being delivered into cells by glucose transporters of the cell membrane, is captured inside cells, and is not further metabolized. It has been reported that most malignant tumors show higher glucose consumption and, consequently, higher ^{18}F-FDG uptake on PET than non-tumor cells. ^{18}F-FDG PET is widely used in oncology for diagnosis, staging, monitoring, and recurrence determination [7]. Typical primary small-bowel adenocarcinoma shows increased ^{18}F-FDG metabolism with intestinal wall thickening (Fig. 3a).

Lymphoma

Among small-bowel lymphomas, diffuse large B-cell lymphoma, Burkitt's lymphoma, mantle cell lymphoma, and enteropathy associated T-cell lymphoma are known to show ^{18}F-FDG intake (Fig. 3b). In contrast, mucosa-associated lymphoid tissue lymphoma is known to show diverse ^{18}F-FDG intake. ^{18}F-FDG PET is used for staging, assessment of treatment effectiveness, and determination of recurrence.

GI Stromal Tumors (GISTs)

^{18}F-FDG PET can predict the early response of tyrosine kinase inhibitors such as imatinib mesylate (Gleevec™) in metastatic or unresectable GISTs (Fig. 3c). On quantitative analysis, it is known that if ^{18}F-FDG intake is reduced by >25% in posttreatment PET, the 1-year progression-free survival rate reaches up to 92%. Further, it may help assess secondary resistance.

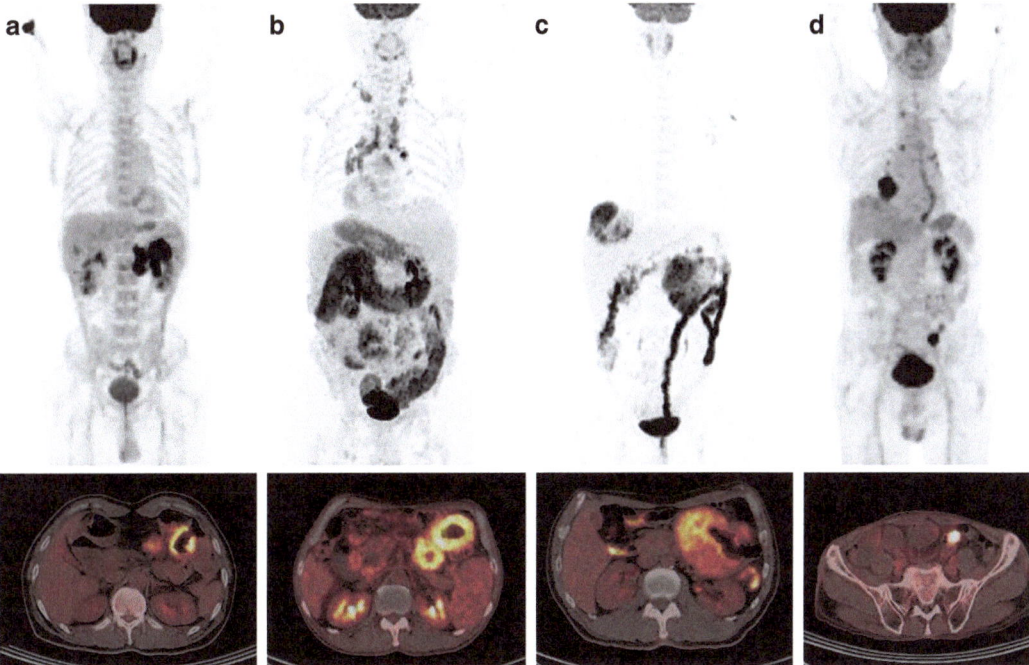

Fig. 3 ^{18}F- fluorodeoxyglucose positron emission tomography scans of small-bowel tumors. (**a**) Adenocarcinoma. (**b**) Lymphoma. (**c**) Gastrointestinal stromal tumors. (**d**) Small-bowel metastasis

Small-Bowel Metastasis

Colorectal cancer, ovarian cancer, and gastric cancer invade the small intestine through direct invasion or transmission inside the abdominal cavity. On the other hand, breast cancer, lung cancer, and melanoma invade the small intestine through remote metastasis. Generally, small-bowel metastasis shows ^{18}F-FDG metabolism similar to that of the primary tumor (Fig. 3d). Especially, malignant melanoma can extensively metastasize to the small intestine, mesentery, and lymph nodes. According to a meta-analysis, ^{18}F-FDG PET shows 92% sensitivity and 90% specificity for recurrent metastatic melanoma carcinoma.

Somatostatin Receptor Imaging

Somatostatin receptor is a kind of membrane glycoprotein manifesting from neuroendocrine cells such as islet cells of the pancreas or neural crest with amine precursor uptake and decarboxylation. Most neuroendocrine tumors grow slowly and are well differentiated. Therefore, it would be better to perform assessment with somatostatin receptor scintigraphy with ^{111}In-DTPA-pentetreotide (Octreoscan™) than with ^{18}F-FDG PET. Easily available radiopharmaceuticals for somatostatin receptor PET imaging are being developed. They show higher additional detection rate and diagnostic accuracy than somatostatin receptor scintigraphy (Fig. 4), and their use for the assessment of neuroendocrine tumors has increased [8]. As somatostatin receptor-rich neuroendocrine tumors respond well to radionuclide treatment, it can also be used to select candidates for radionuclide treatment. In Korea, ^{68}Ga-DOTATOC PET is now clinically used after its recognition as a new medical technology that passed the Center for New Health Technology Assessment for the safety and effectiveness in late 2014.

Fig. 4 Somatostatin receptor imaging of a patient with a recurred neuroendocrine tumor. (**a**) Metastases in the liver and retroperitoneal lymph node are shown on ^{68}Ga-DOTATOC positron emission tomography. (**b**) Only retroperitoneal lymph node metastasis is shown on ^{111}In-DTPA-pentetreotide scintigraphy (Octreoscan™)

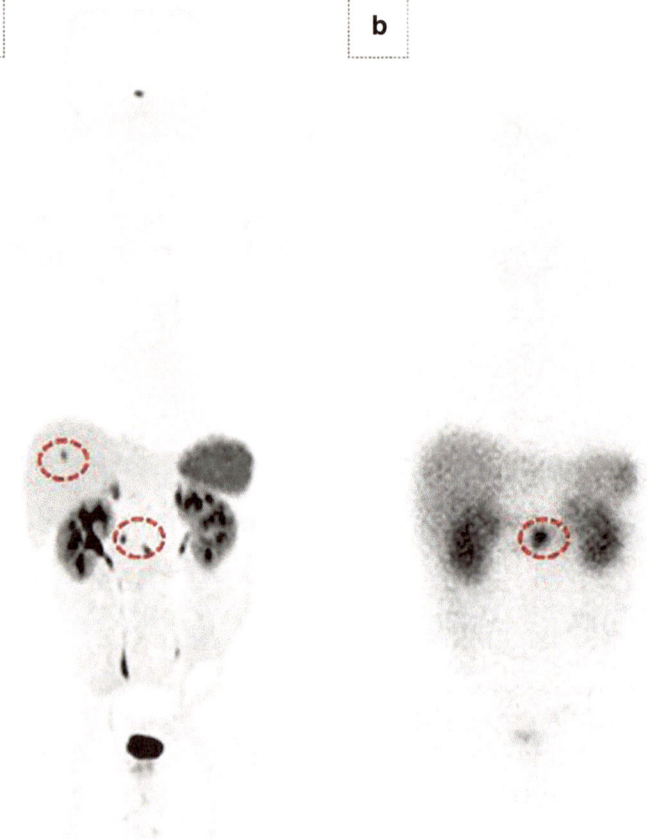

References

1. Bunker S, Lull R, Tanasescu D, Redwine M, Rigby J, Brown J, Brachman M, McAuley R, Ramanna L, Landry A. Scintigraphy of gastrointestinal hemorrhage: superiority of 99mTc red blood cells over 99mTc sulfur colloid. Am J Roentgenol. 1984;143:543–8.
2. Smith R, Copely D, Bolen F. 99mTc RBC scintigraphy: correlation of gastrointestinal bleeding rates with scintigraphic findings. Am J Roentgenol. 1987;148:869–74.
3. Thorne DA, Datz FL, Remley K, Christian PE. Bleeding rates necessary for detecting acute gastrointestinal bleeding with technetium-99m-labeled red blood cells in an experimental model. J Nucl Med. 1987;28:514–20.
4. Grady E. Gastrointestinal bleeding scintigraphy in the early 21st century. J Nucl Med. 2016;57:252–9.
5. Sfakianakis GN, Conway JJ. Detection of ectopic gastric mucosa in Meckel's diverticulum and in other aberrations by scintigraphy: ii. Indications and methods--a 10-year experience. J Nucl Med. 1981;22:732–8.
6. Spottswood SE, Pfluger T, Bartold SP, Brandon D, Burchell N, Delbeke D, Fink-Bennett DM, Hodges PK, Jolles PR, Lassmann M. SNMMI and EANM practice guideline for meckel diverticulum scintigraphy 2.0. J Nucl Med Technol. 2014;42:163–9.
7. Cronin C, Scott J, Kambadakone A, Catalano O, Sahani D, Blake M, McDermott S. Utility of positron emission tomography/CT in the evaluation of small bowel pathology. Br J Radiol. 2012;85:1211–21.
8. Buchmann I, Henze M, Engelbrecht S, Eisenhut M, Runz A, Schäfer M, Schilling T, Haufe S, Herrmann T, Haberkorn U. Comparison of 68Ga-DOTATOC PET and 111In-DTPAOC (Octreoscan) SPECT in patients with neuroendocrine tumours. Eur J Nucl Med Mol Imaging. 2007;34:1617–26.

Part IV

Capsule Endoscopy

History of Capsule Endoscopy

Myung-Gyu Choi

The Birth of a Capsule Endoscope

In 1981, Gavriel Iddan at Raphael, a government defense R&D group in Israel, has established the initial concept of the wireless capsule endoscope using the electronic eye device technology required for missile guidance. Since 1994, animal studies on capsule endoscopy and clinical studies on humans have begun. In 1996, independent research work from Paul Swain groups at the Royal London Hospital succeeded in receiving images from pigs with wireless endoscopes using charged coupled devices and obtained patents in the USA in 1997. Iddan founded Given Inc., commercialized wireless capsule endoscopes, and integrated studies that were conducted separately in England and Israel. In 1999, Paul Swain overcame the technical obstacles and swallowed the first capsule endoscope directly to prove the safety of the test. The two groups combined their efforts and successfully conducted their first study on ten healthy volunteers in 1999. In 2000, the results of ten normal volunteers were published in the Nature [1]. In August 2001, Given's M2A capsule endoscopy was approved by the FDA and earned the Conformité Européenne (CE) mark and became available for clinical use. After the first wireless small bowel capsule by Given Imaging, several types of capsules were developed, including the esophagus, small intestine, and large intestine, depending on the test organ. Since then, different manufacturers of endoscopic capsules in several countries, including Japan, Finland, China, and Italy, have entered the market.

In 2003, a Korean company (Intromedic Ltd., Seoul, Korea) developed a capsule endoscope (MiroCam®) which uses a novel Human Body Communication technology for data transmission, Human Body Communication uses the human body as a conductive medium for data transmission from the capsule endoscope to electrodes attached to the Body. MiroCam® received both Korean market clearance and the CE mark in 2007 [2].

Growth of Capsule Endoscopy

The capsule endoscopy is composed of a capsule for capturing and transmitting images, a recorder for receiving and storing image signals, and a workstation for analyzing and reading stored image data.

Capsule

Capsule endoscopes have been developed as small pills with a size smaller than a maximum dimension of 32 mm in length and 13 mm in

M.-G. Choi (✉)
College of Medicine, The Catholic University of Korea, Seoul, South Korea
e-mail: choim@catholic.ac.kr

© Springer Nature Singapore Pte Ltd. 2022
H. J. Chun et al. (eds.), *Small Intestine Disease*, https://doi.org/10.1007/978-981-16-7239-2_10

diameter for easiness to swallow. Capsule endoscope includes optical systems including LEDs, image sensors, batteries, and communication devices. The lens of the capsule endoscope was equipped with a wide viewing angle of more than 140 degrees. A camera with wider viewing angles has been introduced in the latest versions of the commercial capsules. Capsules with multiple cameras have also been developed and launched on the market. For example, the PillCam COLON® for colonoscopy is equipped with two cameras on both sides to obtain bi-directional images, so that the lesions between the wrinkles are not missed. Newer capsule with a panoramic viewing mode is currently available and might increase the detection rate of bleeding lesions in patients with obscure gastrointestinal bleeding. Conventional wireless capsule endoscopy has a limitation that the capsule moves only by a combination of intestinal peristalsis and gravity. New capsules with active propulsion and orientation control are under development [3].

Storage Device

The image data wirelessly transmitted to the storage device is read through the workstation. Portable devices capable of real-time monitoring have also been developed. Capsule endoscopy may not detect the lesion or capture the area of interest if the capsule progresses faster due to the rapid movement of the small intestine. On the contrary, when the small intestine movement is slow or in a state of resting, repeated capturing of the still image may cause power waste of the capsule. The average operating time of the two oxidized silver cells used in the first capsule endoscope was only 7 ± 1 h, which means that the capsule could not receive all of the data until it entered the large intestine. In recent years, the life span of the battery has been remarkably extended enough to observe the entire small intestine.

Workstation

Reading of the image data stored in the storage device requires substantial periods of training due to inconsistency between capsule and conventional endoscopic images, long recording time, and inter-observer difference. Several reading software have been developed to shorten the image reading time. The function of locating capsule in the intestine, simultaneous viewing of multiple images, enlarging function, and automatic suggestion of suspicious bleeding lesion have been incorporated into the software. The application of deep learning systems and artificial intelligence to detect and diagnose intestinal pathology from computational analysis of video capsule images will be available soon, and we expect to see breakthrough change.

Clinical Application of Capsule Endoscopy

The introduction of capsule endoscopy and device-assisted enteroscopy into the clinic has revolutionized the management of small bowel disease. Evidence-based guidelines on the appropriate use of video capsule endoscopy were published by the European and American Society of Gastrointestinal Endoscopy, respectively [4–8]. The Korean Gut Image Study group was founded in 2003. The Korean Gut Image Study group has established a nationwide database of capsule endoscopy, conducted multicenter clinical studies on capsule endoscopy, established guidelines for appropriate use of capsule endoscopy in Korea. Capsule endoscopy proved superiority of diagnostic yield to other diagnostic modalities in patients with small bowel diseases [9–11]. Since September 2014, capsule endoscopy has been approved and reimbursed for the diagnosis of obscure gastrointestinal bleeding, Crohn's disease, small bowel tumors and other small bowel diseases in Korea [2].

References

1. Iddan G, Meron G, Glukhovsky A, et al. Wireless capsule endoscopy. Nature. 2000;405:417.
2. Group KGIS. Capsule endoscopy. Seoul: Medbook Korea; 2008.
3. Shamsudhin N, Zverev VI, Keller H, et al. Magnetically guided capsule endoscopy. Med Phys. 2017;44:e91–e111.
4. Faigel DO, Baron TH, Adler DG, et al. ASGE guideline: guidelines for credentialing and granting privileges for capsule endoscopy. Gastrointest Endosc. 2005;61:503–5.
5. Ladas SD, Triantafyllou K, Spada C, et al. European Society of Gastrointestinal Endoscopy (ESGE): recommendations (2009) on clinical use of video capsule endoscopy to investigate small-bowel, esophageal and colonic diseases. Endoscopy. 2010;42:220–7.
6. Mishkin DS, Chuttani R, Croffie J, et al. ASGE technology status evaluation report: wireless capsule endoscopy. Gastrointest Endosc. 2006;63:539–45.
7. Rondonotti E, Spada C, Adler S, et al. Small-bowel capsule endoscopy and device-assisted enteroscopy for diagnosis and treatment of small-bowel disorders: European Society of Gastrointestinal Endoscopy (ESGE) technical review. Endoscopy. 2018;50:423–46.
8. Spada C, McNamara D, Despott EJ, et al. Performance measures for small-bowel endoscopy: a European Society of Gastrointestinal Endoscopy (ESGE) quality improvement initiative. Endoscopy. 2019;51:574–98.
9. Park SK, Ye BD, Kim KO, et al. Guidelines for video capsule endoscopy: emphasis on Crohn's disease. Clin Endosc. 2015;48:128–35.
10. Shim KN, Moon JS, Chang DK, et al. Guideline for capsule endoscopy: obscure gastrointestinal bleeding. Clin Endosc. 2013;46:45–53.
11. Song HJ, Moon JS, Do JH, et al. Guidelines for bowel preparation before video capsule endoscopy. Clin Endosc. 2013;46:147–54.

Current Trends in Capsule Endoscopy

Hoon Jai Chun

Types of Currently Used Capsule Endoscopes: Capsule endoscopy can be used to inspect the esophagus, stomach, small intestine, and colon. The currently available capsule endoscopes include the PillCam (Medtronic, USA), MiroCam (Intromedic, Korea), EndoCapsule (Olympus, Japan), OMOM (Jinshan science and technology, China), and CapsoCam (Capsovision, USA).

Efficacy of Capsule Endoscopy: Capsule endoscopy is the first diagnostic method for small bowel examination. In the diagnosis of small intestinal bleeding, capsule endoscopy is superior to push enteroscopy, computed tomography enterography, magnetic resonance enterography, and angiography and is useful for the diagnosis and monitoring of Crohn's disease.

The capsule endoscope is a diagnostic device that is used to observe the inside of the gastrointestinal tract using a camera installed in a pill-like capsule. Capsule endoscopes are made of a wireless endoscopic device, and the current commonly used devices include a capsule endoscope body, external receiver antenna, storage device, and computer and software. Capsule endoscopy can be used to evaluate the esophagus, stomach, small intestine, and colon. When a patient swallows a pill-shaped capsule endoscope, it travels through the esophagus to the stomach, then through the pyloric sphincter to the duodenum, jejunum, and finally the ileum. The capsule endoscope passes through the ileocecal valve and proceeds to the cecum, through the large intestine, and out of the body during defecation. The patient may be able to confirm the passage of the capsule at the time of defecation, but a simple abdominal radiography can be performed to evaluate the complete passage of the capsule endoscope.

The market for capsule endoscopes is growing rapidly in terms of patient convenience, technological advances, and expansion of indications. (Fig. 1).

Types of Capsule Endoscopy

Currently, capsule endoscopes for the esophagus, stomach, small bowel, and colon have been developed and used (Table 1).

H. J. Chun (✉)
Department of Internal Medicine, Korea University College of Medicine, Seoul, South Korea

© Springer Nature Singapore Pte Ltd. 2022
H. J. Chun et al. (eds.), *Small Intestine Disease*, https://doi.org/10.1007/978-981-16-7239-2_11

Small Bowel

The first capsule endoscopy system was produced by Given Imaging (Yokneam, Israel). Currently, the 3rd generation model PillCam SB3 (Medtronic, USA) is being used as a capsule endoscope for the small intestine. In addition, EndoCapsule (Olympus, Japan), OMOM (Jinshan science and technology, China), Mirocam (Intromedic, Korea), and CapsoCam (Capsovision, USA) are also available [1].

Most of these devices use radiofrequency transmission for image transmission, but MiroCam uses human body communication to transmit information. CapsoCam can store the captured images in the capsule endoscope and does not require an external receiver and storage device to be carried during the examination. In addition, CapsoCam provides a 360°

panoramic view with four cameras on the side, unlike conventional capsule endoscopes with a camera at the end of the capsule. However, one disadvantage is that the capsule endoscope must be retrieved from the stool of the patient after the examination to confirm the images taken.

Esophagus

In 2004, Given Imaging developed the esophageal capsule endoscope (PillCam ESO) for esophageal examinations. The second-generation esophageal capsule endoscope PillCam ESO2 is 11 × 26 mm in size and has cameras on each end of both capsules. The PillCam ESO2 captures 18 images per second for a total of 3400 images and provides real-time endoscopic images during the examination. Esophageal capsule endoscopy is used to monitor esophageal diseases, such as esophageal varices, Barrett's esophagus, and esophageal cancer [2]. The esophageal capsule endoscope is operated for about 30 min and then excreted naturally through the intestinal tract with bowel peristalsis. However, to date, the standard method of esophageal examination is upper gastrointestinal endoscopy.

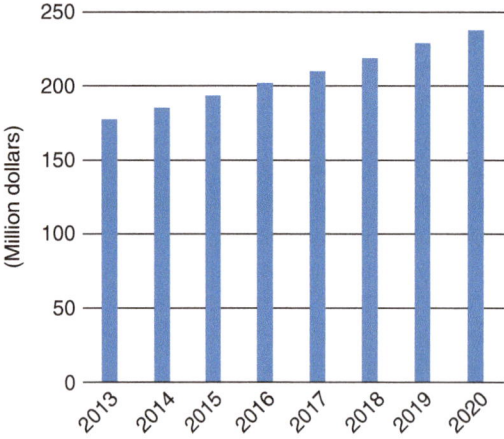

Fig. 1 World Capsule Endoscopy Market Status Forecast. Source: Capsule Endoscopy Domestic and International Market Analysis, Health Industry Brief Vol.25

Colon

Colon capsule endoscopy can be used in colorectal cancer screening, in incomplete colonoscopy, and in patients who refuse colonoscopy or those who cannot receive colonoscopy [3].

Table 1 Currently used capsule endoscopes

System	PillCam SB3	MiroCam	CapsoCam	EndoCapsule	PillCam ESO2	PillCam COLON2
Camera (n)	1	1	4	1	2	2
Field of view	156°	170°	360°	160°	169°	172°
Data transmission	Radiofrequency	Human body communication	N/A	Radiofrequency	Radiofrequency	Radiofrequency
Frame rate (frames/sec)	2–6	3	12–20	2	18	4–35
Dimensions (mm)	11 × 26	11 × 25	11 × 31	11 × 26	11 × 26	12 × 32
Battery life (h)	11	12	15	12	0.5	10
FDA	Yes	Yes	Yes	Yes	Yes	Yes

FDA Food and Drug Administration, *N/A* not applicable

A second-generation colon capsule endoscope, the PillCam COLON2, is currently used in the clinic. The size of the PillCam COLON2 is 12 × 32 mm, with two cameras and a viewing angle of 172°, thereby providing an almost 360° field of view [4].

The colon capsule endoscopy can capture up to 35 images per second with an adaptive frame rate of 4–35 per second, depending on how fast the capsule moves through the colon. When the capsule enters the small intestine, beeps and vibrations alert the patient to take additional boosters to encourage the capsule to pass through the small intestine. However, colon cleansing is very important because even a few stools can interfere with the detection of colon lesions.

Efficacy of Capsule Endoscopy

Small Bowel Bleeding

Obscure gastrointestinal bleeding accounts for about 5% of total gastrointestinal bleeding, and small bowel bleeding is the most common. Capsule endoscopy is a preferred diagnostic method for patients or clinicians for obscure gastrointestinal bleeding because it can be used to non-invasively observe the small intestine and is widely used as the first diagnostic method.

Capsule endoscopy has a diagnostic yield of 32–83% in patients with obscure gastrointestinal bleeding. It is similar to balloon-assisted enteroscopy and is superior to push enteroscopy, computed tomography enterography, magnetic resonance enterography, and angiography [5]. Capsule endoscopy can improve the diagnosis yield of balloon-assisted enteroscopy, and can be used to guide the insertion route. In addition, repetition of capsule endoscopy may be helpful for diagnosis in some of the patients with negative results of capsule endoscopy. Furthermore, capsule endoscopy is used to identify patients who may benefit from additional tests or interventional procedures.

Crohn's Disease

Capsule endoscopy can be used to establish the diagnosis of Crohn's disease; to assess the degree, severity, and activity of the disease; and to evaluate the extent of mucosal healing after treatment [6]. Capsule endoscopy is superior to enterography or computed tomography enterography and similar to magnetic resonance enterography in the diagnosis of Crohn's disease because it can be used to detect early lesions or fine mucosal lesions of Crohn's disease [7]. Capsule endoscopy helps to determine the treatment strategy in patients with Crohn's disease based on an accurate diagnosis, and provides information about the extent of lesions and disease activity. However, because of the possibility of capsule retention due to intestinal stenosis in Crohn's disease, the presence of intestinal stenosis should be assessed by a radiological examination before capsule endoscopy.

Small Bowel Tumor

Adenomatous and mesenchymal tumors are the most common types of tumors of the small intestine and are found in about 6% of patients with obscure gastrointestinal bleeding [8]. Most small intestinal tumors are incidentally found in patients who undergo capsule endoscopy with other indications. Capsule endoscopy has similar diagnostic yield as balloon-assisted enteroscopy, computed tomography enterography, and magnetic resonance enterography [9]. Small bowel tumor lesions can be easily overlooked by a capsule endoscope as it passes rapidly with peristalsis through the distal part of the duodenum or proximal part of the jejunum where 25–30% of small bowel tumors are located. Submucosal tumors covered with the normal mucosa are difficult to diagnose with capsule endoscopy. The miss rate of capsule endoscopy is 16.7–18.9% for small bowel tumors and other tests may reveal missed lesions after the capsule endoscope [8, 10]. An incomplete bowel cleansing rate up to 10–15% is one of the disadvantages of capsule endoscopy.

Recent Trends of Capsule Endoscopy

In recent years, three-dimensional capsule endoscopes have been developed to acquire distance information of lesions or improve image accuracy, and capsule endoscopes using magnetic fields have been developed to expand the diagnostic field of capsule endoscopes. Moreover, the use of artificial intelligence in the diagnosis of capsule endoscopy is currently being researched.

Since its introduction in 2001, the clinical indication for capsule endoscopy has greatly expanded. Capsule endoscopy is a non-invasive approach to visualize areas that have been difficult to approach and can give satisfactory results to both physicians and patients. In the future, it is expected to evolve into a technology that can be applied to new indications through technological development and that can lead to minimally invasive diagnosis and treatment.

References

1. Committee AT, Wang A, Banerjee S, et al. Wireless capsule endoscopy. Gastrointest Endosc. 2013;78:805–15.
2. Kwack WG, Lim YJ. Current status and research into overcoming limitations of capsule endoscopy. Clin Endosc. 2016;49:8 15.
3. Han YM, Im JP. Colon capsule endoscopy: where are we and where are we going. Clin Endosc. 2016;49:449–53.
4. Yung DE, Rondonotti E, Koulaouzidis A. Review: capsule colonoscopy-a concise clinical overview of current status. Ann Transl Med. 2016;4:398.
5. Min YW, Chang DK. The role of capsule endoscopy in patients with obscure gastrointestinal bleeding. Clin Endosc. 2016;49:16–20.
6. Yen HH, Chang CW, Chou JW, Wei SC. Balloon-assisted enteroscopy and capsule endoscopy in suspected small bowel Crohn's disease. Clin Endosc. 2017;50:417–23.
7. Yang DH, Keum B, Jeen YT. Capsule endoscopy for Crohn's disease: current status of diagnosis and management. Gastroenterol Res Pract. 2016;2016:8236367.
8. Rondonotti E, Koulaouzidis A, Yung DE, Reddy SN, Georgiou J, Pennazio M. Neoplastic diseases of the small bowel. Gastrointest Endosc Clin N Am. 2017;27:93–112.
9. Cheung DY, Kim JS, Shim KN, Choi MG, Grp KGIS. The usefulness of capsule endoscopy for small bowel Tumors. Clin Endosc. 2016;49:21–5.
10. Han JW, Hong SN, Jang HJ, et al. Clinical efficacy of various diagnostic tests for small bowel Tumors and clinical features of Tumors missed by capsule endoscopy. Gastroenterol Res Pract. 2015;2015:623208.

The Future of Capsule Endoscopy

Yun Jeong Lim

Capsule endoscopes have been used in clinical practice since 2001, and the capsule endoscope made by Given Imaging Company was first introduced in Korea in 2002. Thereafter, MiroCam, which was developed using Korean technology, was introduced in 2007 and is currently being employed. Capsule endoscopy was introduced to observe the small intestine; however, its application has expanded to the esophagus and colon. In the future, a single capsule will enable observation of the entire digestive tract from the mouth to the anus. By that time, people will be able to easily buy a capsule endoscope for the purpose of screening. After the capsule is swallowed, it will move through the alimentary tract and transmit the captured images to the Internet, which will then be automatically read by artificial intelligence. Currently, capsule endoscopy has the following limitations: it is unable to take tissue samples; the movement of the capsule cannot be actively controlled because there is no self-propulsion force, and there is sometimes insufficient power to observe the entire small intestine. In addition, the results take a long time to read, and capsule retention occasionally occurs because of small-intestinal stenosis. In the future, capsule endoscopy will allow a pathologic diagnosis and enable hemostasis and expansion of the gut lumen by injecting air to precisely observe the mucosa. In addition, artificial intelligence will reduce the reading time of the results (Fig. 1).

Perfect Images Without Blind Spots

Capsule endoscopy, through the peristaltic motion of the gastrointestinal tract, was previously able to take two to three images per second; however, nowadays, the frame rate can be automatically adjusted according to the movement speed of the capsule.1 When the capsule moves faster, it can take up to 20 images in 1 s. When the same image is repeatedly obtained because of lack of capsule movement, the device has the function of removing unnecessary duplicated images [1]. To observe the entire mucosa without blind spots, it would be helpful to have the ability to expand the intestinal lumen by discharging carbon dioxide from the capsule and controlling the movement of the capsule through the external device [2, 3].

Identifying the Exact Location of Lesions

In the small intestine, it is difficult to identify the exact location of lesions in the mucosa. Because the small intestine is a very long organ, accurate lesion localization is important in deciding the treatment approach. Research aiming to reduce

Y. J. Lim (✉)
Department of Internal Medicine, Dongguk University Ilsan Hospital, Dongguk University, College of Medicine, Goyang, South Korea

© Springer Nature Singapore Pte Ltd. 2022
H. J. Chun et al. (eds.), *Small Intestine Disease*, https://doi.org/10.1007/978-981-16-7239-2_12

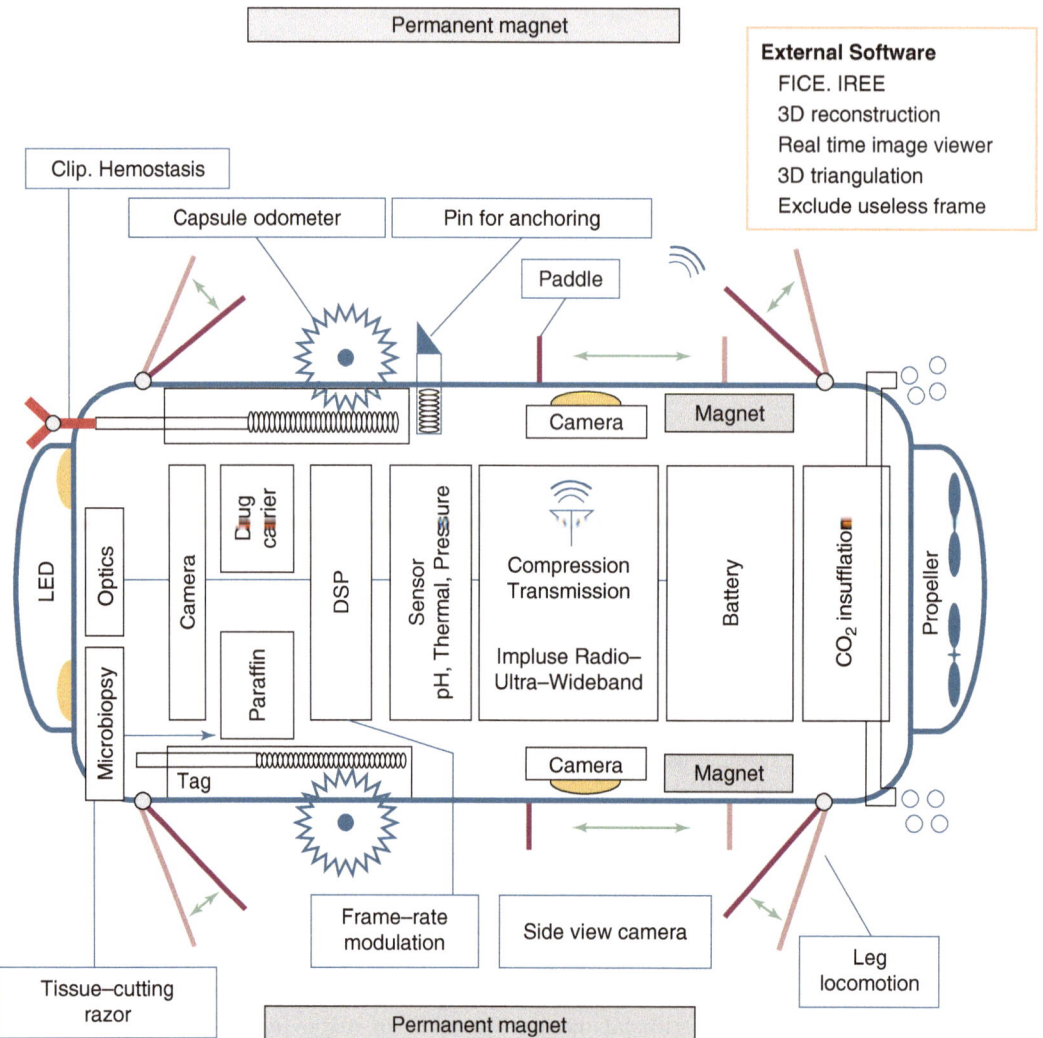

Fig. 1 Future capsule endoscopy. *FICE* Fujinon intelligent chromoendoscopy, *IRFE* infrared fluorescence endoscopy, *3D* three-dimensional, *LED* light-emitting diode, *DSP* digital signal processing. Adapted from Kwack and Lim [1], **with permission from Clinical Endoscopy**

errors in the localization of lesions using three-dimensional triangulation is ongoing [4].

Tissue Biopsy and Therapeutic Endoscopy

One study attempted to obtain biopsy material through the capsule. After tissue biopsy, the specimen was embedded in a paraffin block, stored in the capsule, and collected [1]. However, researchers are also attempting to diagnose lesions by observing the mucosa with a microscope without a tissue biopsy, not only with the wired but also the wireless capsule endoscope [5]. In one animal model, a clip for hemostasis was ejected from the capsule when small-bowel bleeding occurred [1].

Automatic Interpretation Through Artificial Intelligence

The current capsule endoscopy is noninvasive and can monitor the entire small intestine at the same time, unlike the traditional endoscopic examination; however, the long reading time, in which [1, 5] is required to read the numerous acquired images after the patient swallowed the capsule, poses a large burden on endoscopists. Artificial intelligence can reduce the effort and interpretation time of the doctor who reads the results [6]. In the future, artificial intelligence might be able to perform accurate interpretation of capsule endoscopy results, at a level similar to that of a competent doctor or expert.

Active Control of Capsule Endoscopy

Active-locomotion, robotic capsule endoscopy was a long-sought dream [7–9]. However, storing power sufficient to move the capsule in such a small capsule space is very technically difficult. Capsule endoscopy using an external magnetic field to control the movement of the capsule is more realistic. Possible capsule movements using magnetic power are rotation, move forward and backward, jumping, and tilting. Magnetic capsule endoscopy developed from China and Japan requires large space [8]. The capsule can be controlled manually or automatically by a programmed search process. But, another type of magnet capsule endoscopy from Korea requires only an external handheld magnet [9]. Therefore, magnetic capsule endoscopy can be easily used anywhere. Endoscopist should learn complex procedure that require high level of manual dexterity with handheld magnet. This system allows the examination of both the upper GI tract and small bowel using the same capsule. Patient tolerance is better in magnetic capsule gastroscopy than unsedated esophagogastroscopy.

Conclusion

By swallowing the capsule like a pill, examination from the mouth to the anus will be possible. Noninvasive capsule endoscopy can be primarily used to screen for cancers or lesions in the gastrointestinal tract. If abnormal lesions are found by capsule endoscopy, the doctor will make a diagnosis and perform additional treatment steps by referring to the results obtained by artificial intelligence. There are many challenges to be overcomed before the above-described future of capsule endoscopy can be realized. To obtain accurate images, adequate bowel preparation, air inflation, and active image acquisition are needed. Most importantly, it will be necessary to develop a sophisticated reading program that is able to identify the accurate location of lesions and has artificial intelligence functions.

References

1. Kwack WG, Lim YJ. Current status and research into overcoming limitations of capsule endoscopy. Clin Endosc. 2016;49:8–15.
2. Shiotani A, Honda K, Kawakami M, et al. Use of an external real-time image viewer coupled with pre-specified actions enhanced the complete examinations for capsule endoscopy. J Gastroenterol Hepatol. 2011;26:1270–4.
3. Pasricha T, Smith BF, Mitchell VR, et al. Controlled colonic insufflation by a remotely triggered capsule for improved mucosal visualization. Endoscopy. 2014;46:614–8.
4. Marya N, Karellas A, Foley A, Roychowdhury A, Cave D. Computerized 3-dimensional localization of a video capsule in the abdominal cavity: validation by digital radiography. Gastrointest Endosc. 2014;79:669–74.
5. Gora MJ, Sauk JS, Carruth RW, et al. Tethered capsule endomicroscopy enables less invasive imaging of gastrointestinal tract microstructure. Nat Med. 2013;19:238–40.
6. Gan T, Wu JC, Rao NN, Chen T, Liu B. A feasibility trial of computer-aided diagnosis for enteric lesion-smin capsule endoscopy. World J Gastroenterol. 2008;14:6929–35.

7. Valdastri P, Quaglia C, Buselli E, et al. A magnetic internal mechanism for precise orientation of the camera in wireless endoluminal applications. Endoscopy. 2010;42:481–6.

8. Zhao AJ, Qian YY, Sun H, et al. Screening for gastric cancer with magnetically controlled capsule gastroscopy in asymptomatic individuals. Gastrointest Endosc. 2018;88:466–74.

9. Ching HL, Hale MF, Kurien M, et al. Diagnostic yield of magnetically assisted capsule endoscopy versus gastroscopy in recurrent and refractory iron deficiency anemia. Endoscopy. 2019;51:409–18.

Indications and Contraindications of Small-bowel Capsule Endoscopy

Bo-In Lee

Key Points
- The indications of small-bowel capsule endoscopy include obscure gastrointestinal bleeding, Crohn's disease, small-bowel tumors, and polyposis syndrome.
- To maximize the diagnostic yield for obscure gastrointestinal bleeding, capsule endoscopy should be performed as soon as possible after the bleeding episode.
- The risk of capsule retention is increased in patients with Crohn's disease, previous abdominal surgery, intestinal ischemia, volvulus, and previous abdominal radiotherapy.

Indications

Obscure Gastrointestinal Bleeding (OGIB)

OGIB refers to gastrointestinal bleeding of unclear origin that persists or recurs after obtaining negative findings on esophagogastroduodenoscopy and colonoscopy. OGIB accounts for 5% of the total gastrointestinal bleeding, and approximately 80% of OGIB cases are of small-bowel bleeding. Obscure overt bleeding manifests as visible blood (hematochezia or melena), and obscure occult bleeding presents as a positive fecal occult blood test or iron deficiency anemia.

Capsule endoscopy is recommended as the first-line investigation in patients with OGIB. The overall diagnostic yield of capsule endoscopy for OGIB ranges from 30% to 70%, which is higher than that of other diagnostic methods such as push enteroscopy (31%), double-balloon enteroscopy (23%), and small-bowel series (5%) [1–3]. To maximize the diagnostic yield, capsule endoscopy should be performed as soon as possible after the bleeding episode, optimally within 14 days [1]. The capsule endoscopy findings of OGIB are intestinal angiodysplasia, small-bowel ulcers, blood in the small bowel without identified lesions, small-bowel tumors, and small-bowel varices [3, 4]. Approximately one-half to two-thirds of patients taking non-steroidal anti-inflammatory drugs have lesions such as erosions, petechiae, denuded mucosa, bleeding lesions, and ulcers [5]. Capsule endoscopy is a good method for identifying causative lesions once other potential bleeding sources located within the reach of conventional endoscopies have been excluded. Capsule endoscopy is also useful in determining the route of device-assisted enteroscopy [6].

B.-I. Lee (✉)
Division of Gastroenterology, Department of Internal Medicine, The Catholic University of Korea, Seoul, South Korea

© Springer Nature Singapore Pte Ltd. 2022
H. J. Chun et al. (eds.), *Small Intestine Disease*, https://doi.org/10.1007/978-981-16-7239-2_13

Crohn's Disease

Although ileocolonoscopy is one of the first diagnostic procedures for patients with suspected Crohn's disease, capsule endoscopy should be considered in patients without an evidence of small-bowel stricture in the presence of negative ileocolonoscopy findings. Capsule endoscopy is the most sensitive diagnostic modality for detecting mucosal lesions of the small bowel in patients with suspected or established Crohn's disease, and helps in making a differential diagnosis of Crohn's disease in suspected patients by identifying small-bowel involvement proximal to the terminal ileum. It also plays a role in determining the mucosal severity and disease extension in patients with established Crohn's disease [6]. A meta-analysis showed that the diagnostic yield for small-bowel Crohn's disease is higher (50–70%) with capsule endoscopy than with other diagnostic modalities (small-bowel series, 22%; colonoscopy, 48%; push enteroscopy, 8%; and computed tomography [CT] enterography/enteroclysis, 31%) [7].

When stenosis or obstruction is suspected, patency capsule or careful examination using cross-sectional imaging modalities such as magnetic resonance imaging or CT should be considered first. The retention rate was reported to be 13% in patients with known Crohn's disease and 1.6% in patients with suspected Crohn's disease [8].

Small-bowel Tumors and Polyposis Syndrome

Capsule endoscopy is also useful for the detection of small-bowel tumors and polyps. However, device-assisted enteroscopy is preferred over capsule endoscopy in patients with suspected small-bowel tumor in imaging examinations [1]. Whereas, capsule endoscopy has shown significantly better detection than radiologic studies, especially for tumors ≤1 cm in size [9].

The most common presentation of small-bowel tumors is OGIB; the most common histopathological type is adenocarcinoma, followed by neuroendocrine tumor, lymphoma, sarcoma, and hamartoma; and the most common location is the jejunum (40–60%), followed by the ileum (25–40%) and the duodenum (15–25%) [4]. Capsule endoscopy is also useful for the detection of small-bowel polyps and for surveillance in familial adenomatous polyposis and Peutz–Jeghers syndrome [10].

Celiac Disease

Capsule endoscopy is not routinely recommended in patients with suspected celiac disease. The diagnostic hallmark of celiac disease is villous atrophy on endoscopic small-bowel biopsy. Capsule endoscopy can be considered in patients unwilling or unable to undergo conventional endoscopy [1]. It reveals villous atrophy, a loss of Kerckring's folds, notching of folds, and a mosaic pattern, although these findings are not diagnostic.

Abdominal Pain of Unknown Origin

The diagnostic yield of capsule endoscopy in patients with abdominal pain is relatively low (13%). However, it can be increased in patients with chronic abdominal pain accompanied by elevated serum inflammatory markers (C-reactive protein or erythrocyte sedimentation rate), weight loss, or diarrhea [11].

Contraindications

Patients at a Risk of Gastrointestinal Obstruction, Stenosis, or Fistula

Known or suspected stenosis of the gastrointestinal tract increases the risk of capsule retention. Capsule retention can induce a total or subtotal intestinal obstruction, perforation, or capsule disintegration. A systematic review reported that the overall capsule retention rate is 1.4% [12]. The risk of capsule retention should be considered in patients with known Crohn's disease, clinically suspected obstruction, previous radiation treatment, and previous intestinal resection. Known or suspected stenosis is a contraindication until patency is proven (best by patency capsule).

Pediatric Patients

One of the main limitations of capsule endoscopy in children is the ability to swallow the capsule and the fear of capsule entrapment. The Food and Drug Administration (FDA) has approved capsule endoscopy for children aged 2 years or older. Voluntary ingestion may be feasible at ages older than 6–8 years [13]. According to the directions of the manufacturer of PillCam, swallowing a capsule endoscope is not recommended in children under the age of 8 years. When endoscopic delivery is required, the use of a special endoscopic delivery device (AdvanCE®; US Endoscopy, Mentor, OH, USA) is recommended because retrieval nets can cause significant mucosal trauma [14]. There has been no report of capsule aspiration, perforation, or complete small-bowel obstruction in a meta-analysis of more than 1000 capsule endoscopy studies in children [15].

Patients with Swallowing Disorders

Swallowing disorders are a contraindication to the standard procedure of capsule endoscopy. The incidence of capsule aspiration is presumed to be from 1/600 to 1/700 [16]. When there is an increased risk of aspiration, and the capsule can be placed endoscopically into the duodenum. This can be performed through an overtube or with AdvanCE® [17]. A thorough history taking and/or tests for swallowing function are required in patients at risk, such as those with older age, a history of cerebral stroke, bleeding, or trauma.

Pregnant Patients

Theoretically, the risk of capsule retention from prolonged gastrointestinal transit can be increased in pregnancy. In addition, there are no data on the electromagnetic effect of the capsule recorder

device on the fetus. Postponement of elective capsule endoscopy until after delivery should be recommended. Nevertheless, capsule endoscopy may be considered when the maternal condition does not allow diagnostic delay, such as in cases of small-bowel bleeding. The FDA identifies pregnancy as a relative contraindication to capsule endoscopy [18].

Patients with Implantable Cardiac Devices

In vitro and in vivo studies have analyzed the electromagnetic interference between capsule endoscopes and cardiac pacemakers and implantable cardioverter defibrillators [15]. The maximal electromagnetic radiation in close proximity (5 mm) for capsule endoscopes from Medtronic, Olympus, and Jinshan, and the maximal obtainable interference voltage at the input of cardiac devices for capsule endoscopes from IntroMedic are below the safety objectives set by the international product standards for cardiac devices [15].

The European Society of Gastrointestinal Endoscopy states that capsule endoscopy is not contraindicated in patients with a cardiac pacemaker or implantable cardioverter defibrillator [19], whereas the American Society of Gastrointestinal Endoscopy considers cardiac devices as a relative contraindication [20].

References

1. Pennazio M, Spada C, Eliakim R, et al. Small-bowel capsule endoscopy and device-assisted enteroscopy for diagnosis and treatment of small-bowel disorders: European Society of Gastrointestinal Endoscopy (ESGE) clinical guideline. Endoscopy. 2015;47:352–76.
2. Saperas E, Dot J, Videla S, et al. Capsule endoscopy versus computed tomographic or standard angiography for the diagnosis of obscure gastrointestinal bleeding. Am J Gastroenterol. 2007;102:731–7.
3. Shim KN, Moon JS, Chang DK, et al. Guideline for capsule endoscopy: obscure gastrointestinal bleeding. Clin Endosc. 2013;46:45–53.
4. Redondo-Cerezo E, Sanchez-Capilla AD, De La Torre-Rubio P, De Teresa J. Wireless capsule endos-

copy: perspectives beyond gastrointestinal bleeding. World J Gastroenterol. 2014;20:15664–73.

5. Lim YJ, Yang CH. Non-steroidal anti-inflammatory drug-induced enteropathy. Clin Endosc. 2012;45:138–44.

6. Shim KN, Jeon SR, Jang HJ, et al. Quality indicators for small bowel capsule endoscopy. Clin Endosc. 2017;50:148–60.

7. Triester SL, Leighton JA, Leontiadis GI, et al. A meta-analysis of the yield of capsule endoscopy compared to other diagnostic modalities in patients with non-stricturing small bowel Crohn's disease. Am J Gastroenterol. 2006;101:954–64.

8. Cheifetz AS, Kornbluth AA, Legnani P, et al. The risk of retention of the capsule endoscope in patients with known or suspected Crohn's disease. Am J Gastroenterol. 2006;101:2218–22.

9. Cheung DY, Lee IS, Chang DK, et al. Capsule endoscopy in small bowel tumors: a multicenter Korean study. J Gastroenterol Hepatol. 2010;25:1079–86.

10. Syngal S, Brand RE, Church JM, et al. ACG clinical guideline: genetic testing and management of hereditary gastrointestinal cancer syndromes. Am J Gastroenterol. 2015;110:223–62. quiz 263

11. Katsinelos P, Chatzimavroudis G, Terzoudis S, et al. Diagnostic yield and clinical impact of capsule endoscopy in obscure gastrointestinal bleeding during routine clinical practice: a single-center experience. Med Princ Pract. 2011;20:60–5.

12. Liao Z, Gao R, Xu C, Li ZS. Indications and detection, completion, and retention rates of small-bowel capsule endoscopy: a systematic review. Gastrointest Endosc. 2010;71:280–6.

13. Arguelles-Arias F, Donat E, Fernandez-Urien I, et al. Guideline for wireless capsule endoscopy in children and adolescents: a consensus document by the SEGHNP (Spanish Society for Pediatric Gastroenterology, Hepatology, and Nutrition) and the SEPD (Spanish Society for Digestive Diseases). Rev Esp Enferm Dig. 2015;107:714–31.

14. Fritscher-Ravens A, Scherbakov P, Bufler P, et al. The feasibility of wireless capsule endoscopy in detecting small intestinal pathology in children under the age of 8 years: a multicentre European study. Gut. 2009;58:1467–72.

15. Bandorski D, Kurniawan N, Baltes P, et al. Contraindications for video capsule endoscopy. World J Gastroenterol. 2016;22:9898–908.

16. Lucendo AJ, Gonzalez-Castillo S, Fernandez-Fuente M, De Rezende LC. Tracheal aspiration of a capsule endoscope: a new case report and literature compilation of an increasingly reported complication. Dig Dis Sci. 2011;56:2758–62.

17. Holden JP, Dureja P, Pfau PR, et al. Endoscopic placement of the small-bowel video capsule by using a capsule endoscope delivery device. Gastrointest Endosc. 2007;65:842–7.

18. Savas N. Gastrointestinal endoscopy in pregnancy. World J Gastroenterol. 2014;20:15241–52.

19. Ladas SD, Triantafyllou K, Spada C, et al. European Society of Gastrointestinal Endoscopy (ESGE): recommendations (2009) on clinical use of video capsule endoscopy to investigate small-bowel, esophageal and colonic diseases. Endoscopy. 2010;42:220–7.

20. Committee AT, Wang A, Banerjee S, et al. Wireless capsule endoscopy. Gastrointest Endosc. 2013;78:805–15.

Preparation Before Capsule Endoscopy

Jeong Seop Moon

Key Points

- The informed consent form for capsule endoscopy should include the patient's medical history; purpose of the examination; examination procedures; advantage, disadvantage, limitations, and complications of capsule endoscopy; and precautions for the patient.
- On the day before capsule endoscopy, the patient should take a clear liquid diet and plenty of water, as well as fast for 12 h before the test.
- Although there is yet no standardized protocol for capsule endoscopy preparation, simethicone for removing air bubbles, polyethylene glycol for intestinal cleansing, and metoclopramide as a prokinetic drug against infrequent gastric movements have been widely used.

Capsule endoscopy is a painless, noninvasive test. However, it is a long examination that involves difficult-to-repeat steps, including observation, washing, and aspiration. Therefore, capsule endoscopy needs to be performed in an optimal condition. Before the examination, the patient should be provided with a description of the capsule endoscopy procedures. The advantages and disadvantages of capsule endoscopy must be fully explained to the patient, who should provide a signed informed consent form thereafter. Some factors that interfere with diagnosis using capsule endoscopy are food residue, air bubbles, bile fluid, and failure to observe the entire small intestine owing to delayed gastrointestinal transit time [1]. In the early days when the battery of the capsules could not last for >8 h, the failure rate of reaching the cecum was reported to be 19–27%. The manufacturer's recommended preparations for capsule endoscopy include only fasting for 12 h and a clear liquid diet before the examination. However, intake of a purgative preparation as a pretreatment has also been recommended to cleanse the mucosa of the small intestine. The effect of a purgative has been varied. However, many studies have reported that complete or partial cleansing with a purgative increased the small bowel visual quality (SBVQ) [2]. The results of a meta-analysis showed that the use of purgatives such as polyethylene glycol (PEG) or sodium phosphate (NaP) had increased the diagnostic yield and SBVQ compared to that with a clear liquid diet alone. Until now, however, there is no consensus on how to clean the intestines. The American Society of Gastrointestinal Endoscopy previously recommended fasting or drinking only clear liquids for 10–12 h before the examination [2]. In 2017, the clinical guidelines for capsule endoscopy strongly recommended bowel preparation in patients [3].

J. S. Moon (✉)
Department of Gastroenterology, Inje University
Seoul Paik Hospital, Seoul, South Korea
e-mail: moonjs2@unitel.co.kr

© Springer Nature Singapore Pte Ltd. 2022
H. J. Chun et al. (eds.), *Small Intestine Disease*, https://doi.org/10.1007/978-981-16-7239-2_14

Informed Consent Form

Contents of the Informed Consent Form

The consent form for capsule endoscopy is important for the exchange of information between physicians and patients. The demographic information, past and present medical history, and current physical status of the patients should be initially confirmed. These details include idiosyncrasies, concomitant medication, smoking status, any drug allergies, comorbidities such as diabetes mellitus, heart disease, lung disease, bleeding tendency, dysphagia, insertion of a pacemaker or defibrillator, history of abdominal surgery, and history of intestinal obstruction including adhesions. Patients should be informed of the need, purpose, procedures, and benefits and dangers of the examination. The problems and complications that may arise after the examination include incomplete observation of the small intestine, possibility of missed lesions in the small intestine, retention of the capsule, or intestinal obstruction. The consent form should describe the precautions to be followed by the patient before and after the examination, optional examinations that can be performed other than capsule endoscopy, prognosis if the test is not performed, and possibility of changes in the examination process [3].

Precautions in the Consent Form

The patients should maintain daily logs of food intake, activity, and any symptoms during the entire capsule endoscopy duration, and submit them at the end of the examination. After swallowing the capsule endoscope, daily activities can be performed; however, the patient should especially be careful to avoid falls. Bending, sweating, or exercising should also be avoided. The data recorder of capsule endoscopy is mounted on the waist with a belt, and the images are transferred to and stored on the device for approximately 8–12 h. The patient should not remove the belt or the data recorder during the examination, and should avoid shock, vibration, and strong sunlight. Further, the top of the storage device should be checked every 15 min for blinking light which indicates that the device is recording data. If there is no blinking light, the patient should record the time of the discovery in the log and immediately call the hospital. Any place with a strong electromagnetic field (e.g., near a magnetic resonance imaging [MRI] machine or an amateur [ham] radio) should be avoided until the capsule is expelled outside of the body, and MRI should not be performed during the examination. If nausea, vomiting, or abdominal pain occurs during the examination, the patient should immediately contact the hospital because of the possibility of intestinal obstruction. If the capsule does not reach the large intestine at the end of the examination, an abdominal radiography should be performed.

General Preparation

The Week Before Capsule Endoscopy

Vitamins containing iron or iron tablets should be discontinued 7 days before the examination. Anticholinergic agents, antihistamines, and narcotics need to be discontinued 2–3 days before the examination because they can cause gastroparesis. Anticoagulants (including warfarin) do not need to be reduced or discontinued. It has been reported that the diagnosis rate of hemorrhagic lesions increases when anticoagulants promote hemorrhage in patients with suspected small bowel bleeding [4].

The Day Before Capsule Endoscopy

The patient should abstain from smoking 24 h before undergoing capsule endoscopy and avoid antacid suspensions. Patients with diabetes should consult their physician before capsule endoscopy and adjust the dose of oral hypoglycemic agents or insulin injections.

The Day of Capsule Endoscopy

On the day of the examination, the patient can take a bath. However, any lotion, oil, perfume, aftershave, or powder should not be applied on the abdomen. The patient should wear light, loose, and separate top and bottom garments to allow an abdominal belt to be fitted. In principle, the patient should bring a list of medications that had been taken and should not take any medications before the examination. If possible, all medications should be changed to parenteral, liquid, sublingual, or enema form. Any mandatory morning medications should be taken at least 3 h before or 2 h after capsule endoscopy. In general, oral hypoglycemic agents should not be taken on the day of capsule endoscopy before coming to the hospital. Medications should be taken after the completion of the examination, if applicable. The sensor array of the capsule endoscope is attached to the abdomen with an adhesive pad and to the storage device equipped in the abdominal belt. The patient should first take simethicone with a sip of water and swallow the capsule endoscope thereafter.

Diet

Diet Before the Examination

The patient should avoid taking vitamins containing iron or iron tablets, as well as beans, seeded fruits, corn, and popcorn from 7 days before capsule endoscopy. The day before the examination, the patient should take a regular diet until lunch (or until breakfast). After lunch and until 10 pm before the examination, the patient usually should take clear liquids (water, cream-free coffee, tea, sorbet, ginger ale, sports drinks such as Gatorade, or cranberry or apple juice). Solid foods should be avoided. The patient should avoid colored (red, orange, and purple) foods and drinks, as well as alcohol, milk, and dairy products. It is recommended to drink as much water as possible before 10 pm on the day before the examination. The patient should fast for 12 h before the examination. After 10 pm, only necessary medications

should be taken with a sip of water. Thereafter, the patient should not eat or drink anything before capsule endoscopy.

Diet on the Day of Capsule Endoscopy

After swallowing the capsule, the patient should fast for 2 h. Clear liquid should be taken 2 h after swallowing the capsule. After 4 h, the patient may have a light snack while avoiding red-, orange-, and purple-colored foods. After the examination is complete, normal dietary intake is allowed.

Enteric Lavage

The turbid material present in the small intestine, which is composed of small intestinal secretions, bile, and food residues, may obscure the mucosal observation field of the capsule endoscope. The pretreatment protocols for capsule endoscopy are not yet standardized. The manufacturers of capsule endoscopes recommend a clear liquid diet for 24 h and fasting for 12 h as the pretreatment for capsule endoscopy, which is based on the pretreatment for push enteroscopy (performed to observe 80–120 cm below the Treitz ligament) [1]. Because air bubbles and small food residues may interfere with the diagnosis and with the observation of the small intestine, laxatives, or purgatives are used for cleansing. Pretreatment agents, including simethicone to eliminate air bubbles, NaP and PEG to cleanse the small intestine, and prokinetics to accelerate gastrointestinal motility, have been recommended.

Fasting

The manufacturers of capsule endoscopes recommend fasting after a clear fluid diet before the patient undergoes capsule endoscopy. It has been claimed that fasting itself is more physiologically effective than taking laxatives and would avoid the uniform administration of laxatives before capsule endoscopy based on the orocecal transit time for a healthy adult of <2 h. Further, pretreatment with enteric lavage before capsule endoscopy can reduce the patient's compliance with the examination.

Simethicone

Simethicone reduces air bubbles in the lumen by decreasing the surface tension of air bubbles, thus increasing the SBVQ [5]. When simethicone is applied with fasting or PEG pretreatment, it increases the SBVQ without affecting the completion rate of capsule endoscopy. The dose of simethicone used has been reported to range from 80 to 300 mg, and the administration time varies from the day before the examination to 20 min before the capsule endoscopy. Generally, 300 mg simethicone is administered 30 min before capsule endoscopy. Moreover, it has been reported that when concurrent administration of 2 L PEG and 80 mg simethicone is applied, the quality of the observation was increased in the proximal small intestine, except in patients with Crohn's disease.

Polyethylene Glycol Solution

PEG is the most widely recommended solution for capsular endoscopic cleansing as the initial pretreatment. The recommended amount of PEG solution before the examination varies from 500 mL to 4 L, and a method of taking 500 mL PEG after capsule endoscopy has also been introduced. The most common dose of PEG is 2 L because it was confirmed that taking this amount improves the SBVQ as much as taking 4 L of the solution. PEG shortens the gastric transit time, although it has been reported that there is no difference in the small bowel transit time and completion rate of capsule endoscopy. The PEG dosing time was variously reported as 24, 16, 12, 4, and 3 h before swallowing the capsule endoscope and again after swallowing the capsule endoscope. Further studies would be required on

the dosing time and dosing method. According to the guidelines for capsule endoscopy released by the Korean Society of Gastrointestinal Endoscopy in 2013, pretreatment with PEG solution increased the SBVQ and the diagnostic yield of capsule endoscopy but did not affect the overall completion rate of the procedure. Further, 4 L and 2 L of PEG solution have shown similar results with respect to the SBVQ, diagnostic yield, and completion rate of capsule endoscopy [6]. Therefore, concurrent administration of 2 L PEG with 300 mg simethicone is the most commonly used pretreatment in capsule endoscopy. On the other hand, it was discovered that in patients who took a small amount (500 mL) of PEG for 2 h from 30 min after swallowing the capsule endoscope, the SBVQ was well maintained throughout the whole small intestine compared with that in patients in the fasting group. This effect was most significant in the distal ileum [7].

Prokinetic Drugs

Previously, the battery of capsule endoscopes had a short lifespan, and metoclopramide, erythromycin, mosapride, and lubiprostone were used to shorten the transit time and thereby increase the overall observation rate in the small intestine. However, at present, the battery life has increased to up to 12 h, making the effect of prokinetic drugs no longer significant. According to the guidelines released by the Korean Society of Gastrointestinal Endoscopy for capsule endoscopy, prokinetic drugs are not recommended because they do not generally increase the SBVQ, diagnostic yield, and completion rate of capsule endoscopy [6]. However, the use of prokinetic drugs is effective for hospitalized patients or those with limited gastric movement due to disease. The factors that predict incomplete examination in capsule endoscopy are hospital admission, previous abdominal surgery, poor intestinal cleansing, and increased gastric transit time. The most commonly used medication is metoclopramide. If the capsule endoscope is located in the stomach, through the real-time viewer, at 30–60 min after swallowing the capsule endoscope, 10 mg metoclopramide can be administered. Moreover, if the capsule endoscope remains in the stomach for a long time, a method of pushing the capsule through the duodenum is used. However, a study reported that the longer the small intestinal transit time of the capsule endoscope, the higher the diagnostic yield of capsule endoscopy.

Other Pretreatment Methods

Booster Effect with Ingestion of Picolax Purgative After Taking 2 L PEG Solution

For a booster effect with Picolax, 2 L PEG solution should be ingested 12 h before capsule endoscopy. Thereafter, a mixture of 1 packet Picolax (sodium picosulfate, magnesium oxide, and citric acid) in 250 mL water and another 500 mL of water should be ingested 1 h after swallowing the capsule endoscope. Compared with patients who took 2 L PEG alone, this method significantly improved the visibility of the last third of the small intestine (72% vs. 9%, $p = 0.0065$) [8].

Coffee Enema After Ingesting Magnesium Citrate

A coffee enema is known to cause bile duct dilatation and the excretion of bile through the colon wall. The addition of coffee enema to 2 L PEG pretreatment had a more significant cleansing effect than pretreatment with 2 L PEG alone in the middle and distal parts of the small intestine [9].

Gum Chewing

After swallowing the capsule endoscope and gum chewing for 30 min every 2 h, the rate of arrival of the capsule endoscope to the cecum was increased (83.0% vs. 71.7%, $p = 0.19$), with reduced gastric and small bowel transit time of the capsule endoscope (40.8 vs. 56.1 min [$p = 0.045$] and 229.1 vs. 266.2 min [$p = 0.032$], respectively). Gum chewing increases gastric and intestinal motility and stimulates saliva and gastric juice secretion.

Conclusion

Capsule endoscopy should be performed in an optimal condition. Thereby, communication between the physician and the patient is important from the planning stage of the examination. Moreover, the patient should be fully informed about the procedure and should agree to the examination by providing a signed informed consent form. Preparation for capsule endoscopy should start at least 1 week before the examination with detailed instructions including a checklist for daily routine, medications, and food. The patient should review every precaution in the checklist for capsule endoscopy. In particular, training patients on the required preparation on the day before and on the day of the examination is important. Nevertheless, the pretreatment protocol of capsule endoscopy has not yet been standardized. Therefore, capsule endoscopy may be performed in fasting state after taking a clear liquid diet, although purgatives may be used to remove materials that may interfere with small-bowel observation, including air bubbles, food residues, and bile. The recommended pretreatment agents to date include simethicone for eliminating air bubbles, NaP, and PEG for intestinal cleansing, and metoclopramide for gastric retention of the capsule endoscope [10]. Therefore, thorough preparation before the examination, detailed explanation to patients, obtaining written informed consent from patients, dietary control before the examination, and use of pretreatment agents to increase the diagnostic yield of capsule endoscopy are crucial.

References

1. Korean Society of Gastrointestinal Endoscopy Korean Gut Image Study Group. Capsule endoscopy. 1st ed. Seoul: KoreaMedbook; 2008. 255p.
2. ASGE Technology Committee, Wang A, Banerjee S, et al. Wireless capsule endoscopy. Gastrointest Endosc. 2013;78:805–15.
3. Enns RA, Hookey L, Armstrong D, et al. Clinical practice guidelines for the use of video capsule endoscopy. Gastroenterology. 2017;152:497–514.
4. Barkin JA, Barkin JS. Video capsule endoscopy: technology, reading, and troubleshooting. Gastrointest Endosc Clin N Am. 2017;27:15–27.
5. Song HJ, Moon JS, Shim KN. Optimal bowel preparation for video capsule endoscopy. Gastroenterol Res Pract. 2016;2016:6802810.
6. Song HJ, Moon JS, Do JH, et al. Guidelines for bowel preparation before video capsule endoscopy. Clin Endosc. 2013;46:147–54.
7. Endo H, Kondo Y, Inamori M, et al. Ingesting 500 ml of polyethylene glycol solution during capsule endoscopy improves the image quality and completion rate to the cecum. Dig Dis Sci. 2008;53:3201–15.
8. Adler SN, Farkash S, Sompolinsky Y, Gafanovich I, Goldin E, Bar-Gil SA. A novel purgative protocol for capsule endoscopy of the small bowel produces better quality of visibility than 2 l of PEG: timing is of the essence. United European Gastroenterol J. 2017;5:485–90.
9. Kim ES, Chun HJ, Keum B, et al. Coffee enema for preparation for small bowel video capsule endoscopy: a pilot study. Clin Nutr Res. 2014;3:134–41.
10. Song HJ, Shim KN. What is the optimal timing of bowel preparation for video capsule endoscopy? Clin Endosc. 2015;48:183–4.

Procedure and Informed Consent of Patients for Capsule Endoscopy

Byung Ik Jang

Key Points
- When conducting capsule endoscopy for diagnosing small intestinal disease, medical staffs must be fully aware of the entire procedures to ensure quality of capsule endoscopy and improvement of diagnosis.
- When conducting capsule endoscopy, patients must be fully informed of the preparation process before examination, the endoscopy itself, and provisions after the examination. After being informed of all needed information, patients can then sign the consent for capsule endoscopy.

Capsule endoscopy allows the intestinal mucosa of the patient to be examined without discomfort after a patient swallows the capsule for small intestinal examination. However, it also has limitations. First, air insufflation is impossible in capsule endoscopy, making the examination less accurate. In addition, taking biopsy samples and performing therapeutic procedures are not possible with capsule endoscopy. This

B. I. Jang (✉)
Department of Internal Medicine, Yeungnam University College of Medicine, Daegu, South Korea
e-mail: jbi@med.yu.ac.kr

chapter consists of specific procedures needed and informed consents of patient.

Capsule Endoscopy

1. On the examining day, patient's information including personal data, weight, height, and abdominal circumference is collected and entered into a computer system. After connecting portable data storage devices to the computer, patient information is reset.
2. After fastening the belt around the patient's waist, storage device needs to be fixed in place. Patient should be notified that the device can become hot.
3. Attach the sensor array to the patient's abdomen and connect the storage device, making sure that wires are not entangled (Pictures 1 and 2). At this moment, the light in the recording device that flashes turns off as a sign of connection.
4. Now it is time to swallow the capsule. Take out the capsule from the storing case with magnet attached (Picture 3). The capsule endoscopy is now turned on with light starting to flash 2–3 times per second. One needs to check to see if the capsule light and the storage device light are flashing simultaneously.
5. Place the capsule so that the light flashing side is toward the neck. The patient should swallow the capsule with water (Picture 4). The swallowing time is then recorded.

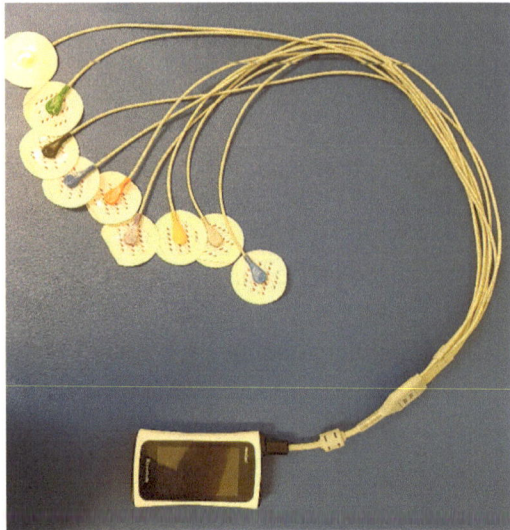

Picture 1   Sensor array and storage device

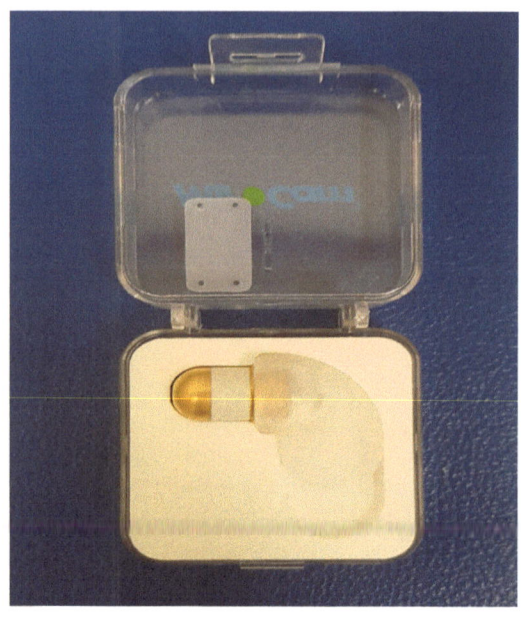

Picture 3   Capsule endoscopy

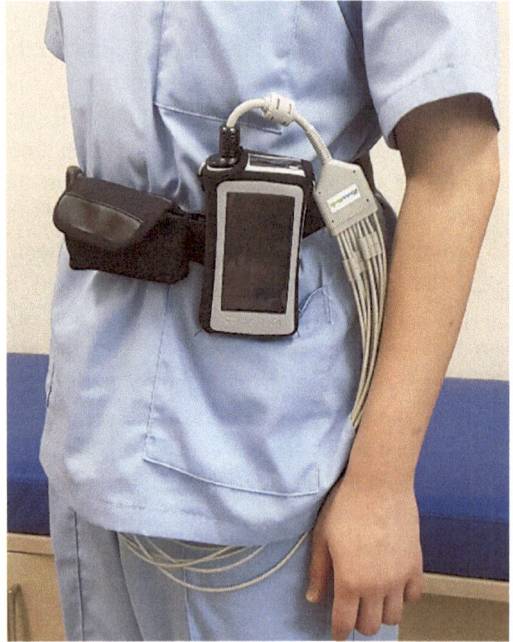

Picture 2   Fasten the belt to the patient's waist, fix the storage device, attach the sensor array to the abdomen, and connect it to the storage device

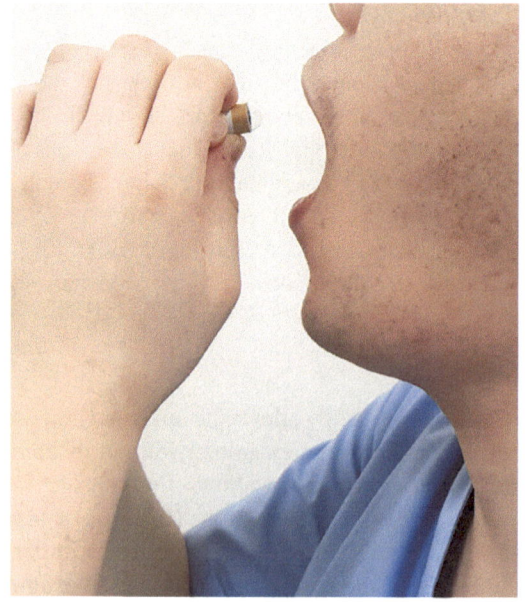

Picture 4   Point the flashing side of the capsule endoscopy to the neck and swallow capsule endoscopy with water

6. Inform the patient to check for the storage device occasionally, making sure that the light is flashing 2–3 times per second. Patient is also asked to record every food consumption, activity, and symptom while the patient is under examination.

7. During capsule endoscopy, storage device, sensor array, and wires should not be touched and the belt should not be removed.

8. When 8–9 h passed after swallowing the capsule, the patient can come back to the examina-

tion room as the process is finished. The belt, storage device, and sensor array are all removed. If the capsule is excreted during the process or if the storage light flashing is ceased, then the examination should be ended immediately.

9. After the process is over, the patient needs to check if the capsule has been excreted. If the capsule has not been excreted within three days, it needs to be checked through an abdominal X-ray.

Informed Consent of Patients

Explain thoroughly the objective, preparation process, procedures, provisions after the examination, and possible complications of capsule endoscopy. After sufficient explanation, the patient can then sign the consent.

Consent form of Capsule Endoscopy

- Capsule endoscopy is conducted in order to observe the mucosa of the small intestine. When the patient swallows a mini camera shaped like a capsule, the camera moves along the digestive canals due to intestinal peristalsis. Images taken by the capsule are sent to the receiver attached at the patient's waist and the computer is used to collect and interpret small intestinal mucosal images.
- Please inform the staff if the patient is taking painkillers or iron pills.
- Iron pills are not to be taken three days prior to capsule endoscopy. Beans, fruits with seeds, corns, popcorns, and red foods should be avoided. Antispasmodic and narcotic agents that can decrease intestine movement should also be avoided if possible.
- No eating is allowed for more than 12 hours prior to capsule endoscopy.
- Check for the storage device occasionally, making sure the light is flashing 2–3 times

per second. If the light is not flashing or if there are unexpected symptoms such as pain in the stomach, contact the hospital immediately.

- Please record every food consumption, activity, and symptom while the patient is under examination.
- Patient can maintain daily routines such as walking, lying down, or driving. However, patient should refrain from working too hard or bending.
- Storage device needs to be secure without sudden movement or shock. It should not be exposed to direct light, heat, or moisture.
- Patient may use a computer, radio, stereo device, and cell phone. However, MRI device and HAM radio that has similar frequency level should not be used.
- Clear liquids such as water and apple juice are allowed 2 hours after swallowing the capsule. Light food consumption and medicine are permitted after 4 hours.
- Capsule endoscopy normally ends after 8–9 hours after swallowing the capsule. After capsule endoscopy ends, patient should come back to the examination room to remove the belt, storage device, and the sensor array.
- Patient must check if the capsule has been excreted during and after the endoscopy each time the patient goes to restroom and inform the medical staff.

Patient address _____
_____.
Name _____
Sign_____.
legal representative address
_____.
Name_____
(relationship with the patient:____)
Sign_____.
Doctor_____
Sign_____.

Closing Remarks

Capsule endoscopy has been established as a primary screening tool for small intestinal diagnosis. It is especially useful for diagnosing obscure gastrointestinal bleeding. Its usage is expected to expand. It can be used not only for examining small intestines, but also for evaluating esophagus, stomach, and large intestine. Medical staff should be fully aware of procedures of capsule endoscopy and inform patients so that both quality and diagnostic yield of capsule endoscopy can be enhanced.

Interpretation of Small Bowel Capsule Endoscopy

Ji Hyun Kim

Key Points
1. Accurate comprehension of the reading software is essential for adequate interpretation in small bowel capsule endoscopy.
2. Approximate review and lesion localization can be performed with the QuickView, suspected blood indicator, tissue color bar, and localization functions.
3. Trainees should begin using frame rates of 5–10 fps and the DualView or QuadView mode for optimal interpretation.

Owing to the anatomical characteristics, conventional endoscopic examination of the entire small bowel remains difficult to perform. Small bowel capsule endoscopy has been proven to be an effective diagnostic modality for small bowel disorders, despite its disadvantages of impossibility of air insufflation/suction and detailed examination of the suspected lesion. The degree of bowel preparation and the interpreter's experience are essential for enhancing the diagnostic quality. The reading time and low interobserver agree-

J. H. Kim (✉)
Inje University College of Medicine,
Busan, South Korea
e-mail: zep2000@hanafos.com

ment were major problems in the earlier version of the reading program. However, the reading time has been made shorter with software upgrades that reduce the number of repeatedly taken images during the examination. The interpretation of capsule endoscopic images is usually composed of three phases: preview, review, and report:

Development of Reading Software

History of the RAPID Program

RAPID® software, which was developed by Given Imaging Company, is the most popular software worldwide. To date, RAPID 8.3 version, which is integrated with the PillCam SB3 system, is available.

The RAPID 1 system was characterized by a speed control function that can control the examination speed of transferred images and a localization function that can approximately localize the capsule endoscope. The suspected blood indicator (SBI) and multiview functions and the standard reporting system were introduced in the RAPID 2 system. Examination of esophageal images was feasible with the RAPID 3 system. In addition, a tissue color bar function, which analyzes the average color of the small bowel lumen, and the QuadView and My GI dictionary functions are also available in the RAPID 3 system (Fig. 1).

© Springer Nature Singapore Pte Ltd. 2022
H. J. Chun et al. (eds.), *Small Intestine Disease*, https://doi.org/10.1007/978-981-16-7239-2_16

Quick Access Toolbar

Information about the open study

Video image

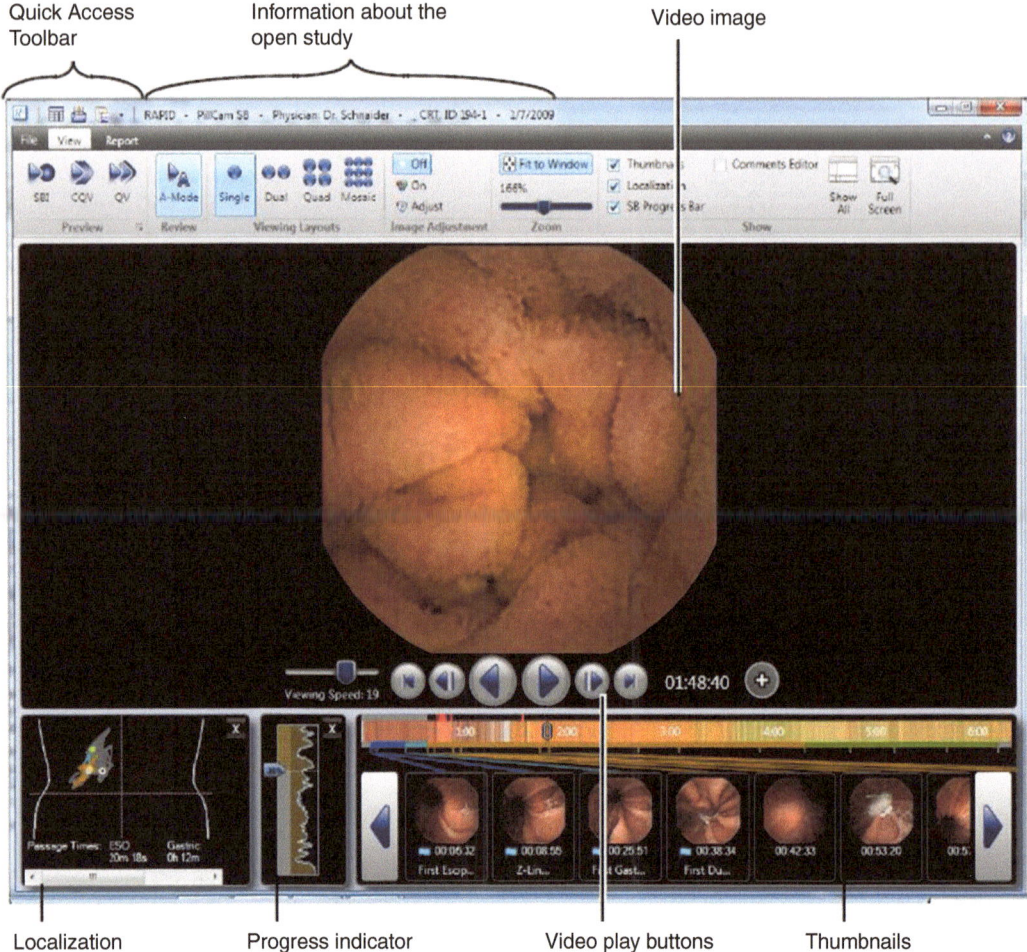

Localization   Progress indicator   Video play buttons   Thumbnails

Fig. 1 Control panel of the RAPID® program for small bowel capsule endoscopy. Courtesy of Medtronic®

Interpretation

The interpretation of capsule endoscopic images is usually composed of three phases: preview, review, and report. In the preview phase, determination of whether or not the examination was complete; determination of the degree of bowel preparation; rough examination of the whole image with the QuickView function; localization of the stomach, duodenum, ileocecal (IC) valve, and cecum; and activation of the SBI, tissue color bar, and localization functions are performed. In case of gastrointestinal bleeding, the presence of bleeding can be approximately identified with the SBI function

beforehand, and accurate examination of the suspected area can reduce the interpretation time. In the review phase, a detailed examination of whole images is performed using the automatic mode. In this phase, the interpretation time is essential for the quality of interpretation, such as the detection rate. Usually, completing the first review takes 45 min to 2 h with a frame rate of 10–25 frames per second (fps). Suspicious images during the review phase should be preserved as thumbnails with brief comments on the location and characteristics of the lesion. Detected lesions are described according to Capsule Endoscopy Structured Terminology in the report phase.

Lesion Localization

The location and characteristics of the lesion provide important clues for further management strategies. However, localization of the lesion with capsule endoscopy is difficult because anatomical landmarks in the small bowel are limited. To date, several approaches for approximate lesion localization are used. First, the total examination time is divided into three, according to separate localization in the proximal, mid, and distal small bowel. Second, localization is made based on the organ landmarks in the gastrointestinal tract, such as the esophagus, duodenum, small bowel, and terminal ileum, as well as on the anatomical landmarks of each organ, such as the Z-line, pylorus, ampulla, and IC valve. Finally, the localizing function of the interpreting software is used, which localizes the lesion based on four compartments of the abdomen. Although the error range of the localizing function was reported to be 6 cm, the validity of the software function for lesion localization is not very practical. The time interval from the localization of the pylorus or IC valve to that of the lesion also can be used for localizing the lesion [1].

Quality Indicators for Interpretation

Although capsule endoscopy is a relatively non-invasive modality that can visualize the entire small bowel mucosa, it has the disadvantage of impossibility of air suction/insufflation and detailed examination of the suspected lesion. In addition, a certain degree of interpreter experience is essential for adequate diagnostic accuracy. For performing adequate capsule endoscopy, the interpreter's ability should be enhanced and effective communication between interpreters is important. Moreover, interpreters should be concerned about the quality control indicators.

Frame Rate

Capsule endoscopy images are taken at a rate of 2 pictures per second. The frame rate (fps) means the number of images that are displayed in a video file by the software for the interpretation of capsule endoscopy results, and could be determined based on the interpreter's experience. Currently, the reading software provides the function of controlling the frame rate from 1 to 40 fps. Naturally, as the frame rate becomes slower, the reading time and detection rate become higher [2, 3]. According to the panel consensus in the 2002 International Conference of Capsule Endoscopy, the fastest acceptable frame rate for review is 15 fps [4]. Trainees should begin using frame rates of 5–10 fps for optimal interpretation [5].

View Mode

The PillCam SB software also has a function of controlling the image number shown in one monitor during the interpretation, from the single image view mode up to 18 images (MosaicView mode). Theoretically, multiple view modes, such as the DualView or QuadView mode, can reduce the reading time as well as enhance the detection rate through a longer single-frame exposure [2, 3]. The detection rates were reported to be 56%, 83%, and 85% with the SingleView, DualView, and QuadView modes, respectively, at 10 fps [2]. However, multiple view modes have the drawback of making the interpreters rely on their peripheral vision because of simultaneously focusing on multiple images [3]. Because the appropriate view mode for the highest detection rate during the review phase has not been determined, the Korean guidelines recommend the DualView mode or QuadView mode rather than the SingleView mode during the interpretation [6].

References

1. Fischer D, Schreiber R, Levi D, Eliakim R. Capsule endoscopy: the localization system. Gastrointest Endosc Clin N Am. 2004;14:25–31.
2. Nakamura M, Murino A, O'Rourke A, Fraser C. A critical analysis of the effect of view mode and frame rate on reading time and lesion detection during capsule endoscopy. Dig Dis Sci. 2015;60:1743–7.

3. Zheng Y, Hawkins L, Wolff J, Goloubeva O, Goldberg E. Detection of lesions during capsule endoscopy: physician performance is disappointing. Am J Gastroenterol. 2012;107:554–60.

4. Lewis BS. How to read wireless capsule endoscopic images: tips of the trade. Gastrointest Endosc Clin N Am. 2004;14:11–6.

5. Gunther U, Daum S, Zeitz M, Bojarski C. Capsule endoscopy: comparison of two different reading modes. Int J Color Dis. 2012;27:521–5.

6. Shim KN, Jeon SR, Jang HJ, et al. Quality indicators for small bowel capsule endoscopy. Clin Endosc. 2017;50:148–60.

Normal Findings of Capsule Endoscopy

Jae Hyuk Do and Beom-Jin Kim

Key Point

Dissimilar to conventional endoscopy in which inspection and reading are performed simultaneously, images captured by capsule endoscopy are downloaded and retrospectively interpreted by a physician. Accordingly, it is essential for physicians to be familiar with normal capsule endoscopy findings, as various factors should be taken into account for precise reading. This chapter reviews the typical normal capsule endoscopy findings of the gastrointestinal tract.

Introduction

Once swallowed, a capsule endoscope intermittently captures two images per second as it passes through the gastrointestinal tract, including the oral cavity, pharynx, esophagus, stomach, small intestine, and large intestine. As artificial air is not injected and intestinal contents cannot be aspirated for the purpose of examination, endoscopic findings typical of conventional endoscopy can be observed in various forms. The distinction between normal and abnormal may be ambiguous, and the detection of lesion sites may even be challenging. Under most circumstances, capsule endoscopy enables direct visualization of the small intestine and ascending colon. Imaging may occasionally be interrupted because of slow small bowel capsule transit time or the finite lifespan of the capsule battery, resulting in an incomplete test. This chapter reviews the normal capsule endoscopy findings of the gastrointestinal tract (Table 1).

Pharynx and Larynx

The pharynx, which is approximately 13 cm in length, is located between the posterior turbinate and sixth cervical vertebra and is anatomically divided into the nasopharynx, oropharynx, and hypopharynx. As the capsule endoscope immediately passes through the pharynx and larynx, only one or two photos may be obtained. The capsule endoscope may become stagnant at the esophageal entrance, which is the first constriction of the esophagus (Figs. 1, 2, and 3).

Esophagus

The esophagus, which is approximately 20–26 cm in length, is located between the hypopharynx and stomach. The average esophageal capsule transit time is 6 seconds, which is sufficient to

J. H. Do (✉) · B.-J. Kim
Division of Gastroenterology, Department of Internal Medicine, Chung-Ang University College of Medicine, Seoul, South Korea
e-mail: jhdo@cau.ac.kr; kimbj@cau.ac.kr

© Springer Nature Singapore Pte Ltd. 2022
H. J. Chun et al. (eds.), *Small Intestine Disease*, https://doi.org/10.1007/978-981-16-7239-2_17

Table 1 Normal capsule endoscopy findings of the gastrointestinal tract

Esophagus (gastroesophageal junction)	Palisade longitudinal vessels of the esophagus are seen, with more prominent gastric mucosa being observed distal to the columnar-lined esophagus.
Gastric cardia	Mucosal folds in the greater curvature of the gastric cardia, which are often obscured by ingested water or gastric juice, are the first to be visualized.
Gastric pylorus	The pyloric sphincter usually remains closed, with the longitudinal gastric folds being encircled predominantly near the pylorus ring.
Duodenal bulb	Endoscopic findings of the duodenal bulb include Brunner's glands and villi, along with its characteristic mucosal color change as the capsule endoscope enters the duodenum.
Ampulla of Vater	Kerckring's folds and major duodenal papilla along with bile flow are visualized.
Terminal ileum	Concentrated dark bile juice is noted by capsule endoscopy, whereas lymphoid follicles are sometimes visible.
Ileocecal valve	The transit time slows down, and concentrated bile may be observed. The ileocecal valve is not difficult to recognize as the smooth intestinal mucosa without villi is readily observed.
Cecum	Prominent submucosal blood vessels are noted along with the smooth mucosa without villi.

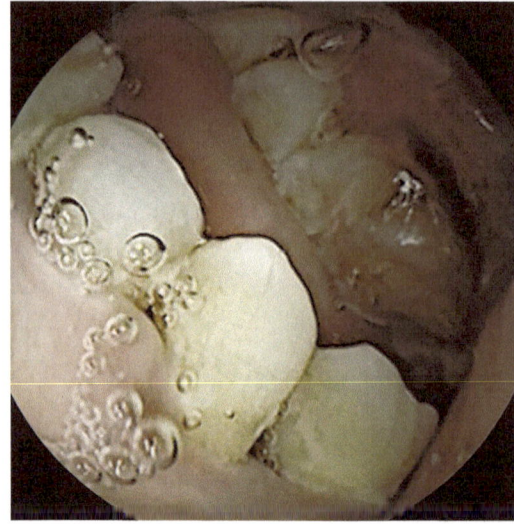

Fig. 1 Teeth

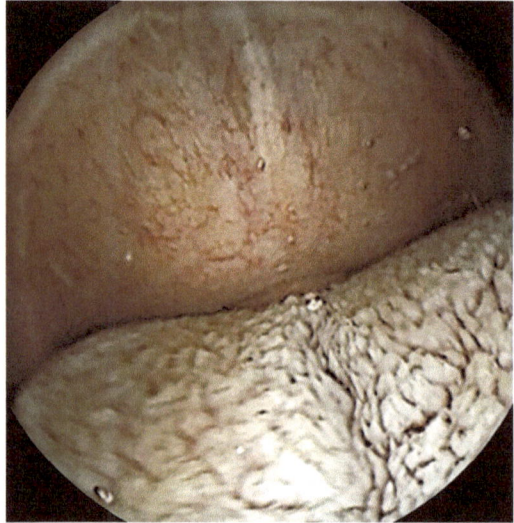

Fig. 2 Tongue and uvula

obtain approximately 10 images. The border between the hypopharynx and esophagus is rarely visualized as the capsule quickly passes through the corresponding structure. Subsequently, the capsule is temporarily stagnated by the lower esophageal sphincter, enabling the Z-line at the esophagogastric junction to be examined. Esophageal contractions elicited by peristalsis and longitudinal vasculature may also be observed (Figs. 4, 5, and 6).

Stomach

The capsule endoscope passing through the esophagogastric junction enters the stomach, reaching the greater curvature of the body where gastric folds can be observed. The average transit time is approximately 1 h, with considerable individual variations [1, 2]. As the stomach can-

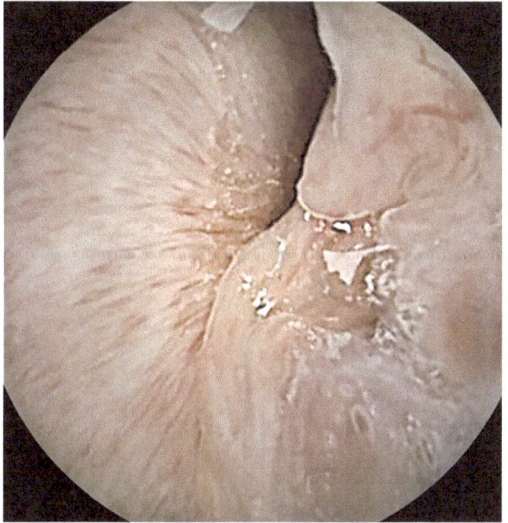

Fig. 3 Normal larynx

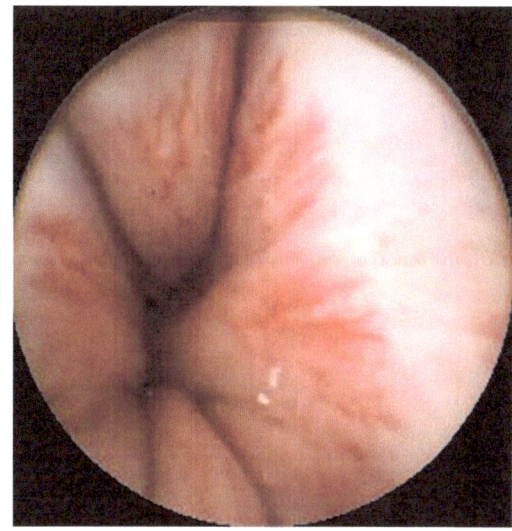

Fig. 5 Lower thoracic esophagus

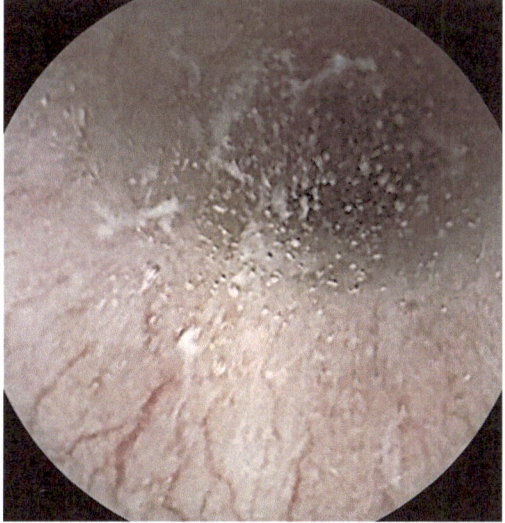

Fig. 4 Middle thoracic esophagus. Longitudinal blood vessels are well observed

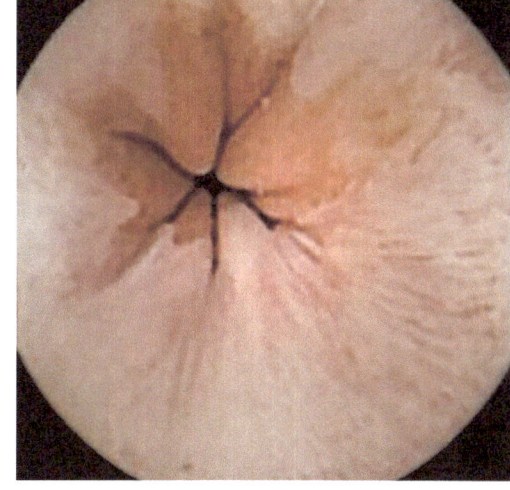

Fig. 6 Gastroesophageal junction

not be artificially inflated with a capsule endoscope, the pylorus generally appears more wrinkled than that observed with a conventional endoscope. The most common and characteristic capsule endoscopy finding of the stomach is the back-and-forth movement of the capsule endoscope, allowing visualization of the gastric folds and distinct gastric parts. If a clear physiologic form of the gastric mucosa is present, the peristalsis of the antrum and pylorus may be well observed with the optical dome of the capsule endoscope pointing to the pylorus (Figs. 7, 8, and 9).

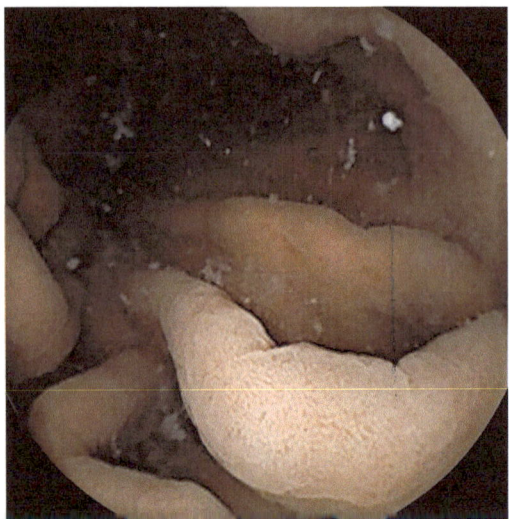

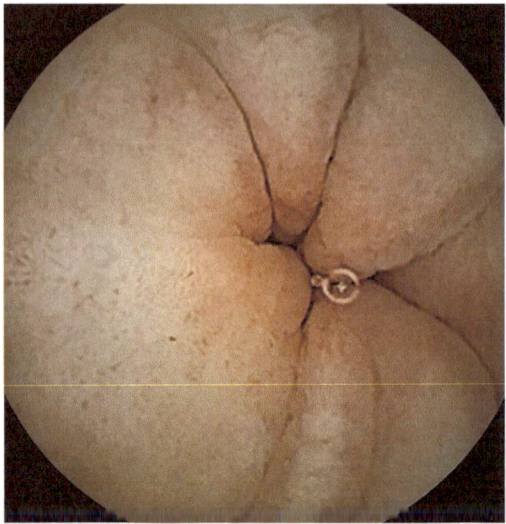

Fig. 7 Gastric cardia. Luminal contraction by the gastric folds and peristalsis of the gastric body are observed

Fig. 9 Gastric pylorus. Longitudinal mucosal folds being encircled predominantly near the pylorus ring are observed

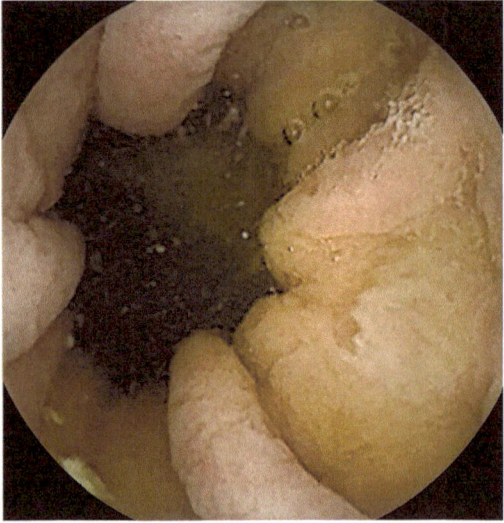

Fig. 8 Gastric antrum

Small Intestine

Duodenum

The capsule endoscope enters the duodenal bulb through the pylorus. The small intestine is approximately 6 m in length, and small intestine capsule transit time is generally defined as the time of passage from the pylorus to the ileocecal valve. The pylorus is well visible when the capsule endoscope enters the duodenal bulb.

Characteristic mucosal color change is noted as the capsule endoscope enters the duodenum. Occasionally, bile juice may be observed to flow from the third portion of the duodenum to the proximal portion. Brunner's glands are distributed mostly near the duodenal bulb and their number gradually decreases below the papilla. The bulb appears non-glossy, with vessels often invisible, and is covered with blunt villi. The capsule endoscope rapidly progresses to the second portion of the duodenum where the villous architecture is evident. The ampulla of Vater lies in the inner wall of the descending duodenum, at 3–6 cm distal to the duodenal bulb. Minor papilla can be observed at 2–4 cm above the major papilla. Kerckring's folds, perpendicular to the long axis of the duodenum, become visible starting from the second portion of the duodenum.

Capsule endoscopy does not expand the lumen with air injection and the capsule itself is partly immersed in intestinal fluid; hence, visualization of the intestinal villi is relatively easier with capsule endoscopy than with conventional endoscopy. Nevertheless, it should be noted that capsule endoscopy frequently fails to visualize the ampulla of Vater, as it is located directly beneath the marginal folds and is often obscured by Kerckring's folds (Figs. 10, 11, and 12) [3].

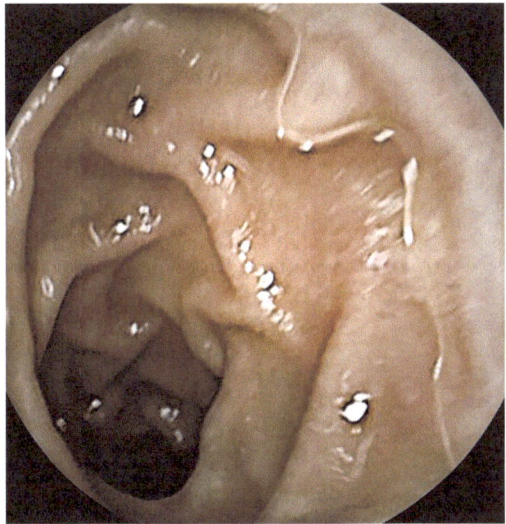

Fig. 10 Duodenum. Kerckring's folds and villi

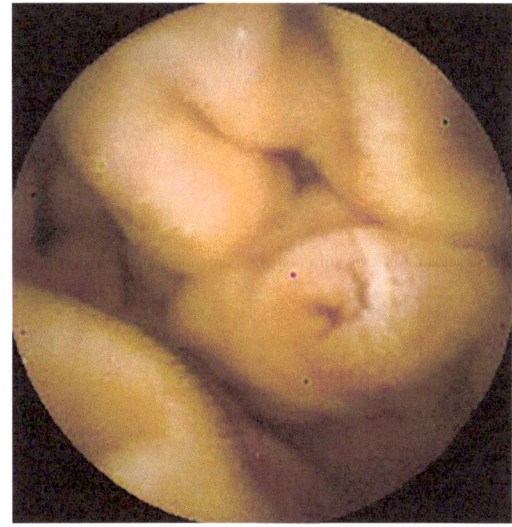

Fig. 12 Ampulla of Vater

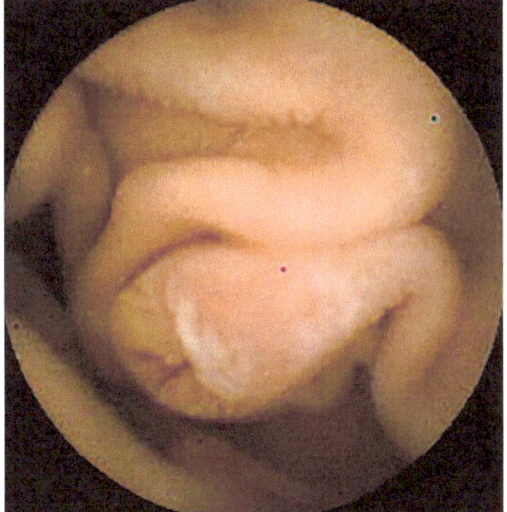

Fig. 11 Ampulla of Vater

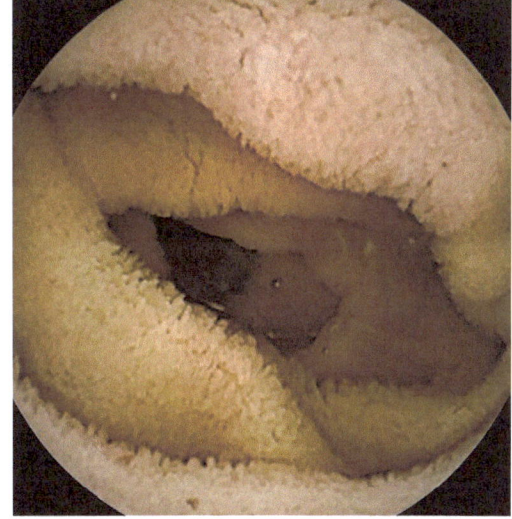

Fig. 13 Jejunum

Jejunum and Ileum

The capsule endoscope now enters the jejunum, distal to the ligament of Treitz. The jejunum, which is predominantly located on the left side of the abdomen, has a thicker wall and larger lumen than the ileum. Nevertheless, the ileum, which is mainly located at the right lower quadrant of the abdomen, has more flexibility than the jejunum. The small intestinal lumen is covered with abundant plicae circulares or Kerckring's folds, which are present throughout the small intestine except in the duodenal bulb and terminal ileum (Figs. 13 and 14).

Lymphoid follicles are present throughout the small intestine but are mostly distributed in the distal ileum. They are more frequently observed in young, immunocompromised patients [4]. Lymphoid follicles extending more than 3 mm into the mucosal layer are referred to as Peyer's patches. Small intestinal villi protruding into the

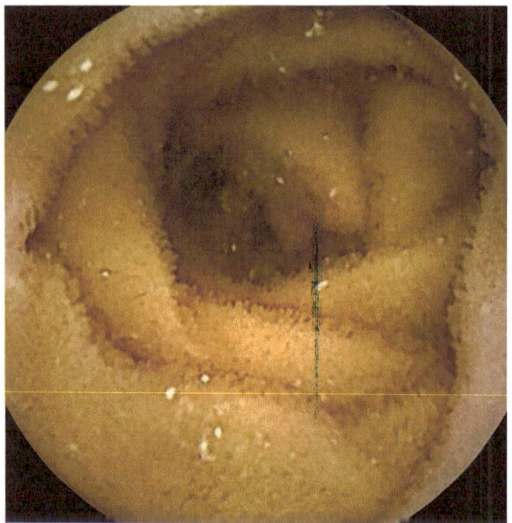

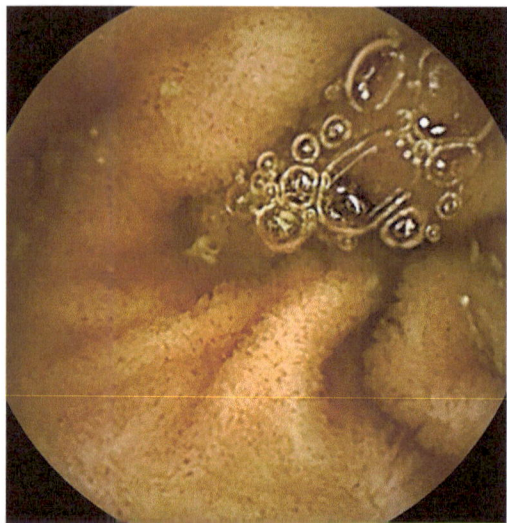

Fig. 14 Jejunum. Kerckring's folds and villi of the jejunum

Fig. 16 Ileum

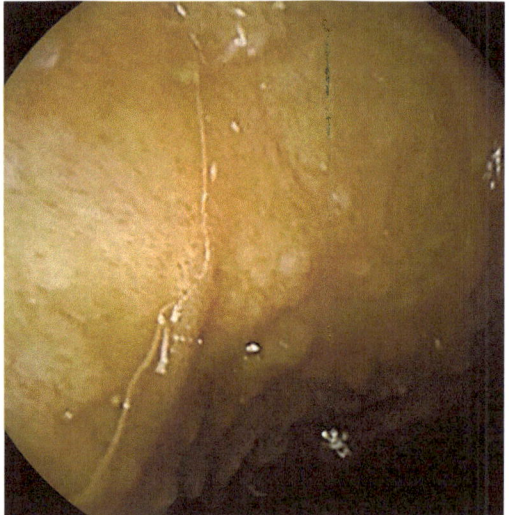

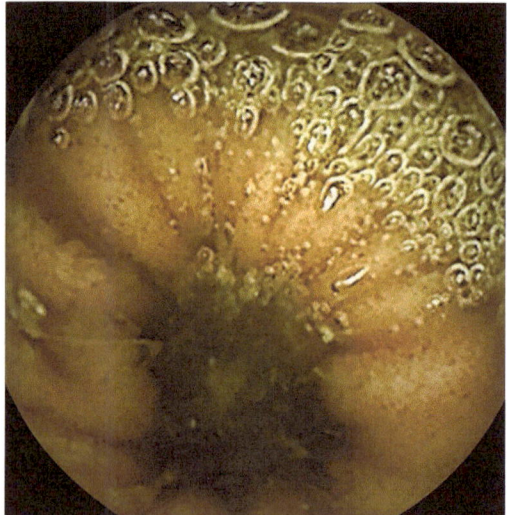

Fig. 15 Lymphoid follicle

Fig. 17 Ileum. Concentrated bile is observed, and villus height is lower in the ileum than in the jejunum

lumen range in length from 0.5 to 1.5 mm and are tallest in the distal duodenum and proximal jejunum (Fig. 15).

The vasculature and architecture of the small intestine become evident as the capsule enters the distal jejunum. Concentrated dark bile juice can be observed by capsule endoscopy as the capsule reaches the distal portion of the duodenum; the villi disappear in the ileum (Figs. 16 and 17).

There is no endoscopically clear distinction between the jejunum and ileum. The ileocecal valve is not difficult to recognize as the smooth intestinal mucosa without villi is readily observed. The capsule occasionally becomes stagnant when the ileocecal valve remains closed. As the capsule passes through the ileocecal valve, the transit time slows down and prominent distribution of vasculature may be observed (Figs. 18 and 19).

Considering that images captured by capsule endoscopy are different from those obtained by conventional endoscopy, distinguishing normal from abnormal endoscopic lesions is essential [5]. Examples include the differentiation between submucosal tumor and bulge caused by extrinsic compression (Figs. 20 and 21); lymphoid follicles and multiple polyposis (Fig. 22); and lymphangiectasia and xanthoma (Fig. 23).

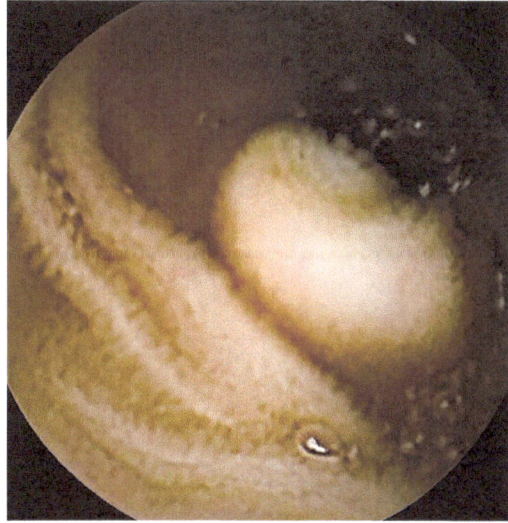

Fig. 20 Submucosal tumor

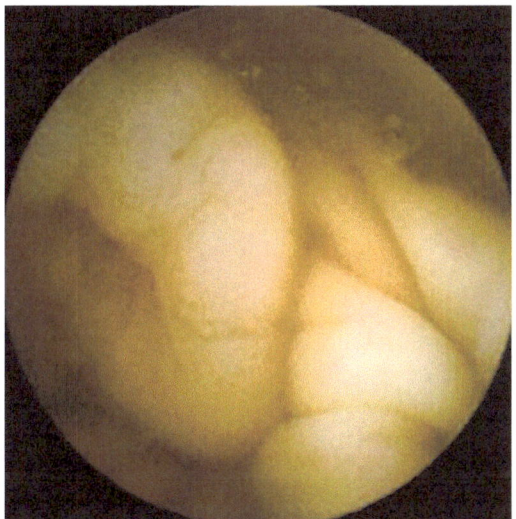

Fig. 18 Ileocecal valve

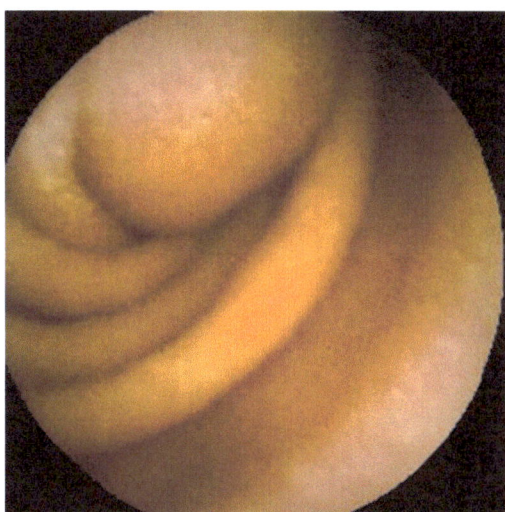

Fig. 21 External compression

Concentrated dark bile juice may be misdiagnosed as gastrointestinal bleeding.

Conclusion

Understanding the nature and endoscopic findings of capsule endoscopy will help improve its diagnostic yield in clinical practice.

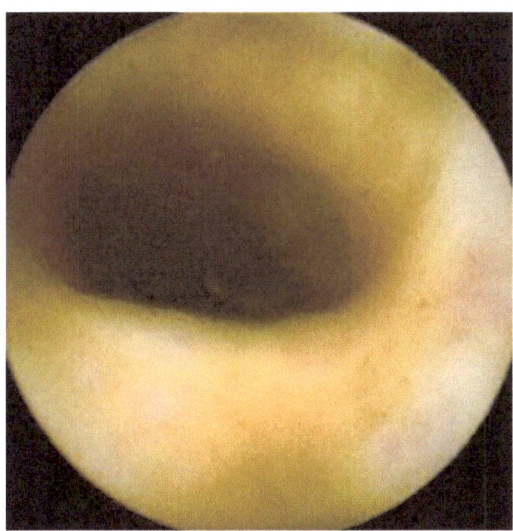

Fig. 19 Ileocecal valve

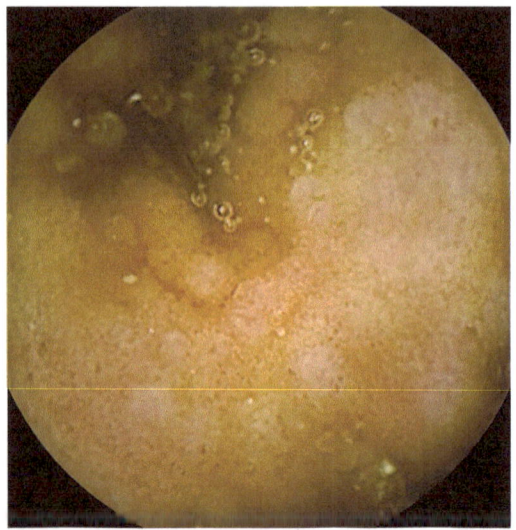

Fig. 22 Lymphoid follicle

References

1. Shim KN, Jeon SR, Jang HJ, et al. Quality indicators for small bowel capsule endoscopy. Clin Endosc. 2017;50:148–60.
2. Eliakim R. Video capsule endoscopy of the small bowel. Curr OpinGastroenterol. 2008;24:159–63.
3. Cheung DY, Kim JS, Shim KN, Choi MG. Korean gut image study group. The usefulness of capsule endoscopy for small bowel tumors. Clin Endosc. 2016;49:21–5.
4. Min YW, Chang DK. The role of capsule endoscopy in patients with ObscureGastrointestinal bleeding. Clin Endosc. 2016;49:16–20.
5. Lim YJ, Joo YS, Jung DY, et al. Learning curve of capsule endoscopy. Clin Endosc. 2013;46:633–6.

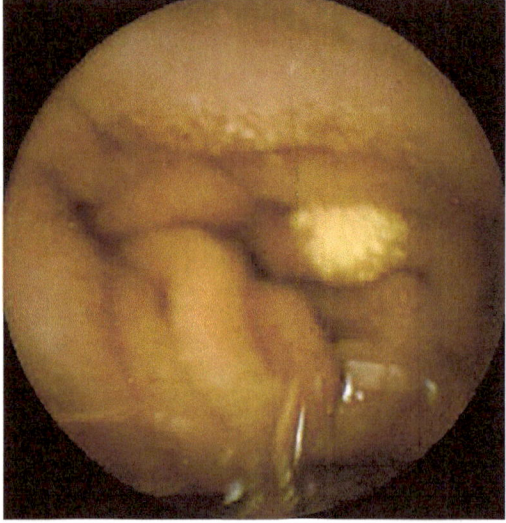

Fig. 23 Xanthoma

Terminology

Chang Mo Moon

Key Points
- Standard terminology is essential for the exact communication of capsule endoscopic results and enhancement of clinical effectiveness.
- The capsule endoscopy report requires patient information and small bowel lesion data (patient data, date of capsule endoscopy, reason for examination, whether examination was complete or incomplete, complications, description of findings, and diagnosis).
- The final diagnosis of capsule endoscopy should be determined after a comprehensive review of the capsule endoscopy images and patient's clinical information.

Standard Terminology

Terms used for capsule endoscopy should be reproducible, so that even a doctor who has not seen the image can readily recognize the small bowel lesion features. Thus, the *Given Capsule Standard Working Group* led by Korman has organized and presented the *capsule endoscopy structured terminology (CEST)* in 2005 [1]. CEST was developed in accordance with the Minimal Standard Terminology guidelines [2].

Description

The report on capsule endoscopy must include patient data and description of the small bowel. Patient data includes patient information, date of examination, reason for examination, whether the examination was complete or incomplete, complications, lesion description, capsule endoscopic findings, and diagnosis (Table 1).

Descriptions

Lesions
CEST consists of clear, distinct, widespread, and common terms. First, the headings for the lesion data based on capsule endoscopy findings are selected. Headings include normal, lumen status, content in the lumen, and mucosa status. When the lesion is observed, it is classified as a flat, protruding, or excavated lesions [3]. The main categorization used for a small bowel lesion includes a presence of a normal lumen (such as presence of stenosis and dilatation), contents (such as blood and bile), mucosa (such as erythema, pale, and granular), flat lesions (such as spot, plaque, and angioectasia), protruding lesions (such as nodule, polyp, and mass), and excavated lesions

C. M. Moon (✉)
The Department of Internal Medicine, Ewha Womans University College of Medicine, Seoul, South Korea

© Springer Nature Singapore Pte Ltd. 2022
H. J. Chun et al. (eds.), *Small Intestine Disease*, https://doi.org/10.1007/978-981-16-7239-2_18

Table 1 Structure of capsule endoscopy report

Data fields
Patient name
Date of birth
Sex
Patient ID
Date of examination
Capsule type
Capsule ID
Physician/provider
Patient history
Clinical indication
ICD indication
Extent of examination
Characteristics of examination
Complication
Findings
Diagnostic impression
Diagnostic ICD
Recommendation

ID identification, *ICD* international statistical classification of diseases and related health problems

(such as aphtha, erosion, and ulcer) [1, 4]. Detailed descriptions, which are added after these headings, include characteristics of the lesion such as its location, shape, and number. After the main categorization is done, the details are described in the order of heading-term-attribute-attribute value [1, 5].

Localization

Discovering the exact location of the lesion is essential for determining the exact location needing treatment. Thus, the location must be included in the capsule endoscopy report. Lesion location can be separated into three parts [5]. First, the small bowel should be divided into three sections (proximal, middle, and distal parts) based on the recording time of the lesion. Second, descriptions should be in the order of the esophagus, stomach, small bowel, and terminal ileum. In this situation, standard anatomical landmarks such as the Z line, pylorus, papilla, and ileocecal valve are used to categorize the location. The third option is included in the interpretation software by which the abdominal region is divided into four parts with the navel in the center (left upper, left lower, right upper, and right lower quadrant) or divided

according to the time required to pass from the pyloric ring to ileocecal valve.

Small Bowel Preparation Quality

A description of the capsule endoscopy procedure itself includes the preparation methods and results, examination time, and final location examined. In particular, since there is no standardized bowel preparation method for capsule endoscopy, various suggestions have been proposed to determine how to conduct quantitative measurement for bowel preparation. For example, examiners measured the bowel preparation quality by inspecting the entire small bowel mucosa or inspecting several images at several recording time points. However, these measurement methods for bowel preparation have limitations in that they are subjective and not quantitative. Accordingly, methods for increasing objectivity and quantitative measurement have been proposed [3].

Diagnosis

The final diagnosis of capsule endoscopy should be decided based on the comprehensive review of capsule endoscopic images and patient's clinical information. CEST diagnosis is divided into major and minor diagnoses depending on the frequency of occurrence. The major diagnosis is categorized as normal, angioectasia, erosion, ulcer, Crohn's disease, celiac disease, NSAID-induced enteropathy, and tumor (benign or malignant) (Table 2) [1, 4]. The capsule endoscopic report should include the final diagnosis based on the capsule endoscopic finding, indication, and medical history. Consequently, not all images have clinical meaning, so the final diagnosis should be determined based on the clinical findings and capsule endoscopic findings.

Closing Remarks

The final diagnosis of capsule endoscopy should be determined after comprehensive review of the capsule endoscopic findings and patient's clinical information. However, standard terminology is

Table 2 Major and minor diagnoses

Major diagnosis	Normal
	Angioectasia
	Erosion
	Ulcer
	Crohn's disease
	Celiac disease
	NSAID enteropathy
	Tumor (benign or malignancy)
	Bleeding of unknown origin
Minor diagnosis	Diverticulum
	Tropical sprue
	Parasite
	Hemobilia
	Phlebectasia
	Varices
	Intestinal lymphangiectasia
	Ischemic enteritis
	Vasculitis
	Radiation enteritis
	Posttransplant lymphoproliferative disease
	Graft-versus-host disease
	Enteropathy (erosive, erythematous, congestive, and hemorrhagic)
	Brunner's gland hyperplasia
	Lipoma
	Neuroendocrine tumor
	Melanoma
	GIST (gastrointestinal stromal tumor)
	Kaposi's sarcoma
	Lymphoma
	Polyps
	Juvenile polyposis
	Familial adenomatous polyposis
	Peutz-Jeghers syndrome

highly recommended to share the data generated by capsule endoscopic images accurately. This will require standardization of the terminology, dissemination, and training. This is ultimately expected to increase the clinical utility of capsule endoscopy and facilitate qualitative improvement.

References

1. Korman LY, Delvaux M, Gay G, et al. Capsule endoscopy structured terminology (CEST): proposal of a standardized and structured terminology for reporting capsule endoscopy procedures. Endoscopy. 2005;37:951–9.
2. Delvaux M, Crespi M, Armengol-Miro JR, et al. Minimal standard terminology for digestive endoscopy: results of prospective testing and validation in the GASTER project. Endoscopy. 2000;32:345–55.
3. Keum B. How to report the capsule endoscopy results. Korean J Gastrointestinal Endoscopy. 2010;40:228–33.
4. Gut Image Study Group, Lim YJ, Moon JS, Chang DK, Jang BI, Chun HJ, Choi M-G. Korean Society of Gastrointestinal Endoscopy (KSGE) guidelines for credentialing and granting privileges for capsule endoscopy. Korean J Gastrointestinal Endoscopy. 2008;37:393–402.
5. Fischer D, Schreiber R, Levi D, Eliakim R. Capsule endoscopy: the localization system. Gastrointest Endosc Clin N Am. 2004;14:25–31.

Capsule Endoscopy in Special Circumstances

Dae Young Cheung

Key Points

- Capsule endoscopy is a noninvasive procedure that can be safely performed in children and elderly patients. However, when patients have difficulty swallowing capsules voluntarily, ancillary measures are needed.
- Capsule endoscopy does not harm the fetus and mother during pregnancy.
- Implanted devices, such as a pacemaker and defibrillator, do not interfere with the operation of the capsule endoscope.

Since its introduction to the clinical field in 2001, more than 1.5 million small bowel capsules had been used in a decade world widely. Several clinically important concerns with capsule endoscopy have been reported, but capsule retention in the small intestine is the only relevant complication. Imperfect test results due to functional or mechanical errors of the capsule are also one of the issues related to the usefulness of the capsule [1]. Therefore, it is necessary to examine various test conditions to predict and prevent possible complications or accidents, such as capsule retention and malfunctions.

In this chapter, we review the results obtained in special circumstances that may affect the safety and performance of the small bowel capsule in capsule endoscopy.

Capsule Endoscopy in Children

The safety of small intestine capsule endoscopy in children was referred to in the manufacturer's safety standards and an announcement by the United States (US) Food and Drug Administration. Since its introduction in 2001 into clinical practice, the indication for small intestine capsule endoscopy has continued to expand and included pediatric patients aged 10–18 years in 2004 [1]. The use of capsule endoscopy was approved in children older than 2 years of age by the US Food and Drug Administration in 2009 [1]. The youngest patient reported was 8 months old [2] and the lowest weight of patients was 7.9 kg [3]. The concerns about capsule endoscopy in children are based on the fact that the diameter of the gastrointestinal tract lumen is smaller in children than in adults, and this factor possibly carries a higher risk of capsule retention in the small intestine of pediatric patients.

The incidence of capsule retention in pediatric patients is approximately 0.5–2.4%, and this is comparable to the 1.4% in adult patients [4–6]. This fact may be due to the shorter transit time in

D. Y. Cheung (✉)
Department of Internal Medicine, The Catholic University of Korea College of Medicine, Seoul, South Korea
e-mail: adagio@catholic.ac.kr

© Springer Nature Singapore Pte Ltd. 2022
H. J. Chun et al. (eds.), *Small Intestine Disease*, https://doi.org/10.1007/978-981-16-7239-2_19

and higher resilience of the small intestine, which are intrinsic characteristics of pediatric patients, even though their intestinal luminal space is smaller than that in adults. The main cause of capsule retention in children is small bowel stenosis due to Crohn's disease. The risk of capsule retention in the small intestine reached 5.2% in pediatric patients with known Crohn's disease. If Crohn's disease was diagnosed with a small bowel series, capsule retention occurred in 35.7% of patients. If the patients were diagnosed with inflammatory bowel disease and had a body mass below the fifth percentile for age, the risk increased by up to 43% [7]. However, small bowel Crohn's disease is the most common clinical indication for small bowel capsule endoscopy in pediatric patients. In contrast, obscure gastrointestinal bleeding is the most common clinical indication for this procedure in adult patients (Table 1) [8]. This explains why the incidence of capsule retention in children (0.5–2.4%) is reportedly higher than that in adults (1.4%). The difference in risk of capsule retention between patients is caused by the disease characteristics of a population rather than structural differences. If Crohn's disease or small bowel obstruction is suspected, the patency or passage of the small intestinal tract should be evaluated with the patency capsule or magnetic resonance (MR) enterography.

The visibility of small intestine capsule endoscopy is another important factor of the examination. The presence of food residue, bile, bubbles, and blood in the stomach and in the small intestine would prohibit visibility of the capsule by covering the camera and reducing clarity of the luminal surface images. Overnight fasting with a clear liquid before the examination is insufficient for ensuring visibility at the distal site during the examination [9]. Proper and active bowel cleansing is a prerequisite in children as well as in adults. Polyethylene glycol (PEG) and simethicone with overnight fasting for 10–12 h have been associated with acceptable visibility during the examination. The most effective doses were 1.75 g/25 mL per kg (up to 1 L) of PEG on the day before the examination and 20 mL (375 mg) of simethicone at 30 min before swallowing the capsules [9].

Difficulty with capsule swallowing is another practical problem in pediatric patients. Children aged 4–5 years are generally considered able to swallow capsules sized 11–13 mm in diameter voluntarily. However, it is common for even children aged 8 years or younger to complain about the difficulty in swallowing the capsule; 1.1–1.5% of adults also experience difficulty in swallowing the capsule [10]. When concerns such as that for aspiration are raised, upper gastrointestinal endoscopy should be used to place the capsule in the stomach or duodenum directly.

Capsule Endoscopy in Pregnant Women

During pregnancy, the gastrointestinal tract undergoes changes. The intestinal transit time is higher, and the loops of the tract are structurally constrained by the growing uterus. Extrinsic compression and delayed transit of the intestinal tract may increase the risk of small bowel capsule retention. However, there has been no reported case of capsule retention during capsule endoscopy associated with pregnancy.

The effect of the electromagnetic field of the capsule endoscope on the fetus has been a topic of interest in clinical practice. Microwaves ranging from 300 to 3000 MHz can increase the risk of miscarriage by 1.28–1.59 times [11]. However, the electromagnetic wave of the capsule endoscope is low at 430 MHz, and the capsule endo-

Table 1 Clinical indications of small intestine capsule endoscopy by different age groups [8]

Indication	Adult patients	Pediatric patients	Age <8 years
OGIB + IDA	66	15	36
CD/UC/IC	10	63	24
Abdominal pain	11	10	14
Polyps/ Neoplasms	3	8	–
Other	10	4	25

CD Crohn's disease, *IDA* Iron deficiency anemia, *OGIB* Obscure gastrointestinal bleeding, *IC* Indeterminate colitis, *UC* Ulcerative colitis

scope has not been reported to have a harmful effect in any case. Considering that there has been no reported case of a cell phone with a high electromagnetic field, it is unlikely that capsule endoscopy would have a negative effect on the fetus.

There is no evidence that capsule endoscopy increases any risk in pregnant women based on previous clinical experience. Capsule endoscopy can be safely performed in pregnant women when clinically required. However, it is desirable to perform capsule endoscopy after childbirth if possible because of lack of sufficient data.

Capsule Endoscopy in Patients with Structural Changes in the Gastrointestinal Tract

Structural changes in the gastrointestinal tract due to surgery or other reasons may affect capsule endoscopy. In the case of gastric bypass or gastrectomy, for example, Roux-en-Y or Billroth II surgery, retention of the capsule endoscope in the gastrointestinal tract can occur. The capsule may not be able to enter the small intestine, or it may have delayed transit in the small intestine [12, 13]. After Billroth II surgery, the time for the capsule to pass the stomach can be delayed. When the inner diameter of the anastomosis is small, the forward movement of the capsule can be prohibited. If the efferent loop and the afferent loop are arranged in the opposite direction, the capsule can be retained in the stomach for a long time. When the capsule is retained for more than one hour in the stomach as assessed based on the real-time transmission image, the occurrence of intragastric retention or incomplete small bowel transit is highly possible. Therefore, it would be better to place the capsule directly into the efferent loop by upper gastrointestinal endoscopy.

The new version of the small bowel capsule has a longer battery life and can work for more than 11 h. The delayed capsule transit owing to an altered structure is now made feasible by the expanded battery life of the new capsule. However, in the case where gastric retention of the capsule endoscope is prolonged, it is helpful to directly place the capsule into the small intestine as aforementioned.

Cicatricial contraction, diverticulum formation, and radiation enteritis are the conditions other than surgery that can cause structural change in the gastrointestinal tract. If the patient has a history of a diverticulum in the small intestine, the retention of the capsule due to the diverticulum should be considered. Zenker diverticulum in the esophagus or epiphrenic diverticulum can also cause retention of the capsule.

Capsule Endoscopy in Patients with Gastrointestinal Motility Disease

Gastrointestinal motility disorders are not an indication for small bowel capsule endoscopy, because they may cause capsule retention in the small bowel and incomplete examination due to delayed transit time. Small bowel capsules now have a longer battery operating time, which reduces the risk of incomplete examination. However, if the patient has a history of gastric evacuation disorders, such as diabetes, or if the capsule is retained in the stomach for more than 60 min after the real-time transmission image, pushing the capsule endoscope directly into the duodenum by using upper gastrointestinal endoscopy is a solution. It is not recommended to directly place the capsule into the duodenum in all patients based on patient's symptom questionnaire because it does not affect the overall result of the examination.

Capsule Endoscopy in Patients with Swallowing Disorders

Aspiration during capsule endoscopy rarely occurs (about 0.1% of cases). Swallowing disorders are the main cause of aspiration [14]. Therefore, dysphagia could be a contraindication to capsule endoscopy. However, swallowing difficulty of the capsule endoscope does not directly mean the presence of dysphagia or swallowing disorder. Swallowing 11–13 mm diameter capsules is not always easy even in patients without dysphagia. In pediatric patients aged 8 years or younger, it is common for them to express anxiety and difficulty with swallowing the capsule, and 1.1–1.5% of adults have difficulty with swallowing the capsule endoscope for the examination [10]. There have been 37 articles about swallowing difficulty in capsule endoscopy from inception until September 2016 [14]. Overall, 94.6% of the patients with aspiration were men aged 79 years on average, and 87.1% had severe comorbidities. The aspirated capsules caused symptoms, such as coughing and dyspnea, in 59.5% of patients, and the capsule was found in the right main bronchus in most cases. There were cases in which spontaneous coughing released the aspirated capsules, but the capsules were removed using a bronchoscope in more than half of the cases.

Therefore, when patients have difficulties with swallowing the capsule endoscope voluntarily, upper gastrointestinal endoscopy can be used to deliver the capsule into the stomach or duodenum directly. To divert the capsule with the endoscope, the capsule is fixed to the fore-end of the endoscope using a mesh or snare and it obscures visibility. In adults, the capsule endoscope can also be pushed into the esophagus using an overtube. The delivery device called AdvanCE (US Endoscopy, Mentor, OH) was developed for capsule endoscopy [15].

Capsule Endoscopy in Patients with Implantable Cardiac Devices

The images captured by the capsule endoscope are mostly transmitted to the external receiver through wireless transmission. The wireless transmission methods use radiofrequency (Pillcam, Medtronic plc, Dublin, Ireland; EndoCapsule, Olympus Medical Systems Corp., Tokyo, Japan; OMOM capsule, Jinshan Science and Technology Co., Ltd., Chongqing, China) or human body conduction (MiRoCam, IntroMedic Co., Ltd., Seoul, South Korea). Accordingly, the concern that the wireless transmission system of the capsule endoscope may affect the functions of electronic devices, such as a pacemaker, defibrillator device, and left ventricular assist device, that are inserted into the human body has been raised.

The radiotransmission of the capsule endoscope uses a 430-MHz band, which is similar to the frequency of a mobile phone (450 MHz). About 22.4–30.7% of electromagnetic interference occurs between a mobile phone and an artificial pacemaker. However, there has been no reported functional abnormality in artificial pacemakers caused by mobile phones. Furthermore, the output of the capsule endoscope is only one of dozens in comparison with that of the cellular phone. Ex vivo experiments mimicking the physiological environment in the human body failed to demonstrate any interference due to electrical interactions between the capsule endoscope and implantable pacemakers and defibrillators [16].

In a study of MiRoCam capsule endoscopy using the human body conduction method, the implantable pacemaker and defibrillator did not interfere with the image signals or affect the operation of the heart device [17].

Capsule endoscopy manufacturers and the US Food and Drug Administration advise physicians not to perform capsule endoscopy in patients with cardiac devices. The American Society of Gastrointestinal Endoscopy guidelines considers cardiac devices as a contraindication to capsule endoscopy [18]. However, guidelines of the European Society of Gastrointestinal Endoscopy state that capsule endoscopy is not contraindicated in patients with cardiac devices, such as pacemakers and defibrillators [9], Cardiac device manufacturers Biotronik and the Medtronic Cardiovascular Group also allow for the use of capsule endoscopy in patients with internal electronic equipment [19, 20]. Based on the available technical data about the maximum effective radiated power or output current and transmitter frequency, the maximum electromagnetic radiation within a 5-mm proximity can be calculated for capsule endoscopes by Medtronic plc, Olympus Medical Systems Corp., and Jinshan Science and Technology Co., Ltd. Likewise, the maximum interference voltage at the input of cardiac devices can be calculated for the capsule endoscope by IntroMedic Co., Ltd. The calculated values were sufficiently low below the safety objectives set by the international product standard for cardiac devices (ISO 14117) by a factor of 8–85 [21]. Data to date prove only negligible interference between the capsule endoscope and the implantable cardiac devices, and there has been no evidence to support a clinically relevant risk of the capsule endoscope on the implantable cardiac devices [21]. Contrarily, the wireless cardiac monitoring device may obstruct the images from the capsule endoscope, and it is preferable to use a wired monitoring device during capsule endoscopy.

Conclusion

Capsule endoscopy is a noninvasive procedure that can be safely performed in children, adults, and elderly patients. However, it is necessary to use the appropriate supplementary approach in consideration of the patient's voluntary swallowing and controlling ability, gastric evacuation and gastrointestinal transit time, and structural change of the gastrointestinal tract. The effect of capsule endoscopy on pregnancy remains unclear, but there is no evidence of harm. Regarding the electromagnetic interference between implantable cardiac devices, especially pacemakers or defibrillators, and the capsule endoscope, the magnitude of interference is sufficiently small and safely negligible. However, it is preferable to use a wired monitoring device because interference with the capsule endoscope image transmission may be expected when using a wireless monitoring device.

References

1. Swaminath A, Legnani P, Kornbluth A. Video capsule endoscopy in inflammatory bowel disease: past, present, and future redux. Inflamm Bowel Dis. 2010;16:1254–62.
2. Nuutinen H, Kolho KL, Salminen P, et al. Capsule endoscopy in pediatric patients: technique and results in our first 100 consecutive children. Scand J Gastroenterol. 2011;46:1138–43.
3. Oikawa-Kawamoto M, Sogo T, Yamaguchi T, et al. Safety and utility of capsule endoscopy for infants and young children. World J Gastroenterol. 2013;19:8342–8.
4. Gralnek IM, Cohen SA, Ephrath H, et al. Small bowel capsule endoscopy impacts diagnosis and management of pediatric inflammatory bowel disease: a prospective study. Dig Dis Sci. 2012;57:465–71.
5. Cohen SA, Ephrath H, Lewis JD, et al. Pediatric capsule endoscopy: review of the small bowel and patency capsules. J Pediatr Gastroenterol Nutr. 2012;54:409–13.
6. Cohen SA, Klevens AI. Use of capsule endoscopy in diagnosis and management of pediatric patients, based on meta-analysis. Clin Gastroenterol Hepatol. 2011;9:490–6.
7. Atay O, Mahajan L, Kay M, Mohr F, Kaplan B, Wyllie R. Risk of capsule endoscope retention in pediatric patients: a large single-center experience and review of the literature. J Pediatr Gastroenterol Nutr. 2009;49:196–201.
8. Oliva S, Cohen SA, Di Nardo G, Gualdi G, Cucchiara S, Casciani E. Capsule endoscopy in pediatrics: a 10-years journey. World J Gastroenterol. 2014;20:16603–8.
9. Ladas SD, Triantafyllou K, Spada C, et al. European Society of Gastrointestinal Endoscopy (ESGE): recommendations (2009) on clinical use of video capsule endoscopy to investigate small-bowel, esophageal and colonic diseases. Endoscopy. 2010;42:220–7.
10. Rondonotti E, Herrerias JM, Pennazio M, Caunedo A, Mascarenhas-Saraiva M, de Franchis R. Complications, limitations, and failures of capsule endoscopy: a review of 733 cases. Gastrointest Endosc. 2005;62:712–6. quiz 752, 754
11. Ouellet-Hellstrom R, Stewart WF. Miscarriages among female physical therapists who report using radio- and microwave-frequency electromagnetic radiation. Am J Epidemiol. 1993;138:775–86.
12. Parikh DA, Mittal M, Mann SK. Incomplete capsule endoscopy examinations after Roux-en-Y gastric bypass. Clin J Gastroenterol. 2011;4:347–50.
13. Spera G, Spada C, Riccioni ME, Perri V, Costamagna G. Video capsule endoscopy in a patient with a Billroth II gastrectomy and obscure bleeding. Endoscopy. 2004;36:931.
14. Yung DE, Plevris JN, Koulaouzidis A. Short article: Aspiration of capsule endoscopes: a comprehensive review of the existing literature. Eur J Gastroenterol Hepatol. 2017;29:428–34.
15. Holden JP, Dureja P, Pfau PR, et al. Endoscopic placement of the small-bowel video capsule by using a capsule endoscope delivery device. Gastrointest Endosc. 2007;65:842–7.
16. Nasseri-Moghaddam S, Mofid A, Nouraie M, et al. The normal range of duodenal intraepithelial lymphocytes. Arch Iran Med. 2008;11:136–42.

17. Chung JW, Hwang HJ, Chung MJ, Park JY, Pak HN, Song SY. Safety of capsule endoscopy using human body communication in patients with cardiac devices. Dig Dis Sci. 2012;57:1719–23.
18. Wang A, Banerjee S, Barth BA, et al. Wireless capsule endoscopy. Gastrointest Endosc. 2013;78:805–15.
19. Medtronic. Medizinische Verfahren und EMI-Vorsichtsmaßnahmen für implantierbare Kardioverter-Defibrillatoren und Defibrillatoren zur kardialen Resynchronisationstherapie, Handbuch für medizinisches Fachpersonal 2014. Available from: http://www.medtronicheart.com/wcm/groups/mdt-com_sg/@emanuals/@era/@crdm/documents/documents/contrib_193764.pdf.
20. Biotronik. Elektromagnetische Verträglichkeit von Herzschrittmachern, ICDs und CRT-Implantaten von BIOTRONIK. 2015 Available from: https://www.biotronik.com/files/75891733AA975C3AC1257F16 003351D8/$FILE/Stoerbeeinflussungen_Implantate_BIOTRONIK.pdf.
21. Bandorski D, Kurniawan N, Baltes P, et al. Contraindications for video capsule endoscopy. World J Gastroenterol. 2016;22:9898–908.

Complications

Hyun Seok Lee

Key Points
- Asymptomatic capsule retention could first be conservatively observed.
- Device-assisted enteroscopy is considered the first-choice method for capsule retrieval. If needed, surgical treatment can be indicated.
- The medical history of a patient should be assessed before capsule endoscopy to minimize the risk of capsule retention.
- Patency capsule examination should be applied in patients at an increased risk of capsule retention.

Capsule endoscopy is usually a safe procedure. However, capsule retention is a complication that should be cautiously considered. Capsule retention is defined as the retention of the capsule in the gastrointestinal tract for at least 2 weeks. Hence, the patency capsule, which could check for small bowel stricture before capsule endoscopy examination, has been developed.

H. S. Lee (✉)
Division of Gastroenterology, Department of Internal Medicine, School of Medicine, Kyungpook National University, Kyungpook National University Hospital, Daegu, South Korea

Capsule Retention

It has been well known that certain underlying conditions predispose patients to capsule retention. A recently published meta-analysis found that the capsule retention rate was 2.1% in patients with suspected small bowel bleeding and 2.2% in those with abdominal pain or diarrhea. The capsule retention rate in patients with suspected inflammatory bowel disease was reported to be 3.6%, whereas that in patients with established inflammatory bowel disease was 8.2% [1].

Capsule retention is usually asymptomatic. The capsule can be retained in the small bowel without symptoms for several months, and capsule retention can be naturally resolved during subsequent follow-up [2]. In a recent study, only 2 of 104 cases (1.9%) of capsule retention progressed to symptomatic bowel obstruction [1, 2]. Therefore, if a malignant disease is not strongly suspected, conservative observation could be an adequate therapeutic option for the management of capsule retention in most cases. During this period, targeted treatment with medications, including corticosteroids, may promote capsule excretion in up to 20–30% of patients with capsule retention [3].

When capsule retrieval is required, both device-assisted enteroscopy and surgery can be performed. Device-assisted enteroscopy could be the first-choice method. In the past, surgery was used in many cases. The increasing availability of device-assisted enteroscopy has reduced the need for surgical intervention. If surgical treatment is required or device-assisted enteroscopy is unsuccessful, capsule retrieval by surgery is indicated. Particularly, surgical intervention is primarily indicated in all cases in which the presence of neoplastic disease is suspected [4].

Patency Capsule

As mentioned above, the overall capsule retention rate is low and associated with the clinical indication. Thus, routine measures to prevent capsule retention are not necessary for every patient undergoing capsule endoscopy. However, the presence of a combination of symptoms including abdominal pain, abdominal distension, and nausea or vomiting before capsule endoscopy has been found to be related to a significantly higher rate of capsule retention. Moreover, previous small bowel resection, abdominal or pelvic radiation therapy, and chronic use of high-dose nonsteroidal anti-inflammatory drugs have all been reported to increase the risk of capsule retention [5, 6]. Thus, before capsule endoscopy examination, it is important to carefully assess the medical history of a patient to identify the requirement for a preliminary workup for preventing capsule retention [4].

In this setting, small bowel follow through is unreliable, whereas patency capsule and small bowel cross-sectional imaging techniques have both been shown to be effective [7]. A recent meta-analysis on the accuracy of patency capsule examination found that the sensitivity was 97% (95% confidence interval [CI] 93–99%) and the specificity was 83% (95% CI 65–94%) [8]. However, studies comparing patency capsule testing and small bowel cross-sectional imaging techniques are limited, and the results have been conflicting. A previous study showed that patency capsule testing and small bowel cross-sectional imaging techniques were similarly effective [9], whereas another study reported that the retention rate was significantly lower (0.7%) in high-risk patients with negative patency capsule results

than in those with negative results from prior small bowel cross-sectional imaging (8.3%) [10]. Patency capsule testing is less likely to expose the patient to ionizing radiation and has a high negative predictive value. However, in some cases, bowel obstruction occurred after patency capsule ingestion [4].

Summary

It is important to obtain the complete medical history (e.g., previous abdominal surgery, current medications, and symptoms of bowel obstruction) of a patient before the application of capsule endoscopy. Patency capsule examination should be applied to patients at an increased risk of capsule retention, not to all patients, before capsule endoscopy.

Asymptomatic capsule retention could be conservatively observed. If capsule retrieval is needed, device-assisted enteroscopy can be considered the first-choice method. However, when surgical treatment is required, or device-assisted enteroscopy is unavailable or has failed, capsule retrieval by surgery can be indicated. Surgical intervention could enable both capsule retrieval and treatment of the underlying disease.

References

1. Rezapour M, Amadi C, Gerson LB. Retention associated with video capsule endoscopy: systematic review and meta-analysis. Gastrointest Endosc. 2017;85:1157–1168.e1152.
2. Fernandez-Urien I, Carretero C, Gonzalez B, et al. Incidence, clinical outcomes, and therapeutic approaches of capsule endoscopy-related adverse events in a large study population. Rev Esp Enferm Dig. 2015;107:745–52.
3. Vanfleteren L, van der Schaar P, Goedhard J. Ileus related to wireless capsule retention in suspected Crohn's disease: emergency surgery obviated by early pharmacological treatment. Endoscopy. 2009;41(Suppl 2):E134–5.
4. Rondonotti E, Spada C, Adler S, et al. Small-bowel capsule endoscopy and device-assisted enteroscopy for diagnosis and treatment of small-bowel disorders: European Society of Gastrointestinal

Endoscopy (ESGE) technical review. Endoscopy. 2018;50:423–46.

5. Hoog CM, Bark LA, Arkani J, Gorsetman J, Brostrom O, Sjoqvist U. Capsule retentions and incomplete capsule endoscopy examinations: an analysis of 2300 examinations. Gastroenterol Res Pract. 2012;2012:518718.

6. Al-Bawardy B, Locke G, Huprich JE, et al. Retained capsule endoscopy in a large tertiary care academic practice and radiologic predictors of retention. Inflamm Bowel Dis. 2015;21:2158–64.

7. Spada C, Spera G, Riccioni M, et al. A novel diagnostic tool for detecting functional patency of the small bowel: the Given patency capsule. Endoscopy. 2005;37:793–800.

8. Zhang W, Han ZL, Cheng Y, et al. Value of the patency capsule in pre-evaluation for capsule endoscopy in cases of intestinal obstruction. J Dig Dis. 2014;15:345–51.

9. Yadav A, Heigh RI, Hara AK, et al. Performance of the patency capsule compared with nonenteroclysis radiologic examinations in patients with known or suspected intestinal strictures. Gastrointest Endosc. 2011;74:834–9.

10. Rondonotti E, Soncini M, Girelli CM, Russo A, de Franchis R. Short article: Negative small-bowel cross-sectional imaging does not exclude capsule retention in high-risk patients. Eur J Gastroenterol Hepatol. 2016;28:871–5.

History of Small-Intestinal Enteroscopy

Moon Sung Lee

Scientific advances in modern society have encouraged significant progress in the field of medicine. In particular, the internal structure of the human body had long been a gray area until the discovery of X-ray (i.e., roentgen examinations), which have enabled doctors to diagnose and understand diseases to a much greater extent than before. Nevertheless, the desire to realistically visualize the inside of the human body, not only with radiographic shadows, grew stronger, leading to the development of endoscopy.

With the recent development of glass fibers, endoscopy has highly evolved and has been used in various fields. For example, endoscopy can be used to observe not only the digestive tract but also the peritoneal cavity, joints, nose, ears, urinary tract, and even blood vessels.

Likewise, endoscopy has been playing a crucial role in medicine, especially in the area of digestive diseases. However, there are a number of difficulties in evaluating the full length of the small intestine with endoscopy. The small intestine is a long organ up to 6 m; is located far from both the mouth and the anus, which are the entry points of the endoscope; is supported only by the mesentery, making the organ freely floating; and forms many complex and curvy loops, which, in addition to the extensive peristalsis, complicate endoscope insertion.

Over the past several decades, several attempts were made to obtain a closer view of the small intestine with an endoscope. In the early 1970s, Hiratsuka et al. [1] introduced the first successful total enteroscopy procedure, called the ropeway method. The patients swallowed a weight attached to the distal end of a long guide string, and the weight was excreted 2–5 days later through the patients' own peristalsis. Thereafter, the guide string was replaced with a slightly stiffer Teflon tube. The endoscopes were then inserted both antegradely (through the oral route) and retrogradely (through the anal route), and the entire small intestine was observed. At around the same time, Tada et al. [2] introduced a method called the sonde-type method. A long thin endoscope with an inflatable balloon at its distal tip was inserted through the nose, passed through esophagus, and placed in the duodenum. Thereafter, the endoscope reached the colon via intestinal peristalsis with the help of its own weight and that of the balloon. Endoscopic examination was carried out upon the withdrawal of the endoscope; that is, the entire small intestine was examined while the endoscope was on its way out. However, both the ropeway and sonde methods have multiple drawbacks: they require extensive preparation time, cause discomfort during endoscopic insertion, and cause pain when the inserted small intestine becomes tight. Additionally, it is difficult to reinsert the

M. S. Lee (✉)
Department of Internal Medicine, Soonchunhyang University College of Medicine,
Bucheon, South Korea

endoscope to and from to confirm the lesion of interest. Further, the methods which require extremely skilled hands and the high durability of the devices restricted their widespread use. In the late 1990s, these small bowel enteroscopic procedures were partially implemented by Lee et al. [3] in Korea.

Radiologic examinations had been the primary tool for the diagnosis of small bowel disease until the development of capsule endoscopy and double-balloon enteroscopy (DBE) in the 2000s. On radiologic examination, when the lesion is located in a proximal area not far from the lower part of ligament of Treitz, antegrade push enteroscopy with a long pediatric colonoscope or a small intestine enteroscope is used to confirm the lesion. Thereafter, biopsy specimens are obtained or therapeutic enteroscopy is performed. When the lesion is located in a distal area, only a small part of the small intestine is observed through colonoscopy. Additionally, another method that has been attempted is intraoperative enteroscopy, in which an endoscope is inserted to observe the entire intestine during an open operation.

Hence, the development of capsule endoscopy and DBE in the 2000s had brought profound progress in small bowel enteroscopy. Capsule endoscopes were first developed by Given Imaging in Israel. The capsule, which can be swallowed, is 11 mm in diameter and 26 mm long with a camera at its tip. As the capsule passes through the gastrointestinal tract, its camera takes two photographs per second (i.e., >50,000 images in about 8 h). These images are wirelessly transmitted and collected in an external data receiving device and analyzed for diagnosis. After its first clinical implementation by Appleyard et al. [4] in 2000, the European and US Food and Drug Administration subsequently approved capsule endoscopy and the method has gained widespread acceptance since then. In particular, capsule endoscopy is a convenient and noninvasive examination, unlike the ropeway and sonde-type methods. Patients do not feel pain and are able to continue their daily life routines after capsule intake. Moreover, capsule endoscopy allows complete small intestine enteroscopy, the

main barrier that could not be previously overcome with push enteroscopy. Owing to its effectiveness and accessibility, capsule endoscopy has now become one of the most established small-intestinal diagnostic methods to date. Since 2002, when capsule endoscopy was initially introduced in Korea, the method has been widely used in many institutions. Multicenter clinical studies have been actively conducted through the Gastrointestinal Imaging Research Association (now called Capsule Endoscopy Research Group) established in 2003. Recently, efforts to improve capsule endoscopy, including the operation time, size of the capsule, resolution of the collected images, and readability of the results, have led to the invention of various types of capsule endoscopes, such as MiroCam in Korea in 2007 and EndoCapsule manufactured by Olympus in Japan. Nevertheless, one of the main disadvantages of capsule endoscopy is its inability to obtain biopsy specimens or perform further therapeutic maneuvers. Hence, many trials are ongoing to overcome this drawback.

The development of capsule endoscopy has prompted the introduction of many accessory devices that facilitate endoscope insertion into the small intestine. The most representative method among these device-assisted enteroscopy techniques is DBE, which was first introduced by Yamamoto et al. [5] in 2001. DBE involves the use of an endoscope and a flexible overtube, both with inflatable balloons attached at their distal ends. While alternately inflating and deflating each balloon, the two balloons grasp and pleat the small intestine over the endoscope like an accordion, thus simplifying endoscope insertion. This method can be applied with either an antegrade or a retrograde approach, or both. When attempted through both approaches, complete enteroscopy can be achieved in 40–70% of patients. The DBE device was marketed by Fujinon in 2003 for the first time and has been used in Korea since 2003. DBE facilitates not only the examination of the entire small intestine but also biopsies and therapeutic maneuvers such as hemostasis, polypectomy, stricture dilation, and foreign body removal. Moreover, DBE is widely applied in cases in which colonoscopy and endoscopic retrograde cholangiopancreatography cannot be performed owing to postoperative anatomical abnormalities, such as in patients with a history of obesity surgery or Roux-en-Y hepaticojejunostomy.

With the successful implementation of DBE, more studies for improving endoscope insertion have been actively conducted. Single-balloon enteroscopy (SBE) [6] was introduced by Olympus in 2007, in which a single balloon is attached on the endoscope. This method allows bending of the endoscope to eliminate bowel slippage. SBE is easier to perform and accelerates the preparation and procedure times. However, there are some reports that SBE has limited ability to deeply insert the endoscope in contrast to DBE, resulting in decreased completion rate of the examination of the entire small intestine. In addition, a spiral enteroscopy device was manufactured by Spiral Medical in 2008. It adopts an overtube with a spiral-like bump on the outer wall instead of a balloon [7]. The overtube turns clockwise like a screw and advances into the small intestine. Spiral enteroscopy is also simple to perform and requires a short procedure time; however, it carries the disadvantage of insufficient insertion depth compared with that of DBE. Recently, a technique with automatic spinning of the spiral overtube is also being developed to simplify the enteroscopy procedure [8].

Moreover, a method of using a balloon catheter instead of an overtube that could readily work as in DBE has also been developed [9]. In recent years, NaviAid balloon-guided enteroscopy [10] was developed by Smart Medical System, in which an add-on balloon catheter is employed through the channel of the endoscope during enteroscopy.

Conclusion

Capsule endoscopy and device-assisted enteroscopy, which were developed in the early 2000s, have revolutionized the research of small bowel diseases. Capsule endoscopy provides a more comprehensive and safer method to observe the entire small intestine; however, the false-negative rate is high and simultaneous biopsy and therapeutic endoscopy is not possible. Conversely, device-assisted enteroscopy allows biopsy and therapeutic endoscopy but it is still relatively invasive and has an unsatisfactory completion rate of the evaluation of the entire small intestine. Further studies are expected in the future to develop safer and more advanced enteroscopy procedures.

References

1. Hiratsuka H, Hasegawa M, Ushiromachi K, Endo T, Suzuki S, Nishikawa F. Endoscopic diagnosis in the small intestine. Stomach Intestine. 1972;7:1679–968.
2. Tada M, Akasaka Y, Misaki F, Kawai K. Clinical evaluation of a sone-type small intestinal fiberscope. Endoscopy. 1977;9:33–8.
3. Lee EH, Kim JH, Kim DH, et al Usefulness of small bowel enteroscopy. Korean J Med 2002;1(\):93(Abstr)
4. Appleyard M, Fireman Z, Glukhovsky A, et al. A randomized trial comparing wireless video capsule endoscopy with push enteroscopy for the detection of small-bowel lesions. Gastroenterology. 2000;119:1431–8.
5. Yamamoto H, Sekine Y, Sato Y, et al. Total enteroscopy with a nonsurgical steerable double-balloon method. Gastrointest Endosc. 2001;53:216–20.
6. Tsujikawa T, Saitoh Y, Andoh A, et al. Novel single-balloon enteroscopy for diagnosis and treatment of the small intestine: preliminary experiences. Endoscopy. 2008;40:11–5.
7. Akermann PA, Agrawal D, Cantero D, Pangtay J. Spiral enteroscopy with the new DSB overtube: a novel technique for deep peroral small-bowel intubation. Endoscopy. 2008;40:974–8.
8. Neuhaus H, Beyna T, Schneider M, Deviere J. Motorized spiral enteroscopy: first clinical case. Gastrointestinal Endoscopy. 2016;83(Suppl):637(Abstr).
9. Adler SN, Bjarnason I, Metzger YC. New balloon-guided technique for deep small-intestine endoscopy using standard endoscopes. Endoscopy. 2008;40:502–5.
10. Kumbhari V, Storm AC, Khashab MA, et al. Deep enteroscopy with standard endoscopes using a novel through-the-scope balloon. Endoscopy. 2014;6:685–9.

Types of Enteroscopy

Namyeong Baek and Dong Kyung Chang

Key Points
- Enteroscopy can be used to diagnose and treat small intestinal lesions while observing the small intestine in real time.
- *Types of enteroscopy*: Double balloon enteroscopy, single balloon enteroscopy, spiral enteroscopy, and balloon-guided endoscopy.
- *Enteroscopy commonly used in Korea*: Double balloon enteroscopy and single balloon enteroscopy.

Types of Enteroscopy

Double Balloon Enteroscopy

Double balloon enteroscopy was developed in the early 2000s, and two double balloon enteroscope models, EN-450 T5 and EN-450P5 (Fujinon Inc., Saitama, Japan), were introduced in Korea in 2004. Recently, two new models, EN-580 T and EN-580XP, have been developed

N. Baek · D. K. Chang (✉)
Division of Gastroenterology, Department of Internal Medicine, Sungkyunkwan University School of Medicine, Seoul, South Korea
e-mail: dkchang@skku.edu

(Table 1) [1]. Figure 1 shows the structure and components of double balloon enteroscopy. The double balloon enteroscopy procedure utilizes two latex balloons, one attached to the enteroscope and one attached to the end of the overtube. The inflated overtube balloon holds the small intestine in place and prevents the intestinal loop from being excessively stretched while the enteroscope is advanced deeper. The enteroscope balloon is then inflated to hold the small intestine as the overtube is advanced. A push-and-pull method is repeated as necessary to bring the enteroscope and overtube together, shortening the small intestine and further advancing the enteroscope (Fig. 2) [2].

In comparison with capsule endoscopy, double balloon enteroscopy has the advantage of enabling the endoscopist to observe lesions in real time, and perform biopsies and therapeutic intervention, if necessary. However, double balloon enteroscopy is highly labor intensive and requires a long procedure time, usually more than 1 h. Both antegrade and retrograde double balloon enteroscopic insertions are necessary to observe the entire small intestine.

Double balloon enteroscopy allows for deeper insertion and has a higher completion rate than single balloon enteroscopy or spiral enteroscopy. However, the higher completion rate of small intestine enteroscopy does not necessarily guarantee higher diagnostic and therapeutic yields. It has been reported that the diagnostic and therapeutic yields are similar in all three enteroscopy

© Springer Nature Singapore Pte Ltd. 2022
H. J. Chun et al. (eds.), *Small Intestine Disease*, https://doi.org/10.1007/978-981-16-7239-2_22

Table 1 Comparison of DBE and SBE Specifications [1]

	DBE (Fujinon)		SBE (Olympus)	
	EN–450T5	EN–450P5	EN–580T	SIF–Q260
Obervation range (mm)	3–100	5–100	2–100	5–100
Angle of view (degree)	140	120	140	140
Distal end diameter (mm)	9.4	8.5	9.4	9.2
Overtube diameter (mm)	9.3	8.5	9.3	9.2
Angulation range (degree) Up/down	180/180	180/180	180/180	180/180
Right/left	160/160	160/160	160/160	160/160
Channel diameter (mm)	2.8	2.2	3.2	2.8
Working length (mm)	2000	2000	2000	2000

DBE double balloon enteroscopy, *SBE* single balloon enteroscopy

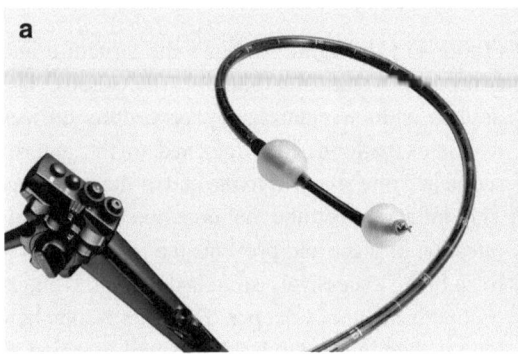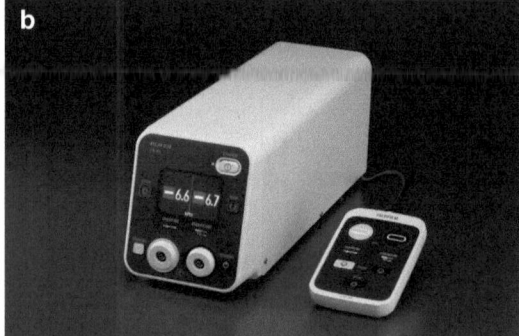

Fig. 1 The structure and components of double balloon enteroscopy. (**a**) Enteroscope with balloon and balloon-equipped overtube. (**b**) Balloon controller

methods [3–6]. The double balloon enteroscopy complication rate is about 1%, which is identical to that of single balloon enteroscopy and spiral enteroscopy (Table 2) [6].

Single Balloon Enteroscopy

Single balloon enteroscopy was developed in 2006 with the introduction of the SIF-Q260 Single Balloon Enteroscope (Olympus Optical Co, Tokyo, Japan). The single balloon enteroscope is equipped with a balloon at the distal part of overtube but not at the enteroscope (Fig. 3 and Table 1). The insertion principle is similar to double balloon enteroscopy, but the distal end of the enteroscope can be bent to hook and hold the intestine in place (Fig. 4) [1].

In contrast to double balloon enteroscopy, single balloon endoscopy has a lower completion rate, but requires less preparation time and has a simpler operation method. Recently, single balloon enteroscopy become widely used, because both the diagnostic yield and therapeutic yield are similar to those of double balloon enteroscopy (Table 2) [7, 8].

Spiral Enteroscopy

Spiral enteroscopy was developed in 2007 with the introduction of the Endo-Ease Discovery SB system (Spirus Medical, LLC, West Bridgewater, MA, USA). This device features a spiral structure at the tip of the overtube (Fig. 5). Turning the spiral overtube clockwise as the screw is tightened shortens the intestine and allows for easier advancement of the enteroscope (Fig. 6). Spiral enteroscopy has the advantage of a shorter procedure time than double balloon or single balloon

Fig. 2 Schematic insertion principle of double balloon enteroscopy. (**a** and **b**) The enteroscope is advanced to the small intestine, and the enteroscope balloon is inflated. (**c**) The overtube is advanced closer to the enteroscope balloon, and the overtube balloon is inflated. (**d** and **e**) The inflated overtube balloon holds the intestine in place, the balloon of the enteroscope is deflated, and the enteroscope is advanced. (**f**) Steps a through c are repeated. (**g**) The two inflated balloons stabilize the intestine, which is shortened by pulling the overtube and enteroscope backward simultaneously

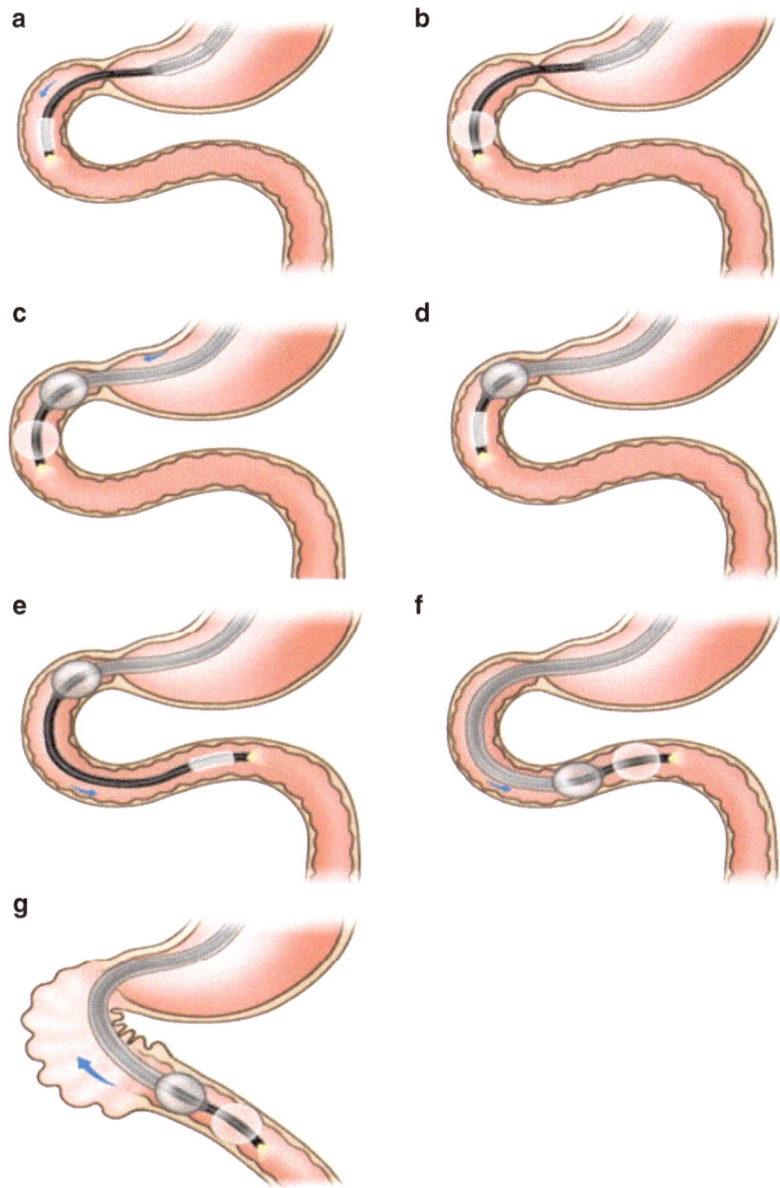

Table 2 Comparison of DBE and SBE clinical features [7, 8]

	DBE	SBE
Depth of insertion	Longer	Shorter
Procedure time	Longer	Shorter
Completion rate	Higher	Lower
Diagnostic yield	Comparable	Comparable
Therapeutic yield	Comparable	Comparable
Complication rate	Comparable	Comparable

DBE double balloon enteroscopy, *SBE* single balloon enteroscopy

enteroscopy, but the device cannot be inserted any deeper than the double balloon enteroscope. This method has not yet been introduced in Korea [4].

Balloon-Guided Endoscopy

Balloon-guided endoscopy was developed in 2008 with the introduction of the NaviAid AB device (SMART Medical Systems Ltd., Ra'anana,

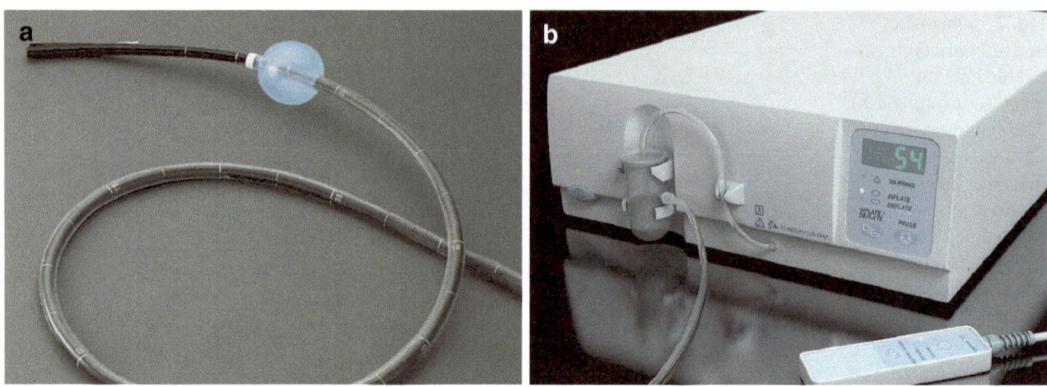

Fig. 3 The structure and components of single balloon enteroscopy. (**a**) Enteroscope with a balloon-equipped overtube. (**b**) Balloon controller

Fig. 4 Schematic insertion principle of single balloon enteroscopy. (**a**) The enteroscope and overtube are advanced into the small intestine, and after the overtube balloon is inflated, the enteroscope is advanced even further. (**b**) The tip of the enteroscope is bent to hold the position of the intestinal loop, and the overtube balloon is deflated. (**c** and **d**) The overtube is advanced to the tip of the enteroscope, and the balloon is reinflated. (**e**) The enteroscope and overtube are pulled backward, shortening the small intestine

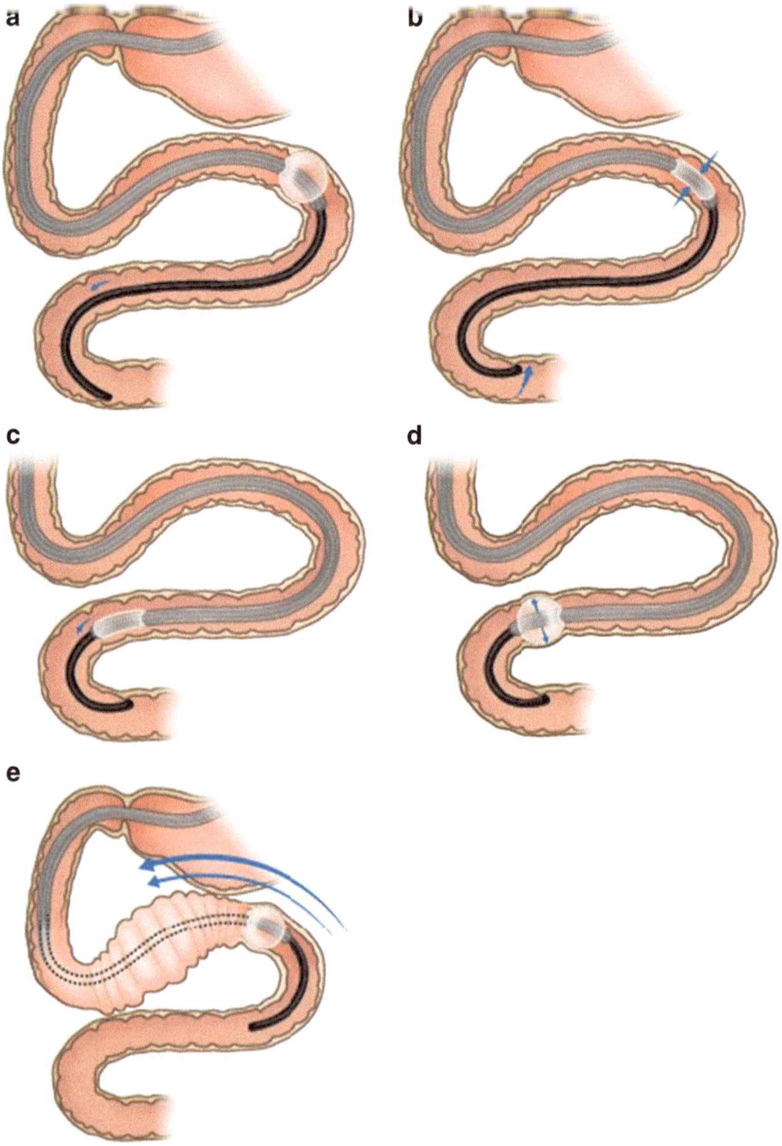

Fig. 5 Spiral enteroscopy

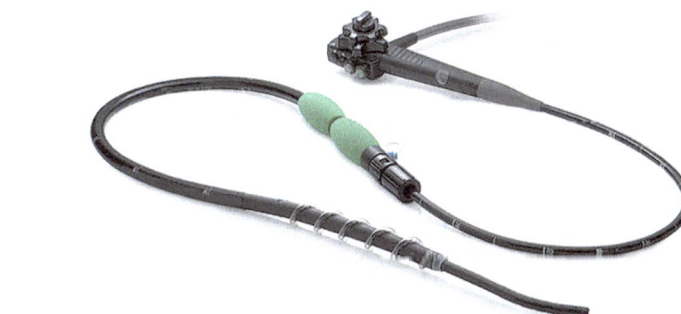

Fig. 6 Schematic insertion principle of spiral enteroscopy. (**a**) After the enteroscope and overtube are inserted in the duodenum, the spiral overtube is turned clockwise to insert it to the tip of the enteroscope. (**b**) When the enteroscope and the spiral overtube are simultaneously turned clockwise, the small intestine is shortened, and the enteroscope can advance

a   b

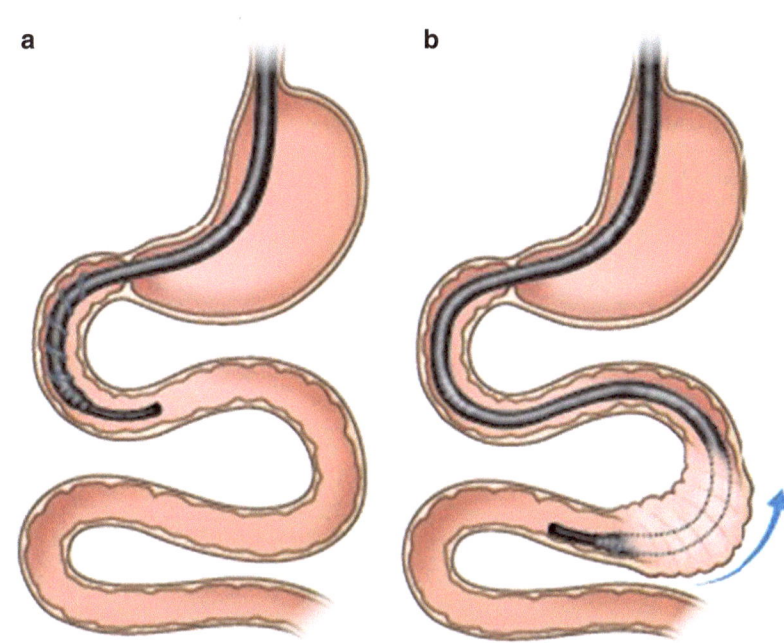

Israel). This method inserts an endoscope through the lower gastrointestinal tract into the small intestine, and a special catheter with a balloon attached is inserted through the endoscope's tool channel (Fig. 7). Once inserted, the catheter balloon is inflated to anchor the small intestine (Fig. 8). In other words, the principle of examination is similar to that of a double balloon enteroscopy. The advantage of this method is that once the endoscope is in place, the balloon catheter can be removed, allowing tools required for histopathologic examinations to be inserted [9]. However, it is difficult to advance the balloon-guided endoscope deeper than other enteroscopy devices, and this method has not yet been introduced in Korea.

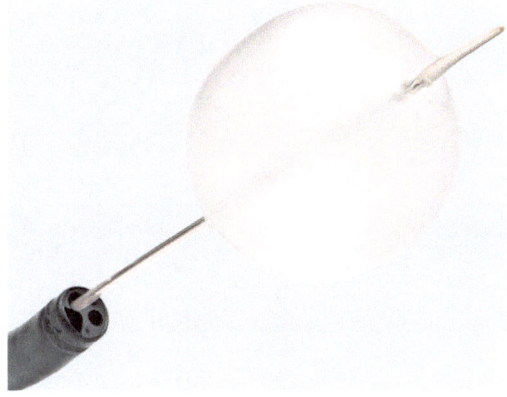

Fig. 7 Balloon-guided endoscopy device

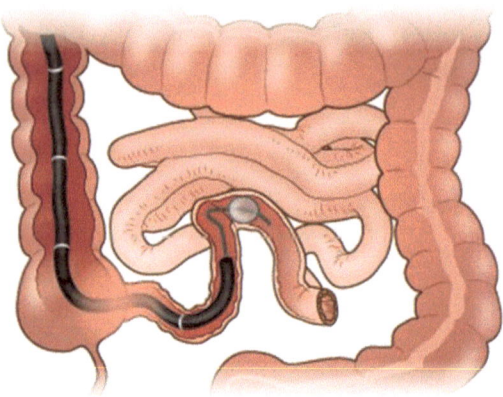

Fig. 8 Schematic insertion principle of balloon-guided endoscopy. After the endoscope is inserted into the small intestine, the balloon catheter is advanced as far as possible. The catheter balloon is expanded to anchor the intestine. The endoscope is pushed forward as the catheter is pulled backward to advance the endoscope. The push-and-pull step is repeated, as necessary

References

1. Kawamura T, Yasuda K, Tanaka K, et al. Clinical evaluation of a newly developed single-balloon enteroscope. Gastrointest Endosc. 2008;68:1112–6.
2. Yamamoto H, Kita H. Double-balloon endoscopy: from concept to reality. Gastrointest Endosc Clin N Am. 2006;16:347–61.
3. Takano N, Yamada A, Watabe H, et al. Single-balloon versus double-balloon endoscopy for achieving total enteroscopy: a randomized, controlled trial. Gastrointest Endosc. 2011;73:734–9.
4. May A, Manner H, Aschmoneit I, Ell C. Prospective, cross-over, single-center trial comparing oral double-balloon enteroscopy and oral spiral enteroscopy in patients with suspected small-bowel vascular malformations. Endoscopy. 2011;43:477–83.
5. Jeon SR, Kim JO. Deep enteroscopy: which technique will survive? Clin Endosc. 2013;46:480–5.
6. Rondonotti E, Spada C, Adler S, et al. Small-bowel capsule endoscopy and device-assisted enteroscopy for diagnosis and treatment of small-bowel disorders: European Society of Gastrointestinal Endoscopy (ESGE) technical review. Endoscopy. 2018;50:423–46.
7. May A, Nachbar L, Schneider M, Ell C. Prospective comparison of push enteroscopy and push-and-pull enteroscopy in patients with suspected small-bowel bleeding. Am J Gastroenterol. 2006;101:2016–24.
8. Kim TJ, Kim ER, Chang DK, Kim YH, Hong SN. Comparison of the efficacy and safety of single versus double-balloon Enteroscopy performed by endoscopist experts in single-balloon Enteroscopy: a single-center experience and meta-analysis. Gut Liver. 2017;11:520–7.
9. Pennazio M, Spada C, Eliakim R, et al. Small-bowel capsule endoscopy and device-assisted enteroscopy for diagnosis and treatment of small-bowel disorders: European Society of Gastrointestinal Endoscopy (ESGE) clinical guideline. Endoscopy. 2015;47:352–76.

Indications and Contraindications of Device-Assisted Enteroscopy

Hyun Joo Jang

Introduction

The device-assisted enteroscope can be inserted through an oral route or anal route and is used to observe the entire small intestine. It enables tissue biopsy and therapeutic endoscopic procedures. This chapter deals with the indications and contraindications of device-assisted enteroscopy.

Main Indications of Device-Assisted Enteroscopy (Table 1) [1]

Small Intestinal Bleeding or Suspected Small Intestinal Bleeding

Suspected small intestinal bleeding is the most important and common indication for device-assisted enteroscopy. Suspected small intestinal bleeding is defined as gastrointestinal bleeding from a source that cannot be identified on upper or lower gastrointestinal endoscopy. Suspected small intestinal bleeding accounts for approximately 50–70% of the cases indicated for device-assisted enteroscopy.

Crohn's Disease

Device-assisted enteroscopy can be performed for the purpose of endoscopic inspection, biopsy,

Table 1 Indications of device-assisted enteroscopy

Diagnostic indications
Suspected small intestinal bleeding
Abnormal findings on radiologic studies or capsule endoscopy
Suspected small intestinal tumors
Suspected small-bowel Crohn's disease
Suspected NSAID-induced small intestinal injury
Evaluation of refractory celiac disease
Detection of polyps in patients with polyposis syndromes such as familial adenomatous polyposis or Peutz-Jeghers syndrome
Examination of the gastric remnant in patients who have undergone roux-en-Y gastric bypass
Diagnostic endoscopic retrograde cholangiopancreatography (ERCP) in patients with roux-en-Y anatomy
Therapeutic indications
Hemostasis of small intestinal bleeding
Polypectomy or endoscopic mucosal resection of small bowel polyps or tumors
Balloon dilatation
Retrieval of foreign body
Stent insertion of small bowel obstruction
Placement of percutaneous endoscopic jejunostomy tube
Therapeutic procedures in roux-en-Y reconstructions

and therapeutic procedures in patients with suspected or established Crohn's disease. Suspected or established Crohn's disease account for 11–22% of enrolled patients in the studies evaluating the performance of double-balloon enteroscopy.

H. J. Jang (✉)
Hallym University of College of Medicine, Division of Gastroenterology, Hwaseong, Korea
e-mail: jhj1229@live.co.kr

© Springer Nature Singapore Pte Ltd. 2022
H. J. Chun et al. (eds.), *Small Intestine Disease*, https://doi.org/10.1007/978-981-16-7239-2_23

Small Intestinal Polyps or Tumor

Device-assisted enteroscopy can detect small intestinal polyps or tumors and facilitate tissue sampling, polypectomy, and tattooing for surgery.

Strictures or Inflammatory Lesions of Small Intestine

Device-assisted enteroscopy is helpful in histologic and endoscopic evaluation for patients with suspected small intestinal stenosis or inflammatory lesions of various causes. Balloon dilatation can be applied for short and fibrous stenosis of the small intestine.

Therapeutic Endoscopic Procedures

Device-assisted enteroscopy is available for most therapeutic endoscopic procedures (Table 1). If lesions requiring endoscopic therapy are found in capsule endoscopy, CT enterography, or MR enterography, device-assisted endoscopy can be performed.

Therapeutic procedures include various endoscopic hemostasis methods for bleeding lesions, dilation of strictures, snare polypectomy of polyps or small intestinal tumors, retrieval of retained capsules and removal of foreign bodies, and biopsy of abnormal tissue.

ERCP for the Patients with Surgically Altered Anatomy

Device-assisted enteroscopy enable ERCP for pancreatobiliary lesions in patients with surgically altered anatomy such as that occurring from Billroth II or Roux-en-Y surgery.

Difficult Colonoscopy

A successful colonoscopy can be performed using balloon-assisted endoscopy in patients with failed or difficult colonoscopy. In several recent studies, successful cecal intubation using DBE was achieved in 88–100% of patients with previously failed colonoscopy.

Diagnostic Yields of Device-Assisted Enteroscopy

Although the diagnostic yields of device-assisted enteroscopy vary depending on the indication, several studies report a 60–80% diagnostic yield in small intestine diseases by double-balloon enteroscopy and therapeutic yields of 70–73% [2–4].

In a large-scale study [5], the diagnostic yield for Peutz-Jeghers syndrome was 82%, obscure gastrointestinal bleeding was 53%, Crohn's disease was 47%, diarrhea was 19%, and abdominal pain was 19%. The application of device-assisted enteroscopy should be determined carefully considering the relative invasiveness and variable diagnostic yields depending on indications.

Contraindications of Device-Assisted Enteroscopy

The contraindications for DBE are the same as those of gastroscopy and colonoscopy. These are severe cardiovascular or respiratory dysfunction, fulminant colitis, acute perforation and peritonitis, and impending perforation. High-grade intestinal obstruction, high risk of perforation such as that in patients who have undergone recent intestinal surgery or chemotherapy for gastrointestinal lymphoma, or tendency for severe bleeding are considered relative contraindications for device-assisted enteroscopy due to the risk of complications [6]. Intraabdominal adhesions limit deep insertion in device-assisted enteroscopy, but they are not considered a contraindication.

Summary

Device-assisted enteroscopy has been developed and used for the diagnosis and treatment of small intestine diseases. They can be applied when various therapeutic endoscopic procedures are required or if small intestinal diseases are suspected because of the advantages of direct observation of small intestine lesion, facilitation of tissue sampling and various therapeutic procedures, and localization of the lesion for surgery.

References

1. Rondonotti E, Sunada K, Yano T, Paggi S, Yamamoto H. Double-balloon endoscopy in clinical practice: where are we now? Dig Endosc. 2012;24:209–19.
2. Hong SN, Kim ER, Ye BD, et al. Indications, diagnostic yield, and complication rate of balloon-assisted enteroscopy (BAE) during the first decade of its use in Korea. Dig Endosc. 2016;28(4):443–9.
3. May A, Nachbar L, Ell C. Double-balloon enteroscopy (push-and-pull enteroscopy) of the small bowel: feasibility and diagnostic and therapeutic yield in patients with suspected small bowel disease. Gastrointest Endosc. 2005;62:62–70.
4. Gross SA, Stark ME. Initial experience with double-balloon enteroscopy at a U.S. center. Gastrointest Endosc. 2008;67;890–7.
5. Moschler O, May A, Muller MK, Ell C, German DBESG. Complications in and performance of double-balloon enteroscopy (DBE): results from a large prospective DBE database in Germany. Endoscopy. 2011;43:484–9.
6. Gerson LB, Flodin JT, Miyabayashi K. Balloon-assisted enteroscopy: technology and troubleshooting. Gastrointest Endosc. 2008;68:1158–67.

Common Preparation for Device-Assisted Enteroscopy

Hong Jun Park

Key Points

- *Fasting and Bowel preparation*: Patients undergoing antegrade (peroral) device-assisted enteroscopy (DAE) are required to fast (8–12 h following a regular diet and 4–6 h following a liquid diet). Retrograde (peranal) DAE requires the administration of laxatives similar to the administration of such agents prior to colonoscopy. Recent guidelines established by ASGE recommend a split-dose bowel preparation regimen prior to colonoscopy for optimal bowel cleansing.
- *Sedation*: Moderate sedation using benzodiazepines, such as midazolam and opioid analgesics, such as pethidine is adequate for patients undergoing retrograde DAE; however, those undergoing antegrade DAE may need deep sedation to prevent nausea, vomiting, and/or epigastric pain. Deep sedation involves the administration of propofol along with a standard sedation regimen (midazolam + pethidine).
- *Usage of carbon dioxide*: Use of carbon dioxide is recommended for patients undergoing DAE.

H. J. Park (✉)
Department of Internal Medicine, Yonsei University
Wonju College of Medicine, Wonju, South Korea

Fasting and Bowel Preparation

Patients undergoing device-assisted enteroscopy (DAE) are required to fast, similar to those undergoing upper gastrointestinal endoscopy. Patients undergoing antegrade DAE are required to fast for 8–12 h following a regular diet and for 4–6 h following a liquid diet. Poor bowel preparation interferes with endoscope insertion, particularly at the ileocecal valve. Therefore, patients are administered laxatives similar to the administration of such agents in those undergoing colonoscopy. Usually, bowel preparation is recommended only for retrograde DAE. However, patients receiving oral iron supplements or those with a history of Roux-en-Y reconstruction need to be administered laxatives prior to antegrade DAE because they are more likely to show food retention in the small intestine. Patients should be instructed to consume a low-residue diet, or dietary restrictions should be advised. Additionally, a split regimen similar to that used in patients undergoing colonoscopy is recommended (Table 1).

Sedation

The following factors necessitate sedation in patients undergoing DAE: (1) DAE requires a relatively long procedure time. (2) DAE can cause abdominal pain secondary to air insufflation into the small bowel and repeated insertion

© Springer Nature Singapore Pte Ltd. 2022
H. J. Chun et al. (eds.), *Small Intestine Disease*, https://doi.org/10.1007/978-981-16-7239-2_24

Table 1 Preparation and sedation based on the route of scope insertion for device-assisted enteroscopy

	Preparation	Sedation level	Sedative
Antegrade DAE	Fasting is adequate: 8–12 h fast (regular diet) 4–6 h fast (liquid diet)	Deep sedation	Midazolam+opioid analgesic+propofol
Retrograde DAE	Administration of a bowel preparation regimen similar to that used for colonoscopy	Moderate sedation	Midazolam+opioid analgesic+propofol

DAE device-assisted enteroscopy

and withdrawal of the endoscope. To date, there is a lack of research to definitively establish the optimal sedatives to perform successful DAE or to determine the depth of scope insertion. Therefore, no standardized sedative regimen is available for DAE. Nevertheless, moderate sedation using benzodiazepines, such as midazolam and opioid analgesics, such as pethidine is suitable for anal intubation. Patients undergoing antegrade DAE require deep sedation to avoid nausea, vomiting, and/or abdominal pain. Deep sedation usually requires the administration of propofol along with a standard sedation regimen. Compared with monitored anesthesia care (MAC) administered by an anesthesiologist, endoscopist-directed, nurse-administered sedation is safer. However, sedation levels and sedatives depend upon patient-associated factors, including general condition, comorbidities, and procedure time. MAC is preferred in high-risk patients or in those who require deep sedation.

Usage of Carbon Dioxide Insufflator

DAE usually requires >1 h. The procedure involves intra-abdominal insufflation of a large quantity of air, which causes dilatation of the small intestine and invariably causes pain. Carbon dioxide (CO_2) is absorbed faster than other gases, which reduces the patient's discomfort during and after the examination. A meta-analysis that included four randomized trials reported that use of CO_2 during DAE was associated with lesser abdominal discomfort and a lower quantity of sedatives. Moreover, the safety levels did not significantly differ, and the oral insertion depth was significantly increased. Lenz reported that CO_2 use increased the mean oral insertion depth > 60 cm, particularly in patients with a history of abdominal surgery. Several other researchers have proved the effectiveness of CO_2. Therefore, the use of CO_2 insufflation is recommended in such cases.

Preparation of Procedure by Device Type

Bong Min Ko

Double-Balloon Enteroscope

Double-Balloon Enteroscope Components

A double-balloon enteroscope system is consisted of enteroscope, balloon-attached overtube, balloon to be attached to distal end of enteroscope (BS-2), band used to attach the balloon to the enteroscope (FX-01G), air pump system to control deflation and inflation of the balloon (Fig. 1, refer to p. 133 Fig. 1).

Double-Balloon Enteroscope Preparation

1. Clear away moisture inside the enteroscope that can block air flow from air pump by connecting 20 mL syringe to connection part in the proximal end and ventilating the enteroscope.
2. Turn on the pump after connecting connection part of the enteroscope to the pump to check that there is adequate inflow of air to the system.

Balloon Attachment to Distal End of Enteroscope

Steps to attach balloon to distal end of enteroscope are as follows (Fig. 2).

Robust attachment of balloon on the distal end of enteroscope so as not to block the inflow of air is critical for effective inflation and deflation of balloon and prevention of balloon displacement during the procedure. An assistive device (ST-10) that helps with robust attachment of the balloon does exist but is not yet introduced to the domestic market.

Overtube Preparation (Fig. 3)

Overtube inflates the balloon to ensure that there is no air leak. Then the water inflow part and connection part that connects to pressure controller on the overtube are checked. Application of lubricant on overtube before insertion is recommended for effortless insertion of overtube.

Air Pressure Controller Preparation

Connect with overtube to ensure that the balloon on overtube and the balloon on the distal end of enteroscope are inflating and deflating robustly (Fig. 2i–j).

B. M. Ko (✉)
Department of Gastroenterology, Soon Chun Hyang College of Medicine, Bucheon, Republic of Korea

© Springer Nature Singapore Pte Ltd. 2022
H. J. Chun et al. (eds.), *Small Intestine Disease*, https://doi.org/10.1007/978-981-16-7239-2_25

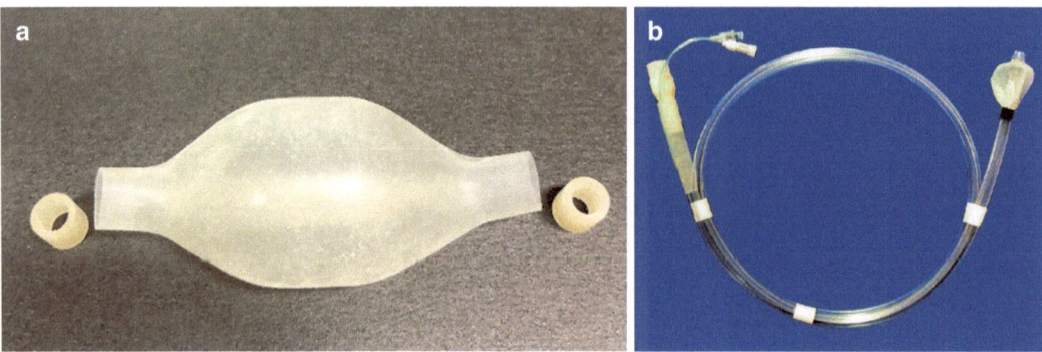

Fig. 1 (**a**) Balloon to be attached to distal end of enteroscope (BS-2). (**b**) Overtube

Single-Balloon Enteroscope (Olympus, Tokyo, Japan)

Preparation for a single-balloon enteroscopy is simpler than that required for a double-balloon enteroscopy.

Single-Balloon Enteroscope Components

Single-balloon enteroscope consists of entero-scope, overtube (ST-SB1), and air pump system (Fig. 4, Refer to p. 135 Fig. 3).

Overtube Preparation

Overtube inflates the balloon to ensure that there is no air leak. Then the water inflow part and con-nection part that connects to pressure controller on the overtube are checked.

1. Connect one end of the air injection channel to reservoir (Fig. 5a).
2. Connect the opposite end of air injection channel connected to reservoir to overtube (Fig. 5b).
3. Inject 10–20 mL of water to overtube lined with hydrophilic lubricant and shake vigorously.

Balloon and Air Pump System Check

1. Turn on the balloon adjusting device.
2. Check that the Inflate/Deflate Switch on the remote controller and overtube balloon opera-tion are in working order.
3. Pump operation check: Make sure that the pump generates a warning sound when the pressure is over the threshold by squeezing the balloon with hands, generating 5.4–8.0 kPa of pressure.
4. Press Inflate/Deflate Switch on the remote controller to ensure that the indicator light flashes and the balloon deflates.
5. Verify that the full deflation pressure is equal to or below −6 kPa.

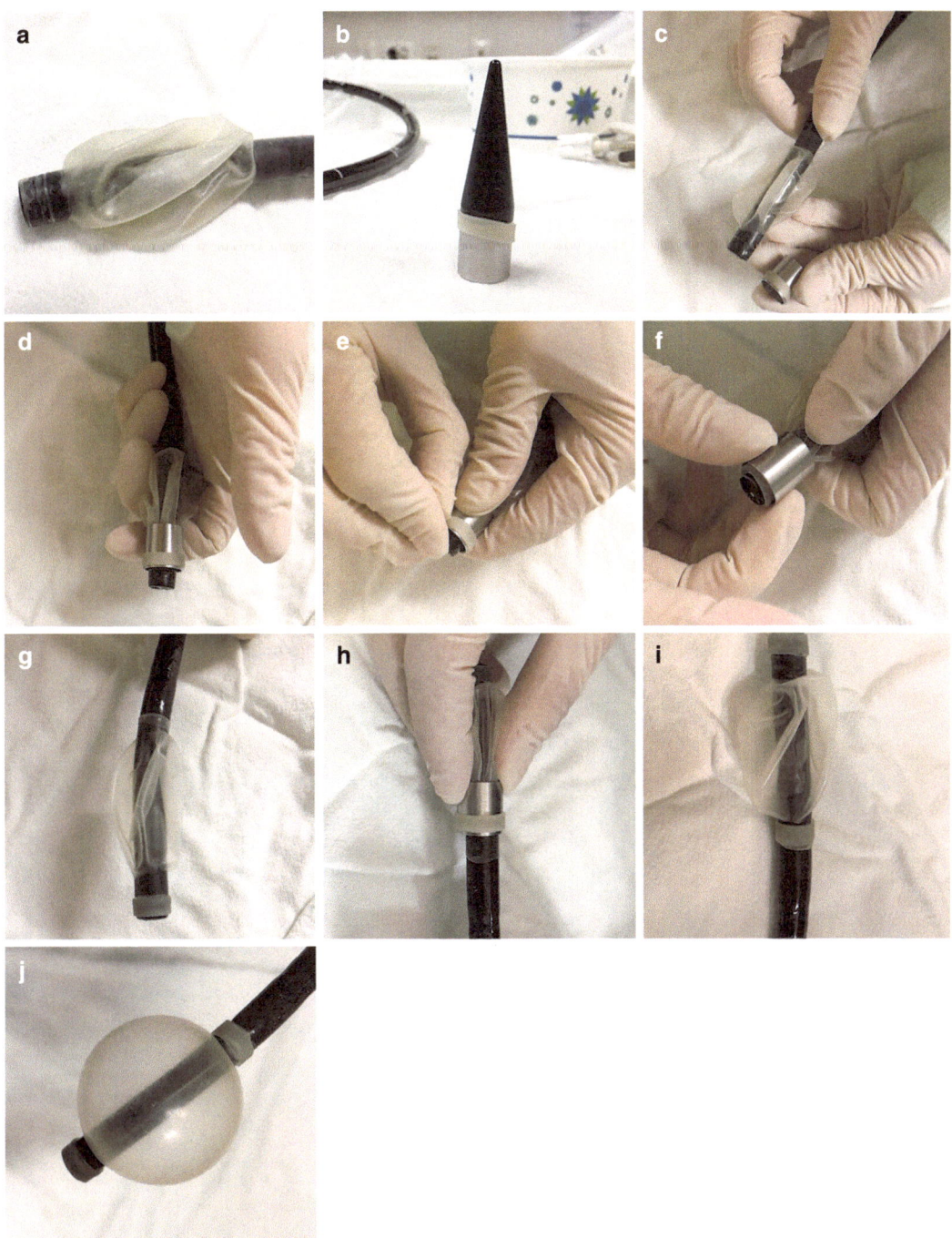

Fig. 2 steps to attach balloon to distal end of double-balloon enteroscope. (**a**) Place the balloon on the distal end of enteroscope. (**b**) Place rubber band on band-holding ring using conical assisting device in order to fix both ends of the balloon. (**c–e**) Place the band-holding ring next to one end of the balloon and roll the rubber band off of the ring using fingers onto the distal end of the enteroscope. (**f**) Remove the band-holding ring. (**g**) Check that the band is properly fixed to that end of the balloon. (**h**) Using the same method, fix the proximal end of the balloon with a rubber band. (**i**) Check that both ends of the balloon are fixed with the rubber bands, (**j**) Inflate the balloon to check for any air leak

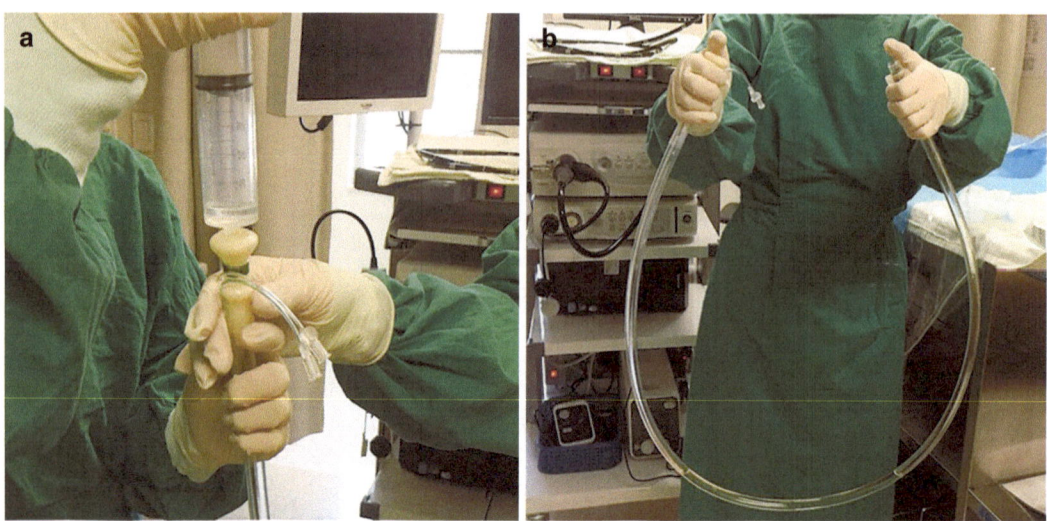

Fig. 3 (**a**) Inject distilled water for lubrication into the overtube. (**b**) While blocking both ends of the overtube with fingers, shake vigorously for uniform application of distilled water on the inner surface

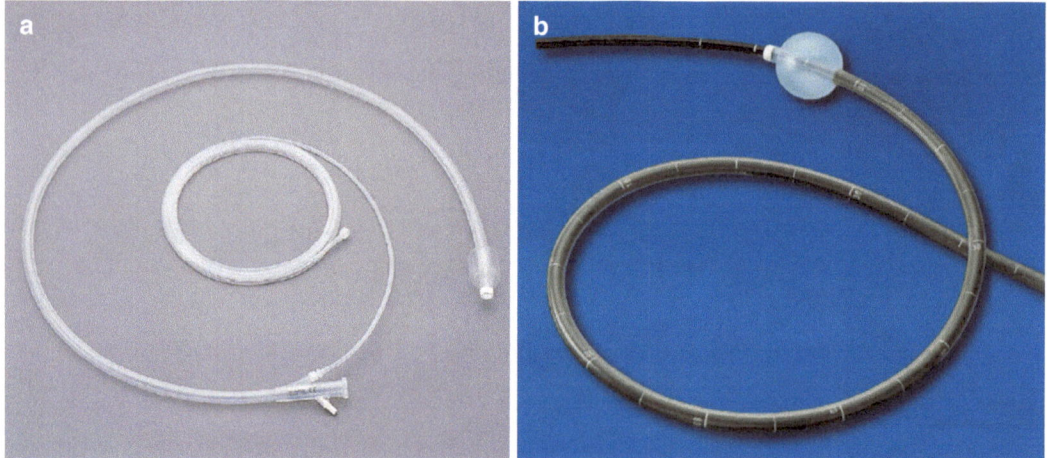

Fig. 4 (**a**) Overtube (ST-SB1), (**b**) Single-balloon enteroscope with overtube inserted

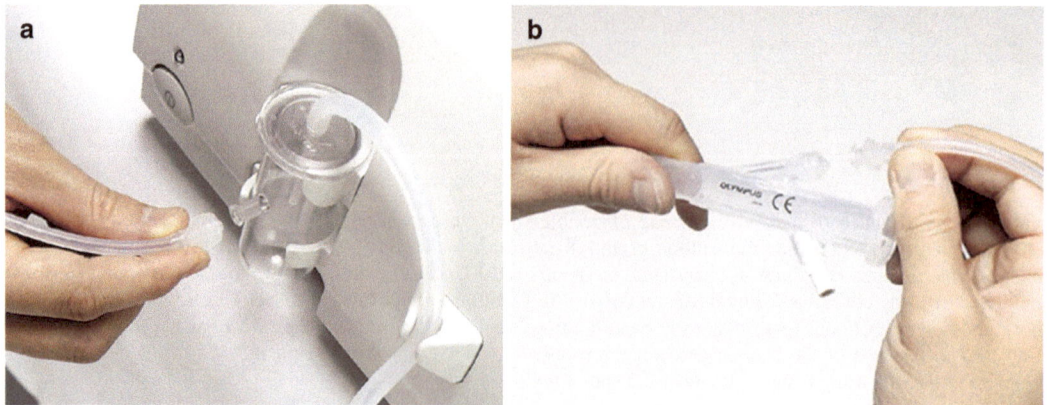

Fig. 5 (**a**) Connect one end of air injection channel to the reservoir. (**b**) Connect air injection channel to Overtube

Insertion Method in Balloon-Assisted Enteroscopy

Beom Jae Lee

Key Points
- Enteroscopy is carried out by repeating the following stages: Insertion of endoscope → Fixation of endoscope (balloon or tip of enteroscope) → Shortening → Proceed with endoscopy.
- Insertion via oral route: After passing through the duodenum, the enteroscope proceeds by making a counterclockwise concentric circle under fluoroscopy.
- Insertion via anus: In the descending colon, the endoscope proceeds with shortening of the intestine by ballooning of the endoscope/overtube. After passing through the terminal ileum, the endoscope enters the small intestine sufficiently and then advances the overtube.
- The use of a clear cap with endoscopy facilitates deep entry of the endoscope into the small intestine.
- Minimizing the injection of air and use of CO_2 is helpful for deep entry of the endoscope into the small intestine and preventing enlargement of the intestine.

B. J. Lee (✉)
Department of Internal Medicine, Korea University College of Medicine, Seoul, South Korea
e-mail: L85210@korea.ac.kr

In the past, endoscopic methods for observing the small intestine included push enteroscopy and ropeway enteroscopy. However, they were not widely used due to their limited view. In 2001, double balloon enteroscopy was introduced by Yamamoto et al. in Fujinon. Subsequently, the single balloon enteroscopy was developed; the small intestine was then no longer called the gastrointestinal blackbox. Small intestine insertion using device-assisted enteroscopy should be performed by an endoscopist who has achieved proficiency in colonoscopy. However, even if medical professionals want to train in enteroscopy, there are limited patients who require enteroscopic evaluation, so an extended period is required to achieve the necessary skill. Therefore, we want to provide information on endoscope insertion and share indirect experiences for beginners.

Basic Operation Methodology

The basic methods of double balloon enteroscopy and single balloon enteroscopy are similar. The small intestine is an unattached organ connected to the interstitial membrane; therefore, it moves around relatively freely in the abdominal cavity. Due to this, the direction of the force exerted on the tip of the endoscope and operating direction do not align, which creates a hyperenlargement of the small intestine, and makes it difficult to insert the endoscope. To overcome

© Springer Nature Singapore Pte Ltd. 2022
H. J. Chun et al. (eds.), *Small Intestine Disease*, https://doi.org/10.1007/978-981-16-7239-2_26

this difficulty with the previous push enteros-copy method, the single and double balloon enteroscopy were developed to position the latex balloon at the overtube and tip of the endoscope to induce shortening of the small intestine and inhibit the organ from hyper-enlargement. This allows the endoscope to be inserted deep within the small intestine. Double balloon enteroscopy involves an endoscope with a balloon attached at the tip and an air pump system that injects air into the balloon-attached overtube and latex bal-loon. Single balloon enteroscopy is similar to double balloon enteroscopy, but the balloon is attached only at the overtube and not at the tip of the endoscope in single balloon endoscopy. Endoscope insertion is carried out by repeating the process of curving the endoscope point, fix-ing the endoscope, proceeding with the overtube, fixing the overtube by balloon extension, and shortening.

Insertion of the Enteroscope

Unlike the stomach and large intestine, the small intestine does not have a particular marker, which makes it difficult to recognize how far the endo-scope has been inserted or what the directional alignment of the endoscope is. Therefore, the assistance of fluoroscopy is required to insert the endoscope deep into the small intestine. Fluoroscopy may not be necessary for profes-sionals with expertise in enteroscopy or cases where the lesions are proximally located. However, fluoroscopy allows cognizance of enteroscopy progress; therefore, even medical professionals with expertise will likely proceed with fluoroscopy. Normally, two enteroscopy assistants are required. One assistant will hold the endoscope and operate the air pump, while the other will observe the patient status and assist with medication and hold the patient when the patient moves badly. Situationally, there can be just one assistant; in such a case, the endoscopist will operate the air pump. Prior to initiating the enteroscopy, the entry path must be decided. The entry path may be decided based on whether the entire small intestine must be observed, signs of

bleeding, and whether the location is proximal or distal within the intestine based on previous imaging tests such as video capsule enteroscopy or abdominal CT.

Oral Insertion

To reach the small intestine, advancement beyond the stomach and duodenum must be performed; however, these organs interfere with deep entry to the small intestine. Therefore, when advancing beyond those organs, it is essential to proceed with the insertion while minimizing enlargement and preventing loops. After the endoscope is advanced beyond the stomach and duodenum and reaches the Treitz, the balloon at the tip of the endoscope is extended. Then, the overtube is advanced to the white boundary area, the balloon is extended, and the endoscope is shortened (Fig. 1). As there is no balloon attached at the tip in single balloon enteroscopy, the endoscope is fixed after curving the endoscope point and extended after proceeding with the overtube

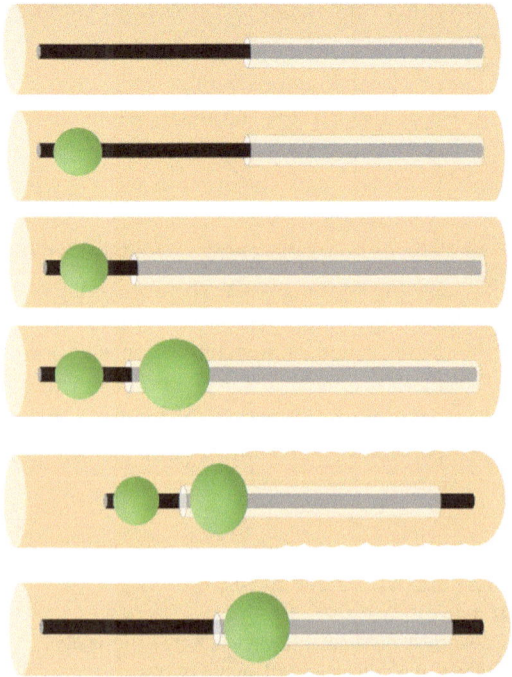

Fig. 1 Insertion method in double balloon enteroscopy

(Fig. 2). The preferable insertion method would be to proceed with the enteroscopy by creating a concentric form under fluoroscopy. Initially, we need to be cautious of the operating direction of the endoscope. Proceeding clockwise will continuously create loops in the stomach and duode-

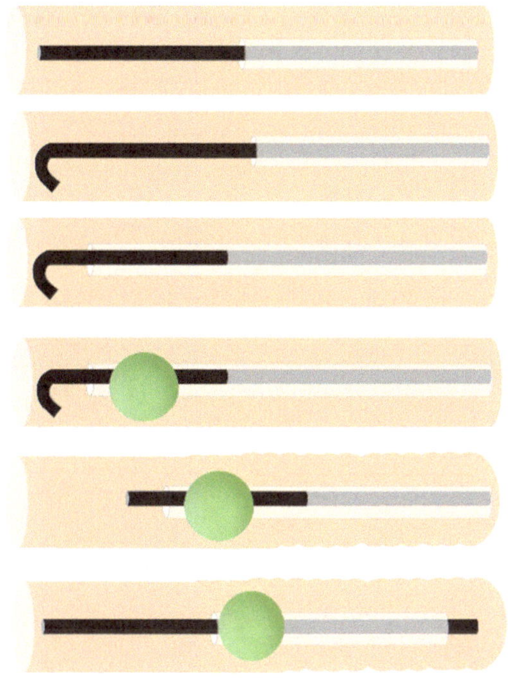

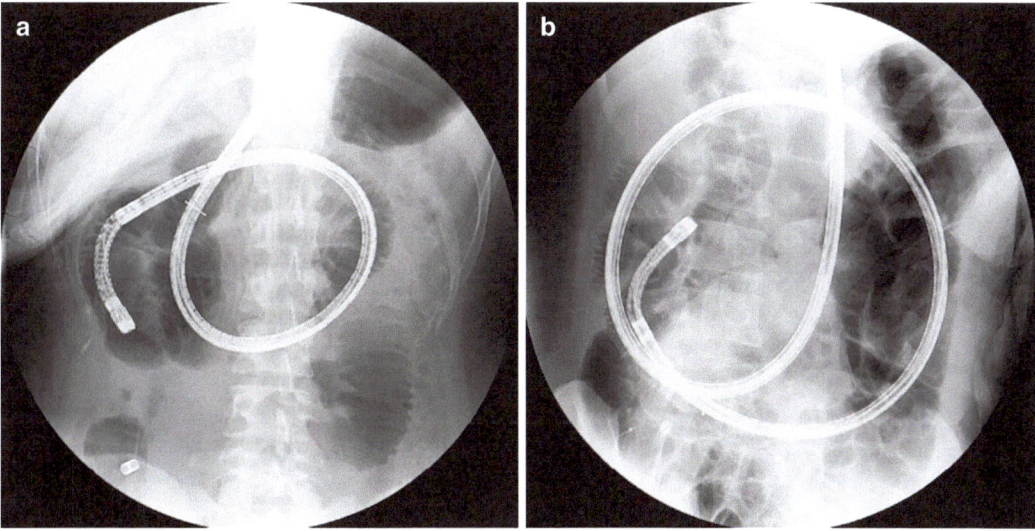

Fig. 2 Insertion method in single ballooan enteroscopy

num, which impedes deep insertion into the small intestine and may lead to complications such as pancreatitis. Therefore, enteroscopy must proceed in a counterclockwise direction under fluoroscopy (Fig. 3a, b). If the entire small intestine needs to be observed or endoscope insertion cannot be continued, the endoscope must be retreated while observing for lesions after marking by a tattoo or an endoscopic clip.

Anal Insertion

When deciding anal insertion as the entry path, a bowel preparation process similar to that in colonoscopy must be performed prior to the procedure. When the endoscope is advanced beyond the sigmoid colon and reaches the descending colon, the balloon is extended after overtube entry. Then, with shortening of the small intestine, we straighten the endoscope with fluoroscopy. With continuous shortening of the small intestine, we can easily reach the appendix. Then, positioning the endoscope to the distal ileum, the overtube is inserted and balloon extended to fix the overtube so that it does not retreat to the large intestine. After shortening of the intestine, enteroscopy is performed by making a counterclockwise concentric circle under

Fig. 3 Fluoroscopic images (**a**) clockwise rotation and (**b**) counterclockwise rotation

fluoroscopy. If insertion is difficult, several measures can be taken such as changing the patient's position (left down position → supine) and applying abdominal pressure while preventing extension of the endoscope by fluoroscopy.

Other Tips for Deep Insertion

The use of the clear cap allows for easier insertion to the deep small intestine by minimizing air injection owing to easier passage through curved areas. Often, the endoscope is inserted with a clear cap attached at its tip. Additionally, the difficulty of endoscope insertion stems from an extensive treatment time lasting over one hour, which causes excessive injection of air. When using CO_2, air absorption is facilitated, and hyper-enlargement of the small intestine is prevented, which allows the endoscope to be easily inserted deep into the small intestine.

Differences in and Characteristics of Insertion Techniques According to type of Balloon-Assisted Enteroscopy

Sung Noh Hong

Key Points

- The insertion technique of double-balloon enteroscopy (DBE) and single-balloon enteroscopy (SBE) is as follows: 1. Advance the enteroscope through the small intestine → 2. DBE: inflate the balloon on the tip of the enteroscope; SBE: anchor the enteroscope in the small intestine by maximally bending its flexible tip → 3. Deflate the overtube (in SBE, the splinting tube) balloon → 4. Advance the overtube (splinting tube) through the enteroscope → 5. Inflate the overtube (splinting tube) balloon → 6. Pull back the enteroscope and overtube (splining tube) → 7. DBE: inflate the balloon on the tip of the enteroscope; SBE: release the bending of the enteroscope flexible tip → 8. Advance the enteroscope into the deeper part of the small intestine.
- DBE and SBE, performed by an experienced endoscopist, are similar in terms of diagnostic and therapeutic yield and complications.

Introduction

To evaluate the small intestine, different balloon-assisted enteroscopes (BAE) are used and each has their own design of the balloon and overtube. Currently, in Korea, DBE and SBE are available; however, spiral enteroscopy is not available [1]. This chapter discusses the differences in and characteristics of the insertion technique according to the type of BAE.

DBE

DBE utilizes two latex balloons attached to the endoscope and overtube. The enteroscope is inserted into the small intestine by alternately inflating and deflating the balloons, and enabling manipulation of the small intestine by the endoscopist by pleating the intestine over an overtube, just like pulling a curtain over a rod. DBE is performed by 2 people, an endoscopist and an assistant, and is often performed under fluoroscopic guidance. Insertion techniques are usually as follows using an endoscope equipped with overtube: 1. Advance the enteroscope through the small intestine → 2. Inflate the balloon on the tip of the enteroscope → 3. Deflate the overtube balloon → 4. Advance the overtube or splinting tube through the enteroscope → 5. Inflate the overtube

S. N. Hong (✉)
Department of Medicine, Samsung Medical Center, Sungkyunkwan University School of Medicine, Seoul, South Korea

© Springer Nature Singapore Pte Ltd. 2022
H. J. Chun et al. (eds.), *Small Intestine Disease*, https://doi.org/10.1007/978-981-16-7239-2_27

balloon → 6. Pull back the enteroscope and over-tube → 7. Inflate the balloon on the tip of the enteroscope → 8. Advance the enteroscope into the deeper part of the small intestine. By repeating these steps, the enteroscope can be inserted into the deeper part of the small intestine (Table 1, Fig. 1) [2].

Table 1 Insertion step of double-balloon enteroscopy

1. Advance the enteroscope through the small intestine
2. Inflate the balloon on the tip of the enteroscope
3. Deflate the overtube balloon
4. Advance the overtube through the enteroscope
5. Inflate the overtube balloon
6. Pull back the enteroscope and overtube
7. Inflate the balloon on the tip of the enteroscope

Fig. 1 Insertion technique in double-balloon enteroscopy

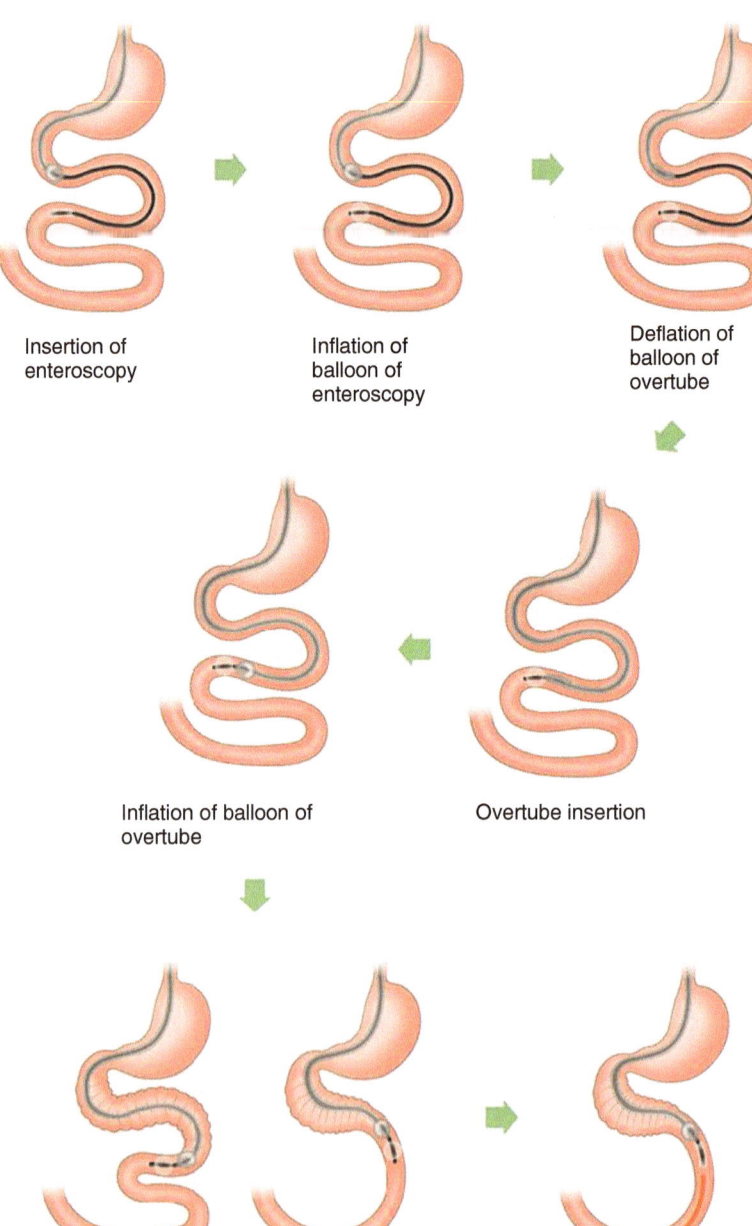

Insertion of enteroscopy

Inflation of balloon of enteroscopy

Deflation of balloon of overtube

Inflation of balloon of overtube

Overtube insertion

Retracting back of enteroscopy and overtube

Deflation of balloon of enteroscopy and insertion of enteroscopy

SBE

Unlike DBE, SBE does not use the balloon on the tip of enteroscope; the balloon is attached only on the silicone overtube, which is called a splinting tube. Instead of the enteroscopy balloon, SBE utilizes bending of the flexible enteroscopic tip to anchor the enteroscope in the small intestine and prevent slipping of the enteroscope. SBE adopted the push and pull technique as with DBE. Insertion techniques are usually as follows using an endoscope equipped with splinting tube: 1. Advance the enteroscope through the small intestine → 2. Anchor the enteroscope in the small intestine by maximally bending its flexible tip → 3. Deflate the splinting tube balloon → 4. Advance the splinting tube through the enteroscope → 5. Inflate the splinting tube balloon → 6. Pull back the enteroscope and splinting tube → 7. Release the bending of the enteroscope flexible tip. By repeating these steps, the enteroscope can be inserted into the deeper part of the small intestine (Table 2, Fig. 2) [3].

SBE was introduced as a simplified and less complex BAE system. Therefore, SBE is thought to have the advantages of shorter preparation, easy to learn, and is accomplished by a single person.

Comparison of Efficacy and Safety Between DBE and SBE

Four previous randomized controlled trials (RCT) were conducted to evaluate the efficacy and safety of SBE versus DBE. The first study included 100 patients with no previous small bowel or colon surgery and used only a Fujinon

Table 2 Insertion step of single-balloon enteroscopy

1. Advance the enteroscope through the small intestine
2. Anchor enteroscope in the small intestine by maximally bending its flexible tip
3. Deflate the splinting tube balloon
4. Advance the splinting tube through the enteroscope
5. Inflate the splinting tube balloon
6. Pull back the enteroscope and splinting tube
7. Release the bending of the enteroscope's flexible tip

DBE system with one or two balloons. There were no significant differences in diagnostic yield and complications, whereas the rate of complete enteroscopy (66% vs. 22%) and therapeutic consequences (72% vs. 48%) were significantly higher in the DBE group than in the SBE group [4]. However, this study mimicked an SBE using a DBE system without attachment of the balloon on the tip of the enteroscope and was performed by less experienced endoscopists in SBE. A subsequent RCT applied the Fujinon DBE system for DBE and Olympus SBE system for SBE. There was no difference in the overall diagnosis rate, complication rate, and therapeutic outcomes. The total enteroscopy rate was significantly higher in DBE compared to that in SBE (0% vs. 57.1%), and the study was terminated early after 38 patients were enrolled [5]. However, endoscopists in this study had experience with 248 DBEs and 10 SBEs. The endoscopist had more experience with DBE than with SBE. BAE is an operator-dependent procedure. The insertion technique and manipulation of instruments for SBE are quite different from that of DBE. Differences in total enteroscopy rates and therapeutic consequences may be due to the "learning curve" of SBE, which might be comparable to the reported learning curve of the DBE technique. The endoscopists enrolled in the European multicenter RCT were more experienced in the SBE technique and endoscopists in each trial center had experienced over 50 SBE procedures before the study although the endoscopists were more experienced in DBE. There was no difference in diagnostic yield, total enteroscopy rate (18% vs. 11%), mean oral intubation depth (253 cm vs. 258 cm), and mean anal intubation depth (107 cm vs. 118 cm) in the DBE and SBE groups [6]. An RCT performed by Efthymiou et al. did not mention the experience in SBE of the enrolled endoscopist. SBE showed diagnostic and therapeutic yields similar to those of DBE. There were no statistically significant differences in insertion depth between SBE and DBE [7].

A retrospective Korean study analyzed the BAE registry to compare the efficacy and safety of SBE vs. DBE as performed by expert endos-

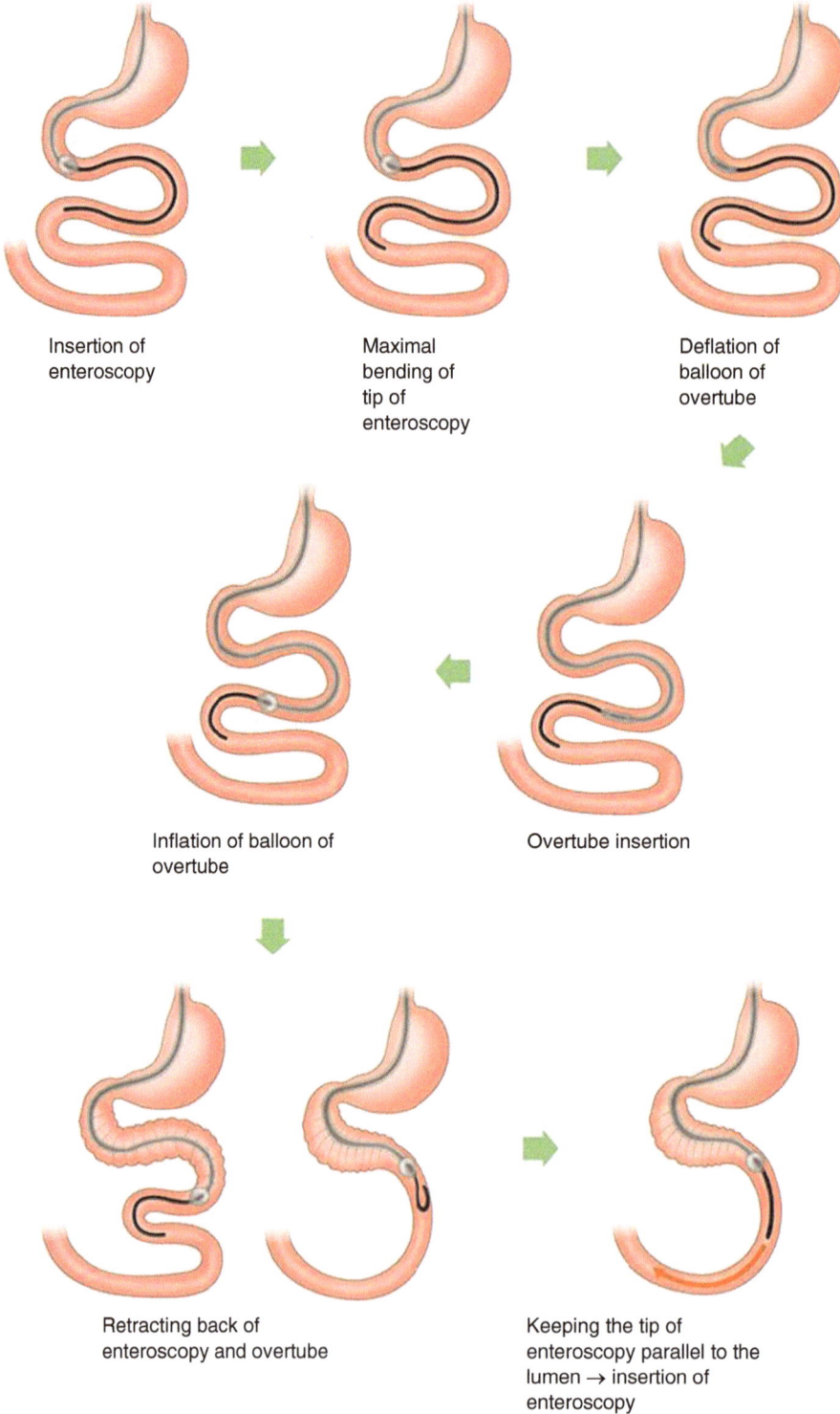

Fig. 2 Insertion technique in single-balloon enteroscopy

copists in SBE. There were no significant differences in diagnostic yield (61.1% vs 77.3%), therapeutic yield (39.1% vs 31.8%), and complication rate (4.4% vs 2.3%). In the meta-analysis, which included four RCT and three observational studies, there were no significant differences in the pooled relative risk and odds ratio for diagnostic and therapeutic yield and complications [8].

Spiral Enteroscopy

Recently, Spiral enteroscopy (SE) has been introduced as an alternative technique for small bowel enteroscopy. A second-generation SE device (Endo-Ease Discovery SB) is a single-use overtube with an overall length of 118 cm. The SB device can be applied with conventional pediatric colonoscopes and any endoscope thinner than 9.8 mm. The internal diameter of the overtube is 9.8 mm, and the external diameter at the distal end is 16 mm. The distal 21 cm of the SE device has a 5.5-mm high hollow spiral that can be rotated both clockwise and counterclockwise via a handle from the proximal end of the device. The SE overtube is engaged to the scope and rotated in a clockwise direction, and the device pleats the small bowel onto the overtube like a corkscrew allowing the endoscope to be advanced into the deeper part of the small intestine. For the ileoscopy, a retrograde SE device (Endo-Ease Vista Retrograde) can be applied for peranal insertion [9]. Although the maximal depth of insertion was shallow compared to that of BAE, SE is easy to learn and shortens the procedure time. Although rare, SE reportedly has a risk of perforation; moreover, SE is not available in Korea [10].

Conclusion

BAE is a novel endoscopic technique that allows deep insertion of the endoscope and permits small bowel mucosa evaluation. There are two forms of BAE: DBE and SBE. DBE was developed in 2001 and has been considered the standard endoscopic technique for small bowel visualization; SBE is a simplified version of DBE. Although both DBE and SBE adopt the push and pull technique, the instruments used and technique details are different as follows: 1. Advance the enteroscope through the small intestine → 2. DBE: inflate the balloon on the tip of the enteroscope; SBE: anchor the enteroscope in the small intestine by maximally bending its flexible tip → 3. Deflate the overtube (in SBE, splinting tube) balloon → 4. Advance the overtube (splinting tube) through the enteroscope → 5. Inflate the overtube (splinting tube) balloon → 6. Pull back the enteroscope and overtube (splinting tube) → 7. DBE: inflate the balloon on the tip of the enteroscope; SBE: release the bending of the enteroscope flexible tip → 8. Advance the enteroscope into the deeper part of the small intestine.

SBE and DBE diagnostic and therapeutic yields and complication rates are not significantly different. DBE and SBE require a learning curve to achieve expertise. Therefore, SBE or DBE would be an appropriate approach for diagnostic and therapeutic requirements in the small bowel based on the experience of the endoscopists and availability.

References

1. Hong SN, Kim ER, Ye BD, et al. Indications, diagnostic yield, and complication rate of balloon-assisted enteroscopy (BAE) during the first decade of its use in Korea. Dig Endosc. 2015;28(4):443–9.
2. Lo SK. Techniques, tricks, and complications of enteroscopy. Gastrointest Endosc Clin N Am. 2009;19:381–8.
3. Hong SN. Insertion technique of balloon-assisted enteroscopy. 58th Seminar of Korean Society of Gastrointestinal Endoscopy 2018.
4. May A, Farber M, Aschmoneit I, et al. Prospective multicenter trial comparing push-and-pull enteroscopy with the single- and double-balloon techniques in patients with small-bowel disorders. Am J Gastroenterol. 2010;105:575–81.
5. Takano N, Yamada A, Watabe H, et al. Single-balloon versus double-balloon endoscopy for achieving total enteroscopy: a randomized, controlled trial. Gastrointest Endosc. 2011;73:734–9.

6. Domagk D, Mensink P, Aktas H, et al. Single- vs. double-balloon enteroscopy in small-bowel diagnostics: a randomized multicenter trial. Endoscopy. 2011;43:472–6.

7. Efthymiou M, Desmond PV, Brown G, et al. SINGLE-01: a randomized, controlled trial comparing the efficacy and depth of insertion of single- and double-balloon enteroscopy by using a novel method to determine insertion depth. Gastrointest Endosc. 2012;76:972–80.

8. Kim TJ, Kim ER, Chang DK, et al. Comparison of the efficacy and safety of single- versus double-balloon enteroscopy performed by endoscopist experts in single-balloon enteroscopy: a single-center experience and meta-analysis. Gut Liver. 2017;11:520–7.

9. Akerman PA, Agrawal D, Cantero D, et al. Spiral enteroscopy with the new DSB overtube: a novel technique for deep peroral small-bowel intubation. Endoscopy. 2008;40:974–8.

10. Akerman PA, Cantero D. Severe complications of spiral enteroscopy in the first 1750 patients. Gastrointest Endosc. 2009;69:AB127.

Therapeutic Enteroscopy (Hemostasis, Polypectomy, Balloon Dilation, and Others)

Jeong-Sik Byeon

Key Points

- The types of therapeutic enteroscopy procedures include hemostasis, polypectomy, and balloon dilation.
- The enteroscopic hemostatic methods include argon plasma coagulation, clip application, and injection hemostasis.
- The indications of enteroscopic polypectomy are premalignant small bowel polyps in Peutz-Jeghers syndrome, sporadic premalignant polyps, and symptomatic polyps.
- The indications of enteroscopic balloon dilation include benign small bowel strictures due to Crohn's disease, nonsteroidal anti-inflammatory drug-associated enteropathy, and anastomosis.
- Other therapeutic enteroscopy procedures such as enteroscopic stent insertion and enteroscopic foreign body removal are also used.

Introduction

Device-assisted enteroscopy methods, such as double-balloon enteroscopy, single-balloon enteroscopy, and spiral enteroscopy, are clinically useful not only for diagnostic purposes but also for therapeutic intent [1]. This review will discuss the types, indications, clinical outcomes, and complications of therapeutic enteroscopy procedures.

Enteroscopic Hemostasis

Indications

The indications of enteroscopic hemostasis include small bowel bleeding from erosions/ulcers of various etiologies, such as idiopathic erosion/ulcer and drug-associated ulcers, vascular abnormalities such as angioectasia and varices, and benign and malignant tumors. In general, capsule endoscopy is performed to find the bleeding lesion in patients with suspected small bowel bleeding before device-assisted enteroscopy. After the localization of the bleeding lesion using capsule endoscopy, the insertion route of enteroscopy can be determined (oral vs. anal) based on the identified location of the bleeding lesion. However, direct per-oral enteroscopy without

J.-S. Byeon (✉)
Department of Gastroenterology, University of Ulsan College of Medicine, Seoul, South Korea
e-mail: jsbyeon@amc.seoul.kr

© Springer Nature Singapore Pte Ltd. 2022
H. J. Chun et al. (eds.), *Small Intestine Disease*, https://doi.org/10.1007/978-981-16-7239-2_28

prior capsule endoscopy can be considered in patients with active ongoing bleeding to increase the diagnostic yield and to conduct timely enteroscopic hemostasis [2].

Types of Enteroscopic Hemostasis

Injection Method

Diluted epinephrine-saline fluid can be injected into the submucosal space to induce a tamponade effect on bleeding vessels and a vasoconstrictive effect, thereby achieving hemostasis. The injection method may be used for hemostasis of bleeding from angioectasia and erosions/ulcers.

Argon Plasma Coagulation

Argon plasma coagulation (APC) is a noncontact hemostatic method in which the probe applies bursts argon gas without making contact with the target tissue. The perforation risk of APC is low because of its noncontact nature. For a safer procedure, APC can be performed after submucosal saline injection around the bleeding area. Because of its safety and technical ease of use, APC is one of the most commonly used hemostatic methods for enteroscopic hemostasis of bleeding from angioectasia and erosions/ulcers.

Clip Application

Clipping is an effective hemostatic method for active pumping or spurting bleeding from the small bowel (Fig. 1) [3]. Another advantage of enteroscopic hemostasis by clipping is that it can help identify the bleeding point when angiography is performed for rebleeding because the clip can show the bleeding site on fluoroscopic observation [4].

Other Hemostatic Methods

Coagulation forceps grasp bleeding exposed vessels, transmit coagulation current, and coagulate the target vessels, thereby achieving hemostasis. Coagulation forceps can be used for immediate bleeding after enteroscopic polypectomy. Heater probe hemostasis is a contact hemostatic method in which the probe makes direct contact with the bleeding site, transmits heat to the bleeding vessels, and coagulates the bleeding vessels. Because of its risk of perforation, a heater probe is rarely used for enteroscopic hemostasis of bleeding angioectasia and erosions/ulcers. Heater probe hemostasis can be performed for enteroscopic hemostasis of bleeding from small bowel tumors for palliative purposes [4].

Clinical Outcome and Complications of Enteroscopic Hemostasis

Initial hemostasis can be achieved in most cases if enteroscopic hemostasis is attempted based on adequate indications. However, rebleeding is common after initial enteroscopic hemostasis of bleeding angioectasia with APC. Therefore, cautious follow-up observation of patients is mandatory after enteroscopic hemostasis of angioectasia [5]. Enteroscopic hemostasis-related complications are rare. One case of enteritis (0.9%) was reported after enteroscopic hemostasis using APC in 108 lesions [6].

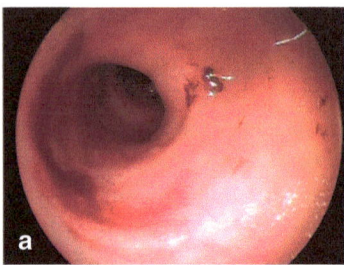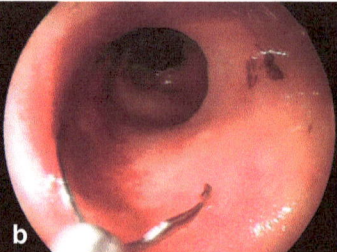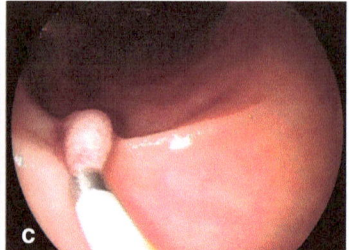

Fig. 1 Enteroscopic hemostasis by clipping of small bowel angioectasia. (**a**) Active bleeding from a small bowel angioectasia. (**b**) Clipping. (**c**) Hemostasis achieved by clipping. To the publisher: The original file names of the following figures are BJS 1, BJS 2, BJS 3

Enteroscopic Polypectomy

Indications

The most important indication of enteroscopic polypectomy is small bowel polyps in Peutz-Jeghers syndrome. For this indication, enteroscopic polypectomy can prevent intussusception with or without obstruction. Enteroscopic polypectomy can also prevent the development of small bowel cancer in patients with Peutz-Jeghers syndrome. Small bowel adenomatous polyps in patients with familial adenomatous polyposis and small bowel benign polyps with symptoms such as bleeding are also indications of enteroscopic hemostasis.

Enteroscopic Polypectomy Methods

The basic principle of enteroscopic polypectomy is similar to that of gastroscopic and colonoscopic polypectomy. Endoscopic mucosal resection (EMR) is usually performed for sessile polyps without a stalk. Enteroscopic polypectomy without submucosal injection is commonly performed for pedunculated polyps (Fig. 2). However, EMR after diluted epinephrine-saline submucosal injection can be performed for large pedunculated polyps with thick stalks, to minimize the risk of immediate postpolypectomy bleeding. A detachable snare may be used to decrease the risk of immediate postpolypectomy bleeding in large pedunculated polyps. Cautious application of preventive hemostatic measures immediately after enteroscopic polypectomy is important because enteroscopic insertion requires a long procedure time and insertion to the target site is not always possible in cases of delayed bleeding.

Clinical Outcome and Complications of Enteroscopic Polypectomy

Successful enteroscopic polypectomy is affected by the size and location of small bowel polyps, maneuverability of the enteroscope, and experience and expertise of the enteroscopist. In a study investigating the outcome of enteroscopic polypectomy of 46 small bowel polyps, 44 polyps (96%) of 1–5 cm diameter were successfully resected using enteroscopic polypectomy. Enteroscopic polypectomy failed in a patient in whom the enteroscopic approach to the adequate polypectomy location was difficult and in another patient with a huge polyp of 8 cm diameter [6]. Laparotomy for the surgical removal of small bowel polyps may be complicated by small bowel adhesion, which can make enteroscopic insertion and manipulation difficult. Therefore, enteroscopic polypectomy in Peutz-Jeghers syndrome is recommended earlier in childhood before surgical laparotomy.

The complication rate of enteroscopic polypectomy is reported to be 0–11%. Bleeding and perforation are the two main complications of enteroscopic polypectomy.

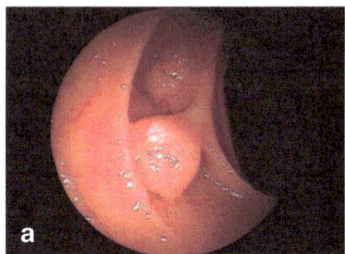 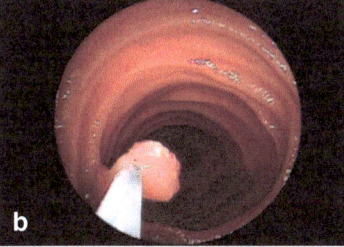 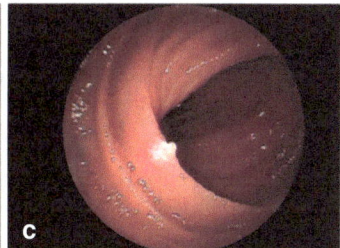

Fig. 2 Enteroscopic polypectomy of small bowel polyps in a patient with Peutz-Jeghers syndrome. (**a**) A 7-mm pedunculated polyp. (**b**) Enteroscopic polypectomy without submucosal injection. (**c**) Postpolypectomy site. To the publisher: The original file names of the following figures are BJS 4, BJS 5, BJS 6

Enteroscopic Balloon Dilation

Indications

Small Bowel Strictures in Crohn's Disease

Chronic fibrotic small bowel strictures in Crohn's disease are the most important indication of enteroscopic balloon dilation. In contrast, inflammatory strictures in Crohn's disease should be initially managed with medications to resolve edema, thereby improving stricture.

Benign Strictures Other than Crohn's Disease

The other indications for enteroscopic balloon dilation include benign small bowel strictures due to non-steroidal anti-inflammatory drug use, surgical anastomosis, small bowel ischemia, and radiation enteritis.

Balloon Dilation Procedures

The balloon diameter is determined by the severity of small bowel strictures. A balloon of 12 mm diameter is commonly selected for initial dilation. After the initial dilation, the diameter of the balloon can be serially increased according to the degree of dilation of the stricture site. In general, the maximum balloon diameter used for enteroscopic dilation is 20 mm. The risk of perforation can increase if a balloon with a diameter > 20 mm is used for enteroscopic dilation. It is not clear whether local injection of a steroid after enteroscopic balloon dilation in Crohn's disease can decrease the risk of stricture recurrence [7].

Clinical Outcome of Enteroscopic Balloon Dilation

Small Bowel Strictures in Crohn's Disease

The technical success rate of enteroscopic balloon dilation in Crohn's disease has been reported to be 89–97%. In a meta-analysis of 13 studies involving 347 patients with Crohn's disease in whom enteroscopic balloon dilation was per-

formed, the surgery-free survival rate was 58% over 33 months of follow-up. The most important prognostic factor for a good clinical course without surgery after enteroscopic balloon dilation in patients with Crohn's disease is small bowel stricture with a length of <4 cm [7]. In other words, Crohn's disease-related small bowel stricture longer than 4 cm is a relative contraindication of enteroscopic balloon dilation. Repeat enteroscopic balloon dilation is required in 50% of patients because of symptomatic recurrence of small bowel strictures after the initial enteroscopic balloon dilation. Surgery is required within 5–6 years in 25% of patients because of symptomatic recurrence of strictures even after repeat enteroscopic balloon dilation [7].

Small Bowel Strictures from Other Etiologies

Only a few small case series have reported the clinical outcomes of enteroscopic balloon dilation in benign small bowel strictures from etiologies other than Crohn's disease, which showed similar performance to that in strictures due to Crohn's disease. Technical success of enteroscopic balloon dilation was achieved in 45 of 47 cases (96%) in which both Crohn's disease and other conditions were included as etiologies [7].

Complications of Enteroscopic Balloon Dilation

The two major complications of enteroscopic balloon dilation are perforation and bleeding. The incidence of these complications was reported to be 0–5% [6, 7]. Small bowel stricture with active ulcer has a high risk of perforation and is a relative contraindication to enteroscopic balloon dilation [4].

Other Therapeutic Enteroscopy Procedures

Stenting

Enteroscopic stenting can be performed for palliation of malignant small bowel obstruction.

Further developments of enteroscopic accessories are necessary to increase the effectiveness of enteroscopic stenting.

Enteroscopic Foreign Body Removal

Foreign bodies in the small bowel can be removed using enteroscopy. The most common indication of enteroscopic foreign body removal is the retrieval of a retained capsule.

Conclusion

Therapeutic enteroscopy procedures such as hemostasis, polypectomy, and balloon dilation have been successfully performed with the aid of various enteroscopy accessories and devices. Enteroscopists should have proper knowledge about the indications, methods, performances, and complications of therapeutic enteroscopy procedures to optimize the clinical outcomes.

References

1. Akyuz U, Akyuz F. Diagnostic and therapeutic capability of double-balloon Enteroscopy in clinical practice. Clin Endosc. 2016;49:157–60.
2. ASGE Standards of Practice Committee, Fisher L, Lee Krinsky M, Anderson MA, et al. The role of endoscopy in the management of obscure GI bleeding. Gastrointest Endosc. 2010;72:471–9.
3. Yano T, Yamamoto H, Sunada K, et al. Endoscopic classification of vascular lesions of the small intestine (with videos). Gastrointest Endosc. 2008;67:169–72.
4. Kaffes AJ. Advances in modern enteroscopy therapeutics. Best Pract Res Clin Gastroenterol. 2012;26:235–46.
5. Jeon SR, Byeon JS, Jang HJ, et al. Small intestine research Group of the Korean Association for the study of intestinal disease (KASID). Clinical outcome after enteroscopy for small bowel angioectasia bleeding: a Korean Association for the Study of intestinal disease (KASID) multicenter study. J Gastroenterol Hepatol. 2017;32:388–94.
6. May A, Nachbar L, Pohl J, Ell C. Endoscopic interventions in the small bowel using double balloon enteroscopy: feasibility and limitations. Am J Gastroenterol. 2007;102:527–235.
7. American Society for Gastrointestinal Endoscopy Standards of Practice Committee, Shergill AK, Lightdale JR, Bruining DH, et al. The role of endoscopy in inflammatory bowel disease. Gastrointest Endosc. 2015;81:1101–21.

Complications Related to Device-Assisted Enteroscopy

Dong-Hoon Yang

Key Points
- The major complications of device-assisted enteroscopy are bleeding, perforation, and acute pancreatitis.
- The incidence of bleeding related to double-balloon enteroscopy (DBE) ranges from 0.2 to 0.3%; however, the risk of bleeding increases with polypectomy and balloon dilation.
- The incidence of perforation ranges from 0.1 to 0.3% in diagnostic DBE procedures and from 0.8 to 2.9% in polypectomy.
- Acute pancreatitis can occur in 0.3% of antegrade (per-oral) DBE procedures and generally presents with abdominal pain within 24 h of the procedure.

Both diagnostic and therapeutic device-assisted enteroscopy (DAE) procedures may pose the risk of various but rare complications, which may be related to prolonged procedure time, deep sedation, or general anesthesia. Because the procedural principle is basically common between double-balloon enteroscopy (DBE) and single-

balloon enteroscopy (SBE), the kinds of procedure-related complications are similar between the two types of enteroscopy. However, complications related to spiral enteroscopy (SE) are not well investigated, as the clinical experience of SE is limited to date.

As DBE is the first clinically applied DAE, most data of DAE-related complications are derived from studies about DBE. The major complications are perforation, bleeding, acute pancreatitis, and sedation-related complications.

Major Complications

Bleeding

Bleeding can occur in approximately 0.2–0.3% of overall DBE procedures [1]. However, the risk of bleeding increases in therapeutic DBE procedures, such as polypectomy (up to 4.3%) [2] and balloon dilation for stenotic Crohn's disease (1.5%) [3]. Mucosal damage due to diagnostic procedures may cause minor bleeding, which resolves spontaneously in most cases [4].

Perforation

The incidence of perforation ranges from 0.1 to 0.3% in diagnostic DAE procedures (Fig. 1) and from 0.8 to 2.9% in polypectomy cases [1, 5–7]. The risk of perforation significantly increases in

D.-H. Yang (✉)
University of Ulsan College of Medicine,
Seoul, South Korea
e-mail: dhyang@amc.seoul.kr

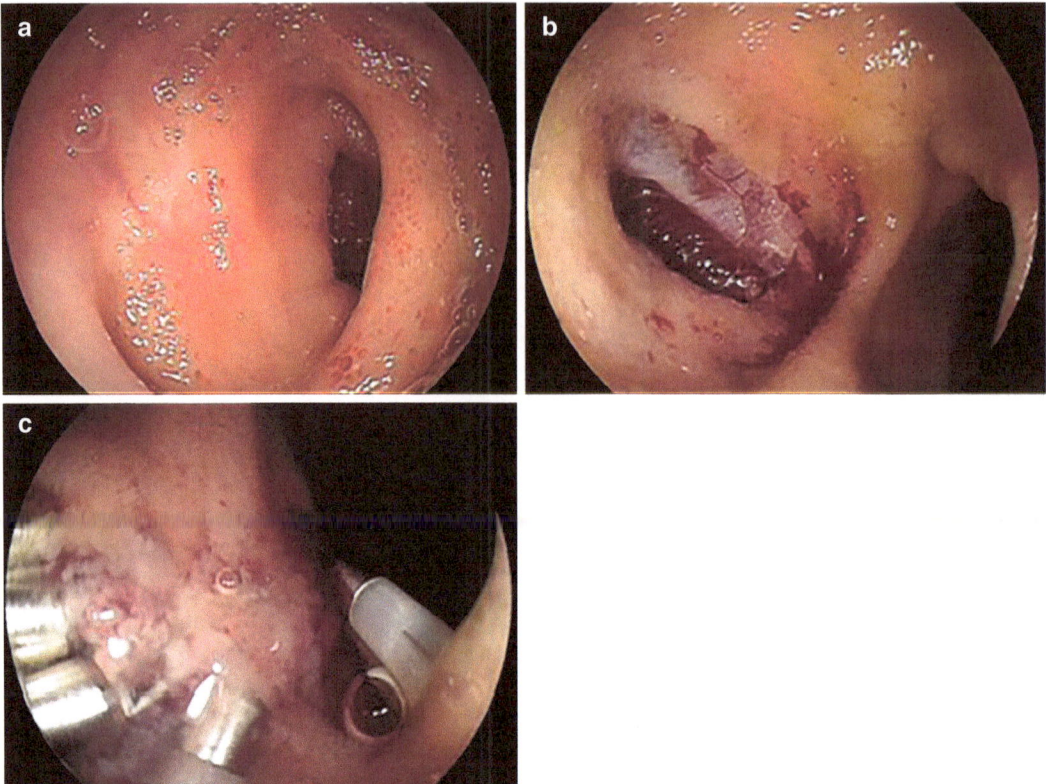

Fig. 1 (**a**) The patient had a history of abdominal surgery and combined radiation enteritis. Per-anal double-balloon enteroscopy was performed for suspected small bowel bleeding. (**b**) A perforation occurred while inserting the enteroscope. (**c**) The perforation site was closed using hemoclips

polypectomy for large polyps and in retrograde (per-anal) enteroscopy procedures in patients with a surgically altered anatomy [2, 7]. To reduce the risk of perforation, piecemeal resection is recommended for large polyps [8]. If a sense of severe resistance is transmitted through the scope, as when it is trapped in an adhesive and fixed bowel segment, the scope should be manipulated very carefully to avoid tearing of the bowel or mesentery [4]. The incidence of perforation related to balloon dilation for strictures in Crohn's disease has been reported as high as 7.7% (1/11) in an earlier small study [9]; however, a subsequent study reported a perforation rate of 1.5% (1/65) [3]. When perform-

ing argon plasma coagulation for hemostasis, perforation can occur in 1% [2, 6].

Acute Pancreatitis

Acute pancreatitis can occur in 0.3% of cases after antegrade (per-oral) diagnostic DBE procedures and mostly presents with abdominal pain within 24 h of the procedure [5, 6]. Given that most pancreatitis after DBE occurs at the tail of the pancreas, physical stress on the duodenum and pancreas during the per-oral insertion procedure is a potential cause of pancreatitis [8]. Acute pancreatitis can occur after antegrade SBE and very rarely after retrograde (per-anal) DBE or SBE [8].

Sedation-Related Complications

To minimize the discomfort of patients in a prolonged procedure, it is common to perform DAE under deep sedation or general anesthesia. As a result, various sedation-related complications, such as decrease or increase in blood pressure, hypoxia, arrhythmia, and aspiration, can occur. It has been reported that the incidence rate of aspiration pneumonia after DBE is 0.07% [1].

Other Complications

There are two reported cases of hemoperitoneum without damages in the small intestine, one in DBE and the other in SE. Both patients had a history of abdominal surgery [4]. Transient pneumobilia without perforation has been reported in a patient with Crohn's disease after DBE and balloon dilation for strictures. Subcutaneous emphysema without a visible intestinal perforation after a retrograde DBE has been observed. The risk of these rare complications that do not show overt perforation may be reduced if carbon dioxide is used instead of air during the procedure and if an excessively long operation is avoided [4]. One case of superior mesenteric artery thrombosis after DBE in a patient with Crohn's disease has been reported [4]. It is known that post-procedural increase in serum amylase level can occur from 17 to 51%; however, it does not require treatment [4].

Conclusions

Various complications can occur in both diagnostic and therapeutic DAE procedures owing to the use of an overtube, physical pressure on the small bowel and adjacent organs during the deep insertion process, prolonged procedure time, and necessity of deep sedation. The risk of bleeding and perforation significantly increases in therapeutic procedures. Endoscopists should make an effort to prevent complications related to DAE, recognize the complications as early as possible, and provide proper treatment.

References

1. Xin L, Liao Z, Jiang YP, Li ZS. Indications, detectability, positive findings, total enteroscopy, and complications of diagnostic double-balloon endoscopy: a systematic review of data over the first decade of use. Gastrointest Endosc. 2011;74:563–70.
2. May A, Nachbar L, Pohl J, Ell C. Endoscopic interventions in the small bowel using double balloon enteroscopy: feasibility and limitations. Am J Gastroenterol. 2007;102:527–35.
3. Hirai F, Beppu T, Takatsu N, et al. Long-term outcome of endoscopic balloon dilation for small bowel strictures in patients with Crohn's disease. Dig Endosc. 2014;26:545–51.
4. Chavalitdhamrong D, Adler DG, Draganov PV. Complications of enteroscopy: how to avoid them and manage them when they arise. Gastrointest Endosc Clin N Am. 2015;25:83–95.
5. Moschler O, May A, Muller MK, Ell C, German DBESG. Complications in and performance of double-balloon enteroscopy (DBE): results from a large prospective DBE database in Germany. Endoscopy. 2011;43:484–9.
6. Mensink PB, Haringsma J, Kucharzik T, et al. Complications of double balloon enteroscopy: a multicenter survey. Endoscopy. 2007;39:613–5.
7. Gerson LB, Tokar J, Chiorean M, et al. Complications associated with double balloon enteroscopy at nine US centers. Clin Gastroenterol Hepatol. 2009;7:1177–1182, 1182.e1–3.
8. Yamamoto H, Ogata H, Matsumoto T, et al. Clinical practice guideline for enteroscopy. Dig Endosc. 2017;29:519–46.
9. Despott EJ, Gupta A, Burling D, et al. Effective dilation of small-bowel strictures by double-balloon enteroscopy in patients with symptomatic Crohn's disease (with video). Gastrointest Endosc. 2009;70:1030–6.

Various Applications of Device-Assisted Enteroscopy

Jin Su Kim

Key Points
- The indications of device-assisted enteroscopy are now expanding into areas such as altered gastrointestinal anatomy, incomplete colonoscopy, and small bowel stenting.
- With the development of devices and techniques, the utilization of device-assisted enteroscopy is expected to increase not only in simple small intestine diseases but also in various gastrointestinal diseases.

Device-assisted enteroscopy (DAE) is commonly used to diagnose and treat obscure gastrointestinal bleeding, and to diagnose small bowel tumors and inflammatory bowel disease. With the development of devices and enteroscopic techniques, the indication of DAE is expanding steadily, and DAE has been applied to various clinical settings, such as endoscopic resection of small bowel tumors, small bowel stenting due to malignant or benign obstruction, and foreign body removal from the small bowel. DAE uses unique attachment devices called an overtube and balloon that can effectively resolve the intestinal loop that occurs when the endoscope enters the small bowel.

Device-Assisted Enteroscopy in Altered Anatomy

The endoscopic approach to a lesion in the small bowel and biliary tract was limited or impossible in patients who underwent various operations, such as Roux-en-Y anastomosis and Billroth II subtotal gastrectomy. This is because the intestinal loop that occurs cannot be properly resolved owing to postoperative adhesions, which make it difficult for the endoscope to enter the deep part of the intestine. In addition, when entering the afferent loop from the jejuno-jejunal anastomotic junction, a V-shaped sharp acute angle is created, which is an obstacle to deep insertion of the enteroscope into the afferent loop due to paradoxical movement of the scope similar to that in the duodenal bulb. DAE can fix and tightly hold the intestine through the overtube and attached balloon, and then pull the endoscope and overtube to resolve the sharp angulated intestinal loop. After the angulated small bowel is straightened, the enteroscope can be pushed into the afferent loop without paradoxical movement. In altered anatomy of the small bowel, endoscopy is often performed for endoscopic retrograde cholangiopancreatography (ERCP). DAE, which is generally used for diagnostic and therapeutic

J. S. Kim (✉)
Department of Gastroenterology, The Catholic University of Korea, Seoul, South Korea

purposes, has a working channel of only 2.8 mm in diameter, which limits the use of instruments for ERCP. A short double-balloon enteroscope (EI-580BT; Fujifilm, Tokyo, Japan) with a length of 155 cm and a working channel of 3.2 mm can be used instead. In addition to using DAE in ERCP, it can be used to diagnose and treat small intestinal hemorrhagic disease or remove foreign bodies in patients with altered anatomy (Fig. 1a–c).

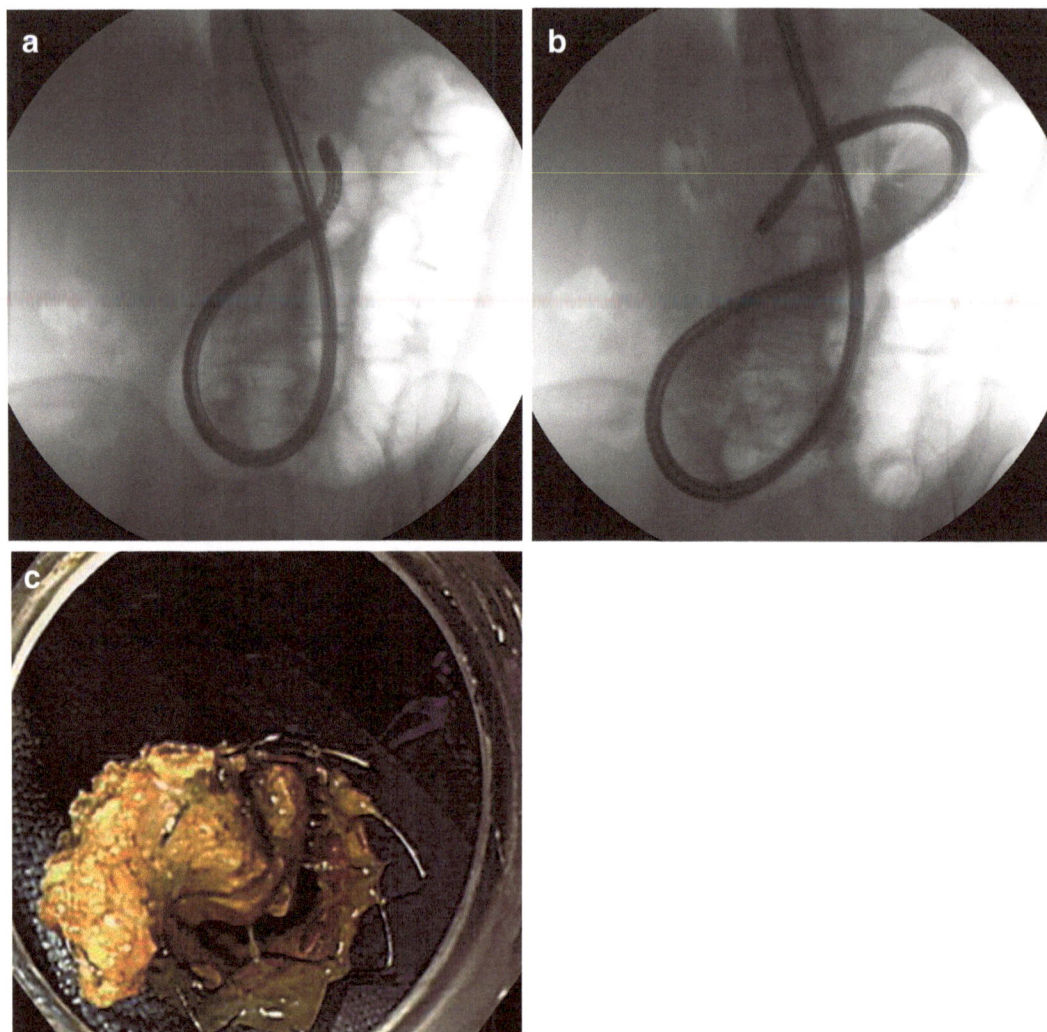

Fig. 1 Removal of a migrated biliary stent in a total gastrectomy state. (**a**) After passing through the jejunum-jejunum anastomosis, it is difficult to enter into the distal end of the afferent loop due to paradoxical movement of the scope during insertion. (**b**) After passing the overtube over the jejunum-jejunum anastomosis and ballooning, the enteroscope is inserted into the distal end of the afferent loop without paradoxical movement. (**c**) The migrated biliary stent is removed with biopsy forceps after the papillary area is reached

Device-Assisted Enteroscopy in Incomplete Colonoscopy

In a colonoscopy, insertion into the cecum is performed in 95–99% of patients, and when the colonoscope cannot reach the cecum, it is called incomplete colonoscopy [1, 2]. A previous history of abdominal surgery, female sex, diverticulosis, a redundant large bowel, history of abdominal radiotherapy, and low body mass index increase the risk of incomplete colonoscopy. The presence of such a risk factor makes it difficult to insert the colonoscope into the cecum because of severe angulation due to adhesion during colonoscopy, formation of the large bowel loop, and severe pain during insertion. In the case of incomplete colonoscopy, a pediatric colonoscope, gastroscope, colonoscope with variable stiffness, and push enteroscope can be used for cecal intubation. When the pediatric colonoscope and push enteroscope were used in patients with incomplete colonoscopy, insertion up to the cecum was possible in 58% and 69% of patients, respectively. However, in 30–40% of patients, insertion into the cecum was still impossible even with the aforementioned method.

Recently, the usefulness of DAE in incomplete colonoscopy has been demonstrated. In one single study, cecum insertion was possible in 88–100% of double-balloon endoscopies and 93–96% of single balloon endoscopies. DAE can effectively control the loop that develops during insertion, making it easy to insert the scope into the cecum. In a multicenter prospective study, cecum insertion was possible in 110 patients using DAE, with an average insertion time of 12 min. Complications related to the procedure were only mild mucosal injury in one patient [3].

Small Bowel Stenting with Device-Assisted Enteroscopy

Unlike gastric, duodenal, and colonic obstruction, the endoscopic approach and treatment of small bowel obstruction due to malignant or benign obstruction is generally impossible. After the development of DAE, endoscopic access to the site of the small bowel obstruction became possible. However, the diameter of the working channel is too small to insert the small bowel stent using the through-the-scope method.

When the stent is inserted using the over-the-wire (OTW) method along the inserted guidewire, it is very difficult to insert the stent into the deep small intestine along the guidewire due to looping of the guidewire in the stomach and small intestine. To overcome such problems, the OTW stent insertion method using the overtube has been reported [4]. This method can suppress the occurrence of loops during insertion of a stent and makes it possible to insert the stent into the deep small bowel (Fig. 2a–f).

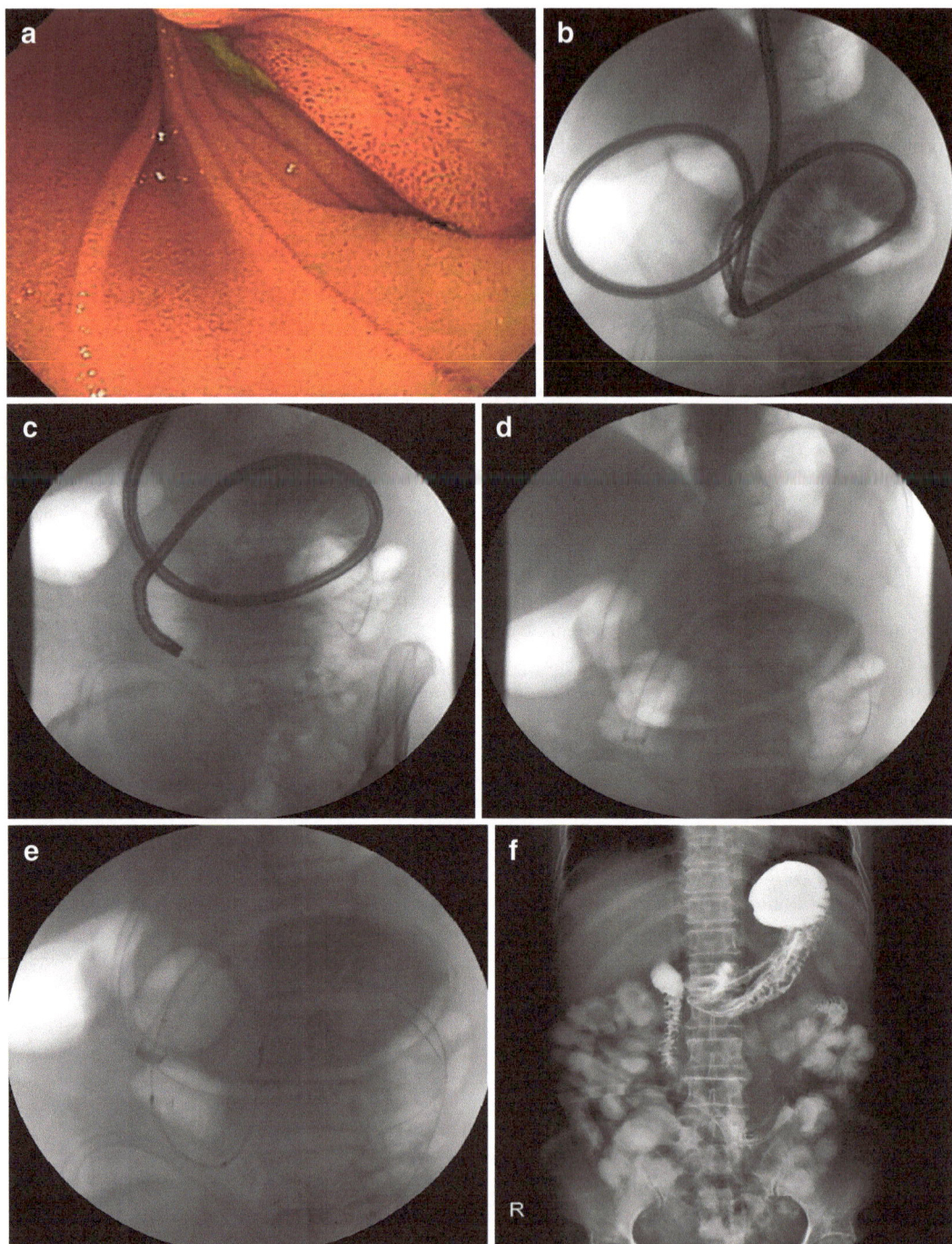

Fig. 2 Small bowel stent using the overtube technique. (**a**) Insertion of the enteroscope into the lesion causing the small bowel obstruction. (**b**) During insertion of the enteroscope, intestinal loops are usually created, and it is crucial to resolve the loop before the procedure and straighten the enteroscope. (**c**) After expanding the balloon attached to the overtube, the enteroscope and overtube are pulled to resolve the loop, and the guidewire is inserted over the lesion. (**d**) Only the enteroscope is withdrawn and the overtube and guidewire remain. (**e**) The stent is inserted along the guidewire using the over-the-wire method. (**f**) In the small bowel series, after the procedure is performed, the contrast agent passes smoothly through the deployed stent

References

1. Shimatani M, Tokuhara M, Kato K, et al. Utility of newly developed short-type double-balloon endoscopy for endoscopic retrograde cholangiography in postoperative patients. J Gastroenterol Hepatol. 2017;32:1348–54.
2. Takahashi Y, Tanaka H, Kinjo M, Sakumoto K. Prospective evaluation of factors predicting difficulty and pain during sedation-free colonoscopy. Dis Colon Rectum. 2005;48:1295–300.
3. Hotta K, Katsuki S, Ohata K, et al. A multicenter, prospective trial of total colonoscopy using a short double-balloon endoscope in patients with previous incomplete colonoscopy. Gastrointest Endosc. 2012;75:813–8.
4. Espinel J, Pinedo E. A simplified method for stent placement in the distal duodenum: enteroscopy overtube. World J Gastrointest Endosc. 2011;3:225–7.

Part VI

Miscellaneous Tests for Small Bowel Disorders

Principle and Clinical Application of the Hydrogen Breath Test

Kwang Jae Lee

Key Points

- There are many bacteria in the large intestine. In contrast, relatively few bacteria live in the small intestine, particularly in the proximal small intestine.
- Bacterial overgrowth of the small intestine may occur in various conditions such as irritable bowel syndrome, inflammatory bowel diseases, gastrointestinal motility disorders, hypochlorhydria, immunosuppressed states, gastrointestinal structural abnormalities, liver cirrhosis, and chronic pancreatitis.
- In the lactulose hydrogen breath test, the criterion that measures an early increase of hydrogen levels in the exhaled air is generally used but may produce false-positive results when the orocecal transit time is short. The glucose hydrogen breath test has the disadvantage that it is not able to diagnose bacterial overgrowth present only in the distal small intestine.
- Lactose or fructose malabsorption can also be diagnosed using the hydrogen breath test.

Recently, many studies have suggested that many microorganisms are present in the gastrointestinal tract and that the gut microbiota is associated with diverse diseases. The upper gastrointestinal tract has a relatively small number of bacteria due to the influence of gastric acid, but the bacterial number increases when reaching the distal part [1, 2]. The small intestine has a relatively small number of bacteria compared to that in the large intestine. Small intestinal bacterial overgrowth (SIBO), in which the number of bacteria is abnormally increased in the small intestine, is associated with a variety of gastrointestinal and hepatobiliary diseases (Table 1) [3]. Invasive and noninvasive tests are used to diagnose SIBO. Culturing the jejunal aspirates is a relatively invasive method and cannot detect SIBO distal to the jejunum. Moreover, only a part of gut microbiota can be detected by culture. The hydrogen breath test is a simpler and noninvasive method and is commonly used.

The hydrogen breath test can be used to diagnose malabsorption or intolerance of lactose or fructose, as well as to confirm SIBO. This chapter reviews the principle, method, and clinical application of the hydrogen breath test.

Principles

When food materials are digested and fermented by intestinal bacteria, gases such as carbon dioxide, hydrogen, and methane are produced. Those

K. J. Lee (✉)
Department of Gastroenterology, Ajou University School of Medicine, Suwon, South Korea
e-mail: kjl@ajou.ac.kr

© Springer Nature Singapore Pte Ltd. 2022
H. J. Chun et al. (eds.), *Small Intestine Disease*, https://doi.org/10.1007/978-981-16-7239-2_31

Table 1 Diseases or conditions related to small intestine bacterial overgrowth

	Disease
Gastrointestinal diseases	Irritable bowel syndrome
	Celiac disease
	Inflammatory bowel disease
	Chronic intestinal pseudo-obstruction
	Connective tissue diseases with small bowel involvement such as systemic sclerosis
	Gastric surgery
	Enteric surgery
	Short bowel syndrome
	Small intestinal diverticula
	Enteric fistula or stricture
	Visceral neuropathy associated with diabetes mellitus or amyloidosis
	Lactose malabsorption
Hepatobiliary diseases	Liver cirrhosis
	Non-alcoholic fatty liver disease
	Spontaneous bacterial peritonitis
	Chronic pancreatitis
Other conditions	Chronic use of proton pump inhibitors
	Immune deficiency states
	Hypothyroidism
	Chronic renal diseases
	Advanced age

gases diffuse into the systemic circulation and are expired through the lungs. Although carbon dioxide is produced during the metabolic processes of cells as well, hydrogen and methane gases are produced only by bacteria. The hydrogen breath test is a method of measuring the amount of hydrogen in the exhaled air by gas chromatography. Generally, anaerobic bacteria in the large intestine produce hydrogen when they encounter sugars or carbohydrates not absorbed in the small intestine. When the processes related to digestion or absorption of sugars or carbohydrates are disrupted in the small intestine, a large amount of hydrogen is generated in the large intestine. In SIBO, an increase in the number of bacteria in the small intestine, in turn, increases the amount of hydrogen produced in the small intestine. The hydrogen is absorbed through the wall of the small intestine or large intestine, enters the blood vessel, moves to the lungs, and is discharged

through exhalation. Therefore, if there are excessive bacteria in the small intestine, the amount of hydrogen gas in the exhaled air increases before the gas reaches the large intestine. If there is absorption failure of a specific carbohydrate, a large amount of hydrogen is produced in the large intestine, causing an abnormal increase of hydrogen in the exhaled air.

To diagnose SIBO in the small intestine, substances such as lactulose, which are not digested or absorbed in the small intestine, are generally used. In the case of SIBO, the increase in the hydrogen level in the exhaled air can be observed before the gas reaches the large intestine or produces two peaks, one in the small intestine and one in the large intestine. However, when the intestinal transit time is short, the increase in hydrogen level can also be observed early after the ingestion of lactulose, causing a false-positive diagnosis of SIBO.

Approximately 15–30% of people have intestinal flora including *Methanobrevibacter smithii*. Because this type of bacteria converts hydrogen gas into methane gas, the presence of SIBO or carbohydrate malabsorption does not increase the amount of hydrogen gas in the exhaled air. Instead, the amount of methane gas increases [4]. Therefore, it is recommended to measure methane gas in addition to hydrogen gas to reduce the false-negative diagnosis rate.

Methods

Slowly absorbed carbohydrates and fiber, such as those in bread, vegetables, fruits, pasta, and soybeans, should be avoided from the evening of the day before the test. Drinking water is generally acceptable, but it is recommended to fast for 8–12 h. Sleep, smoking, and exercise are not permitted for at least 1 h before the test, because they affect respiration and may change the amount of hydrogen in the exhaled air. Antibiotics should be avoided for 4 weeks before the breath test. Prokinetics and laxatives should be stopped at least 1 week prior to the breath test. Conclusive data on the discontinuation or continuation of probiotics, motility-reducing agents, and acid inhibitory agents before the test are lacking.

To prevent the early increase in hydrogen concentration owing to the bacteria present in the mouth, brushing the teeth and rinsing the mouth with mouthwash and tap water are recommended before the breath test. After measuring the basal hydrogen concentration in exhalation, patients are asked to orally ingest 10 g of lactulose, 75 g or 1 g/kg of glucose, 25 g of lactose, or 25 g of fructose mixed with 200–250 mL of water as a test material. Exhalation gas is collected in 15 min intervals for 2 h after the ingestion of glucose and for 2–4 h after the ingestion of lactulose. Subsequently, the amount of hydrogen and methane is measured by a commercially available machine (Fig. 1). Samples are collected for at least 3 h after the ingestion of lactose or fructose. The assessment of symptoms during the test is recommended as well. In the lactose tolerance test, the blood glucose level is generally measured in a fasting state and 30 min after the intake of lactose together with the hydrogen breath test [5].

Results

An average basal hydrogen level in the exhaled air above 16 ppm is considered abnormally high, wherein the test should not be carried out. In that situation, pre-treatment should be performed again before the start of the hydrogen breath test. In the hydrogen breath test, SIBO is diagnosed when the hydrogen level is above 20 ppm from the baseline [6]. In the lactulose breath test, the presence of two peaks above 20 ppm from the baseline value may lead to the diagnosis of SIBO. However, the data on the validity of a double peak are lacking [6]. The sensitivity of the glucose hydrogen breath test is 20–93%, indicating a large difference between the reports. Furthermore, SIBO in the distal small intestine that is not accompanied by SIBO in the proximal small intestine cannot be detected by the glucose hydrogen breath test. The lactulose hydrogen breath test also has a low diagnostic sensitivity for SIBO (31–68%) [7, 8]. The diagnostic criteria for the lactulose hydrogen breath test is a result of 20 ppm or higher above the baseline value within 90 min. However, when the orocecal transit time is less than 90 min, those criteria are not

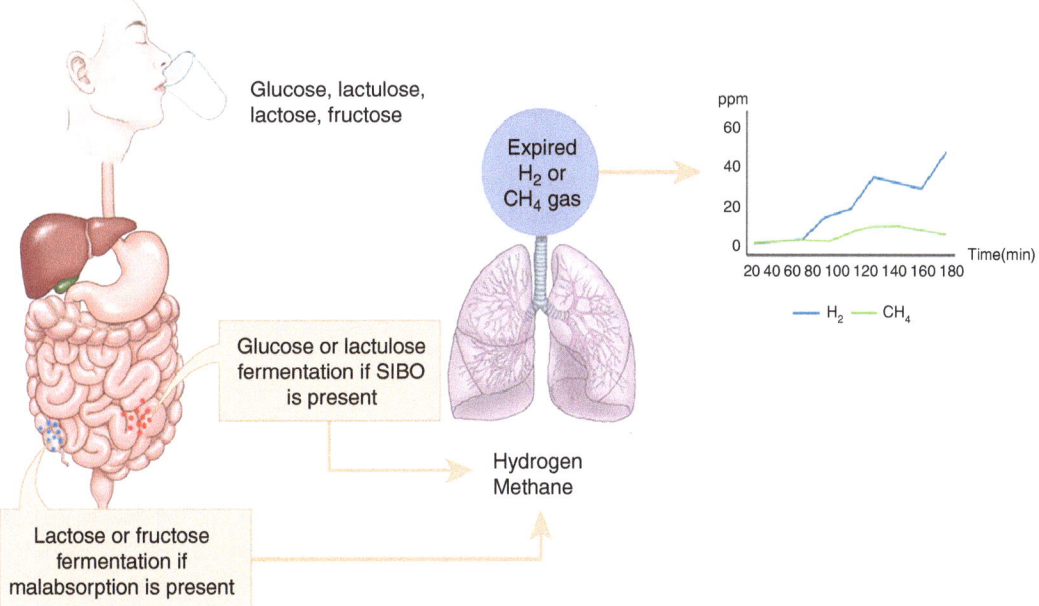

Fig. 1 Principles of the hydrogen breath test to diagnose small intestinal bacterial overgrowth

suitable. Patients exhibiting the diarrhea subtype of irritable bowel syndrome are considered to have a shorter orocecal transit time due to increased intestinal motility. Asian people are also known to have a shorter orocecal transit time than Western populations. Therefore, the diagnostic criteria using the early increase in the hydrogen level are not likely to be appropriate, particularly in Asia, unless the orocecal transit time is measured simultaneously by a radioisotope-labeled scintigraphic method [9, 10]. A level of 10 ppm or higher over the baseline can be considered positive for the methane breath test [6].

When the hydrogen level in the exhaled air is increased above 20 ppm from the baseline, or the methane level is increased above 10 ppm from the baseline in the lactose or fructose hydrogen breath test, it is considered to indicate malabsorption or intolerance. When the blood glucose level is not increased above 20 mg/dL at 30 min after lactose intake, it is also regarded as malabsorption or intolerance. However, a false-negative result is common [5].

Limitations

There are some limitations in diagnosing SIBO using the hydrogen breath test. The lactulose hydrogen breath test shows different diagnostic sensitivity depending on the diagnostic criteria [7, 8]. In addition, the culture test of the jejunal aspiration is not suitable as a standard test, because only 30% of the gut microorganisms can be cultured and the test site is limited to the proximal small intestine. Because glucose is completely absorbed in the proximal small intestine, bacterial overgrowth of the distal small intestine cannot be diagnosed by the glucose hydrogen breath test. Therefore, the glucose hydrogen breath test may underestimate SIBO prevalence. The lactulose hydrogen breath test is affected by the orocecal transit time. If the transit time is long, the increase of hydrogen level in the exhaled air appears late because it requires a long time to reach the cecum. On the contrary, if the transit time is short, the increase of hydrogen concentra-

tion in the exhaled air appears early, which is misdiagnosed as SIBO. Therefore, a combination of the hydrogen breath test with the measurement of the orocecal transit time is desirable. It is suggested that SIBO be diagnosed when the hydrogen level in the exhaled air increases above 5 ppm from the baseline at least 15 min before the radioisotope reaches the cecum when the combination of the lactulose hydrogen breath test and ^{99m}Tc-DTPA small intestine transit time test is performed simultaneously [11]. SIBO cannot be detected through the hydrogen breath test if bacteria in the small intestine produce other gases such as methane or hydrogen sulfide without producing hydrogen. The level of methane gas can be measured, but that of the hydrogen sulfide cannot be measured yet. Methane is known to be associated with constipation [12]. The diagnosis of SIBO by the hydrogen breath test does not always guarantee that the symptoms of the patients are caused by SIBO. If symptoms are improved by the treatment of SIBO, the diagnosis is confirmed.

Clinical Applications

Symptoms associated with SIBO are non-specific and the presence of SIBO can be suspected when symptoms are accompanied by conditions that may cause SIBO. The hydrogen breath test is recommended for patients with chronic abdominal symptoms including bloating, gas, and diarrhea, and particularly in those with conditions such as irritable bowel syndrome, inflammatory bowel diseases, gastrointestinal motility disorders, hypochlorhydria, immunosuppressed states, gastrointestinal structural abnormalities, cirrhosis, and chronic pancreatitis.

Conclusion

The hydrogen breath test is a diagnostic tool for SIBO and is simple and easy to perform. However, its sensitivity and specificity vary according to the materials used and the method of analysis. In the lactulose breath test, the diagnostic criterion using the early increase in the hydrogen concentration in the exhaled air is commonly used but may produce false-positive results when the orocecal transit time is short. The other diagnostic criterion involving the assessment of the two peaks of hydrogen level has the disadvantage of low sensitivity and is not recommended. Simultaneous measurement of small intestinal transit time using the radioisotope with the lactulose breath hydrogen test appears to be ideal. In the glucose breath test, a false-negative result can be a problem when SIBO is present only in the distal small intestine. Each methodology has its own advantages and disadvantages. The choice of methodology may be affected by the suspected location of SIBO and intestinal transit time. If SIBO is suspected to be in the proximal small intestine, the glucose hydrogen breath test is recommended. If SIBO is suspected to be in the distal small intestine, the lactulose breath hydrogen test appears to be more appropriate than the glucose hydrogen breath test; however, in that case, consideration of small intestinal transit time may be necessary. Methane gas measurement is important, particularly in patients with constipation. The diagnostic criteria and test methodology to increase sensitivity, indications for use, and relationship of SIBO with patient's symptoms need to be established.

References

1. Mackie RI, Sghir A, Gaskins HR. Developmental microbial ecology of the neonatal gastrointestinal tract. Am J Clin Nutr. 1999;69:1035S–45S.
2. Gabrielli M, D'Angelo G, Di Rienzo T, et al. Diagnosis of small intestinal bacterial overgrowth in the clinical practice. Eur Rev Med Pharmacol Sci. 2013;17(Suppl 2):30–5.
3. Ghoshal UC, Ghoshal U. Small intestinal bacterial overgrowth and other intestinal disorders. Gastroenterol Clin N Am. 2017;46:103–20.
4. Levitt MD, Furne JK, Kuskowski M, Ruddy J. Stability of human methanogenic flora over 35 years and a review of insights obtained from breath methane measurements. Clin Gastroenterol Hepatol. 2006;4:123–9.
5. Babu J, Kumar S, Babu P, Prasad JH, Ghoshal UC. Frequency of lactose malabsorption among healthy southern and northern Indian populations by genetic analysis and lactose hydrogen breath and tolerance tests. Am J Clin Nutr. 2009;91:140–6.
6. Rezaie A, Buresi M, Lembo A, et al. Hydrogen and methane-based breath testing in gastrointestinal disorders: the north American consensus. Am J Gastroenterol. 2017;112:775–84.
7. Ghoshal UC, Srivastava D, Ghoshal U, et al. Breath tests in the diagnosis of small intestinal bacterial overgrowth in patients with irritable bowel syndrome in comparison with quantitative upper gut aspirate culture. Eur J Gastroenterol Hepatol. 2014;26:753–60.
8. Khoshini R, Dai SC, Lezcano S, Pimentel M. A systematic review of diagnostic tests for small intestinal bacterial overgrowth. Dig Dis Sci. 2008;53:1443–54.
9. Ghoshal UC, Ghoshal U, Ayyagari A, et al. Tropical sprue is associated with contamination of small bowel with aerobic bacteria and reversible prolongation of orocecal transit time. J Gastroenterol Hepatol. 2003;18:540–7.
10. Lu CL, Chen CY, Chang FY, Lee SD. Characteristics of small bowel motility in patients with irritable bowel syndrome and normal humans: an oriental study. Clin Sci (Lond). 1998;95:165–9.
11. Zhao J, Zheng X, Chu H, et al. A study of the methodological and clinical validity of the combined lactulose hydrogen breath test with scintigraphic orocecal transit test for diagnosing small intestinal bacterial overgrowth in IBS patients. Neurogastroenterol Motil. 2014;26:794–802.
12. Ghoshal UC, Srivastava D, Verma A, Misra A. Slow transit constipation associated with excess methane production and its improvement following rifaximin therapy: a case report. J Neurogastroenterol Motil. 2011;17:48–51.

The Principles and Practice of Alpha-1 Antitrypsin Clearance

Eun Ran Kim

Introduction

In healthy individuals, only 1–2% of total daily protein is lost through the gastrointestinal (GI) tract. Protein loss through the GI tract is derived from active intestinal secretions such as pancreatic and biliary secretions, and mucosal turnover. About 10% of albumin metabolism is lost through the GI tract [1].

Even if serum protein loss through the GI tract is increasing, retinol-binding protein, pre-albumin, immunoglobulin E, clotting factors, transferrin, and so on are almost preserved because of their rapid turnover rate. However, albumin, which contributes to approximately 80% of the total colloidal osmotic effect of human serum, is a slow turnover protein with a half-life of about 15–30 days. In case of increased serum protein loss, albumin synthesis is increased by 25%. If serum protein loss is excessive, the balance between protein synthesis and metabolism can be altered in resulting in decreased serum albumin; this situation results in third-spacing of fluid, which generally manifests clinically as peripheral edema, ascites, and pleural effusions.

Protein-losing enteropathy (PLE) is defined as a diverse group of disorders associated with

excessive loss of serum protein through the GI tract. Although the key clinical characteristics of PLE are hypoalbuminemia and edema, hypoalbuminemia and edema can be caused by other diseases such as hepatic synthetic dysfunction, malnutrition, nephrosis, and other benign and malignant chronic diseases. Therefore, the diagnosis of PLE is based on the verification of serum protein loss through the GI tract in addition to hypoalbuminemia, hypogammaglobulinemia, and edema.

PLE is an unusual cause of hypoproteinemia and is characterized by the shedding of large quantities of protein from the GI mucosa. PLE may result from a wide variety of etiologies and can be both, a diagnostic and a therapeutic challenge to the practicing gastroenterologist.

Previously, protein loss through the GI tract was measured by the fecal excretion of labeled protein following intravenous (IV) administration of radioactive materials for an average of 5–12 days. This method markedly limits its clinical utility as it imposes, on the patient, the need to undergo the requisite radioactive exposure and the long experimental period of daily stool collection after infusion of the labeled protein [2]. Currently, the methods used to quantitate the loss of protein through the GI tract are alpha 1-antitrypsin (α_1-AT) clearance measurement, or simply the measurement of fecal α_1-AT concentration (mg/dry weight) or the amount of α_1-AT in stool collected over a given period (e.g., 1 day).

E. R. Kim (✉)
Division of Gastroenterology, Department of Internal Medicine, Sungkyunkwan University School of Medicine, Samsung Medical Center, Seoul, South Korea

α1-Antitrypsin

α_1-AT constitutes 4% of all serum protein and it is similar in size to albumin (50 kDa).

α_1-AT is mainly (over 80%) synthesized and secreted by hepatocytes and in additional quantities by the intestinal macrophages, monocytes, and epithelial cells. α_1-AT acts as the principal inhibitor of neutrophil elastase and other human serine proteases. During acute-phase responses, α_1-AT levels increase up to fourfold; this plays an anti-inflammatory or tissue-protecting role through the reduction of proteolytic activity by free elastase from neutrophils [3]. Because α_1-AT inhibits various proteases, it is neither absorbed nor physiologically secreted into the intestine, and it is resistant to intestinal proteolysis; measurement of its fecal loss should be indicative of the rate of loss of similar-sized serum proteins. However, detecting plasma protein loss from the stomach by measuring fecal α_1-AT clearance is quite difficult. This is because α_1-AT is rapidly destroyed in the gastric juice at pH values below three. Therefore, it is useful for detecting protein-losing gastropathy by measuring fecal α_1-AT clearance and administering a proton pump inhibitor to suppress the acid level [4].

α1-Antitrypsin Clearance

The loss of protein through the GI tract can be detected by increased α_1-AT concentration (or amounts) in a collected stool sample, or by measuring fecal α_1-AT clearance. Fecal α_1-AT clearance is a more reliable marker than fecal α_1-AT concentration because the loss of protein through GI tract is influenced by the type and severity of diseases and the serum protein concentration.

When fecal α_1-AT concentration and fecal α_1-AT clearance were compared between normal subjects and subjects with GI disorders, the fecal α_1-AT concentration showed about 21% errors in both groups. However, when the normal subjects had diarrhea, secondary to the ingestion of poorly absorbed solutes, their fecal α_1-AT clearance and the total amount of α_1-AT in their stool samples increased, while their fecal α_1-AT concentration decreased [5].

By measuring the α_1-AT levels in both serum and a 24-hourly stool sample, α_1-AT clearance can be calculated as follows [6, 7]:

$$\alpha_1 - \text{antitrypsin}\,(AT)\,\text{plasma clearance} = \left(\left[\text{Daily stool volume}\right] \times \left[\text{Stool}\,\alpha_1 - AT\right]\right) / \text{Serum}\,\alpha_1 - AT$$

An elevated α_1-AT clearance >24 mL/day reflects abnormal GI protein loss in patients without diarrhea. Diarrhea, irrespective of the cause, results in some obligate α_1-AT loss and, thus, a higher threshold (>56 mL/day) is considered as abnormal GI protein loss for the diagnosis of PLE in patients with diarrhea.

There is an inverse correlation between serum albumin and α_1-AT clearance; when serum albumin levels fall below 3 g/dL, α_1-AT clearance exceeds 180 mL/day. In case of the presence of intestinal bleeding, α_1-AT clearance is elevated. Therefore, α_1-AT clearance must be interpreted by taking these situations into consideration [6].

Summary or Conclusion

α_1-AT is similar in size to albumin and mainly synthesized in the liver. α_1-AT is neither absorbed nor secreted in the intestine, and resistant to proteolysis. Therefore, α_1-AT is normally present in the stool in low concentrations. Consequently, the measurement of α_1-AT clearance is a reliable indicator of the rate of loss of similar-sized serum proteins, and it is a useful method for the diagnosis and follow-up of PLE.

References

1. Wochner RD, Weissman SM, Waldmann TA, Houston D, Berlin NI. Direct measurement of the rates of synthesis of plasma proteins in control subjects and patients with gastrointestinal protein loss. J Clin Invest. 1968;47:971–82.
2. Levitt DG, Levitt MD. Protein losing enteropathy: comprehensive review of the mechanistic association with clinical and subclinical disease states. Clin Exp Gastroenterol. 2017;10:147–68.
3. de Serres F, Blanco I. Role of alpha-1 antitrypsin in human health and disease. J Intern Med. 2014;276:311–35.
4. Takeda H, Nishise S, Furukawa M, Nagashima R, Shinzawa H, Takahashi T. Fecal clearance of alpha1-antitrypsin with lansoprazole can detect protein-losing gastropathy. Dig Dis Sci. 1999;44:2313–8.
5. Strygler B, Nicar MJ, Santangelo WC, Porter JL, Fordtran JS. Alpha 1-antitrypsin excretion in stool in normal subjects and in patients with gastrointestinal disorders. Gastroenterology. 1990;99:1380–7.
6. Feldman M. Sleisenger and Fordtran's gastrointestinal and liver disease. 10th ed. Philadelphia, PA: Elsevier; 2015.
7. Magazzu G, Jacono G, Di Pasquale G, et al. Reliability and usefulness of random fecal alpha 1-antitrypsin concentration: further simplification of the method. J Pediatr Gastroenterol Nutr. 1985;4:402–7.

Hemodynamically Unstable Patients with Acute Gastrointestinal Bleeding

Chung Hyun Tae and Ki-Nam Shim

Key Points
- Emergency angiography should be considered in hemodynamically unstable patients with acute gastrointestinal bleeding of unknown origin.
- Small-intestine endoscopy or intraoperative small intestine endoscopy could be performed in cases of failure of detection of the bleeding focus on angiography.

Introduction

Obscure gastrointestinal bleeding (OGIB) refers to gastrointestinal (GI) bleeding of unclear origin that persists or recurs after obtaining negative findings on esophagogastroduodenoscopy and colonoscopy. OGIB accounts for approximately 5% of all types of GI bleeding. The ability to detect OGIB in the small bowel has been significantly revolutionized by the introduction of capsule endoscopy, double-balloon enteroscopy, computed tomography enterography, magnetic resonance enterography, and angiography. In approximately 75% of OGIB cases, lesions are detected in the small bowel distal to Vater's papilla. OGIB is classified as "occult" when fecal occult blood tests are positive or iron deficiency anemia is presumed to be caused by GI blood loss, and as "overt" when there are manifestations of bleeding such as hematochezia or melena. In addition, according to clinical manifestations, OGIB is classified as chronic or subacute bleeding in patients in a hemodynamically stable condition and as acute bleeding in patients in a hemodynamically unstable condition. We here describe a systematic approach for hemodynamically unstable patients with OGIB.

Systematic Diagnostic Approach

Clinical Manifestations and Physical Examination

The initial evaluation of a patient with a suspected clinically significant acute GI bleeding includes history taking, physical examination, laboratory tests, and, in some cases, nasogastric lavage. The goal of the evaluation is to assess the severity of bleeding, identify potential bleeding sources, and determine the status of bleeding (ongoing or has stopped). In most cases, hematemesis is highly specific for bleeding proximal to the ligament of Treitz, whereas hematochezia is more suggestive of bleeding distal to the ligament of Treitz. However, these are not reliable indicators of potential bleeding location because they are influenced by the bleeding

C. H. Tae · K.-N. Shim (✉)
Department of Internal Medicine, Ewha Womans University College of Medicine, Seoul, Korea
e-mail: jhtae@ewha.ac.kr; shimkn@ewha.ac.kr

© Springer Nature Singapore Pte Ltd. 2022
H. J. Chun et al. (eds.), *Small Intestine Disease*, https://doi.org/10.1007/978-981-16-7239-2_33

volume or the residence time of blood in the gut. In addition, hematochezia can occur from sites proximal to the ligament of Treitz.

On physical examination, resting hypotension (systemic blood pressure ≤ 100 mmHg) or tachycardia (pulse rate ≥ 120/min) indicates significant blood loss of >1000 mL, whereas hypovolemic shock indicates about 40% (or 2000 mL) blood loss [1]. Hematocrit changes do not show the extent of blood loss because erythrocyte volume demonstrates late changes (after 24–72 h). Therefore, clinical manifestations and physical examination findings are more important components of the assessment of hemodynamic stability than laboratory examination [1].

Hemodynamically Unstable Patients with Acute GI Bleeding

Adequate resuscitation and hemodynamic stabilization are essential before an endoscopy. In particular, patients with coagulopathy or thrombocytopenia should generally be transfused with prothrombin complex concentrate infusions or platelet transfusions. In the presence of orthostatic hypotension, unstable vital signs, ongoing severe hematemesis, a requirement for transfusion, or ongoing bloody lavage, attention should be paid to the patient's hemodynamic stability first. Thereafter, evaluations to identify the causes and potential treatment of the source of bleeding should follow.

Second-Look Endoscopy

If it is difficult to judge whether a complete inspection had been performed during the first endoscopy, owing to poor bowel preparation, poor proficiency, or insufficient inspection time, the first approach for OGIB is to perform a second-look upper endoscopy and colonoscopy. The lesions such as angioplasia, peptic ulcers, and newly detected tumors could be missed during the first endoscopy [2]. In addition, a second-look investigation could achieve a higher diagnostic yield by further approaching the proximal small bowel or distal ileum.

Diagnostic Tools for Patients with Small-Bowel Bleeding

Angiography

In patients with hemodynamic instability due to massive hemorrhage, angiography could not only detect a treatable vascular focus through contrast extravasation but also stop active hemorrhage through selective embolization. Therefore, angiography can be used for medical and endoscopic therapy as a bridge therapy to surgery. However, bleeding rates ≥0.5 mL/min have traditionally been considered necessary for contrast extravasation to be detectable. Therefore, angiography would not be considered if the bleeding rate is slow enough not to require transfusion. There are few studies about angiography for GI bleeding of unknown origin. In one study, the diagnostic yield of angiography for lower GI bleeding was 27–77% [3].

Embolic materials such as microcoils and particles could be used for the management of GI bleeding through super-selective embolization after identifying the source of bleeding. However, if an anatomical approach to the bleeding site is not feasible, embolization using N-butyl cyanoacrylate, glue, polyvinyl alcohol particles, or Gelfoam could be attempted. However, there is a disadvantage to this method in that it is difficult to determine the cause of bleeding only based on the bleeding pattern, and it is challenging to diagnose venous bleeding including esophageal varices and intermittent hemorrhage. In addition, postembolization bowel ischemia/necrosis or rebleeding might occur if super-selective embolization for bleeding vessels is not performed.

Double-Balloon Enteroscopy

One recent study reported that double-balloon enteroscopy could be performed in cases of massive small-bowel bleeding, for the purpose of both diagnosis and treatment [4]. Before double-balloon enteroscopy, stable vital signs should be achieved in the patient. Further studies on double-

Fig. 1 Diagnostic and therapeutic algorithm for acute hemorrhage in patients with gastrointestinal hemorrhage of unknown origin

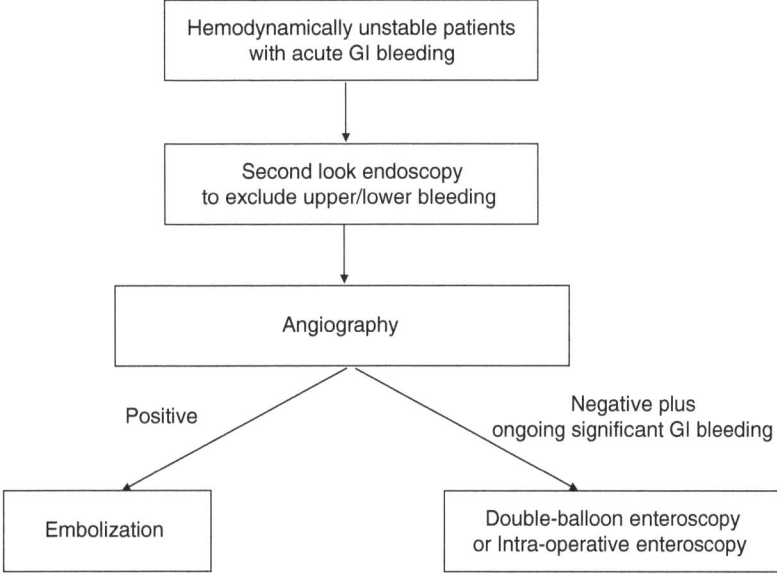

balloon enteroscopy will be needed to confirm its usefulness in the real clinical setting.

Intraoperative Enteroscopy

Intraoperative enteroscopy is one of the most reliable methods for the complete examination of the small intestine; however, it is a highly invasive method with a diagnosis rate of 58–88%. Intraoperative enteroscopy can have complications including intestinal lacerations, tearing of mesenteric vessels, and persistent paralytic ileus, and has a mortality rate of about 17% [5]. Therefore, intraoperative enteroscopy should be performed in cases of severe bleeding that could not be resolved despite overall small-bowel examination, or if the patient cannot undergo deep enteroscopy because of a history of previous surgery or intestinal adhesions [6].

Conclusions

Emergency angiography could detect the bleeding focus and treat hemorrhage through selective embolization. Therefore, it could be performed in hemodynamically unstable patients suspected to have small-bowel bleeding. In addition, if the

cause of hemorrhage is not found on angiography, either small-intestine endoscopy or intraoperative small-intestine endoscopy could be performed (Fig. 1). As there are few studies to date, customized treatment according to the clinical situation may be possible by referring to previous studies and physician experiences.

References

1. Kasper DL, Fauci AS, Hauser SL, Longo DL, Jameson JL, Loscalzo J. Harrison's principles of internal medicine. New York: McGraw-Hill; 2015.
2. Gerson LB, Fidler JL, Cave DR, Leighton JA. ACG clinical guideline: diagnosis and management of small bowel bleeding. Am J Gastroenterol. 2015;110:1265–87.
3. Zuckerman GR, Prakash C. Acute lower intestinal bleeding: part I: clinical presentation and diagnosis. Gastrointest Endosc. 1998;48:606–17.
4. Mönkemüller K, Neumann H, Meyer F, et al. A retrospective analysis of emergency double-balloon enteroscopy for small-bowel bleeding. Endoscopy. 2009;41:715–7.
5. Douard R, Wind P, Panis Y, et al. Intraoperative enteroscopy for diagnosis and management of unexplained gastrointestinal bleeding. Am J Surg. 2000;180:181–4.
6. Leighton JA, Goldstein J, Hirota W, et al. Obscure gastrointestinal bleeding. Gastrointest Endosc. 2003;58:650–5.

Hemodynamically Stable Acute or Chronic Small-Bowel Bleeding

Hyun Joo Song

Key Points
- The most common causes of hemodynamically stable acute or chronic small-bowel bleeding include angiodysplasia in patients aged ≥40 years and inflammatory bowel disease in those aged <40 years.
- For the diagnosis and treatment of hemodynamically stable acute or chronic small-bowel bleeding, upper endoscopy and colonoscopy should first be performed. If the result is negative, second-look endoscopy and capsule endoscopy should follow. If capsule endoscopy is not possible or a small-bowel tumor is suspected, computed tomography (CT) enterography and CT angiography could be performed.

Obscure gastrointestinal bleeding (OGIB) refers to persistent or recurrent bleeding that could not be explained by upper endoscopy and colonoscopy and may be either overt or occult [1]. Eighty percent of cases of OGIB are small-bowel bleeding, and small-bowel bleeding accounts for 5% of the total gastrointestinal bleeding cases.

H. J. Song (✉)
Department of Internal Medicine, Jeju National University College of Medicine, Jeju City, Korea

In this chapter, the following guidelines were consulted: 2013 guidelines for capsule endoscopy for OGIB from the Korean Society of Gastrointestinal Endoscopy [2], the European Society of gastrointestinal endoscopy 2015 guidelines [3], the American College of Gastroenterology guidelines [4], and the American Society of Gastrointestinal Endoscopy 2017 guidelines [5]. The purpose of this study was to evaluate hemodynamically stable acute or chronic hemorrhage in patients with small-bowel bleeding or OGIB and to determine the diagnostic approach based on published literature [3–5].

Etiology

The causes of small bowel bleeding are detailed in Table 1, Part II, chapter "Small-bowel Bleeding" [4]. The etiology of small bowel bleeding differs according to age, and angiodysplasia is the most common cause. The risk factors of angiodysplasia are old age, atherosclerosis, chronic renal failure, left ventricular assist device, and other genetic diseases. Recurrence of angiodysplasia is common and the number of lesions, old age, underlying diseases, and anticoagulant therapy are risk factors for recurrent bleeding [1]. In patients younger than 40 years, the most common cause of small-bowel bleeding is inflammatory bowel disease, including Crohn's disease, followed by Dieulafoy's lesion, tumors, Meckel's diverticulum, and polyps. For patients aged

40 years or older, angiodysplasia is the most common cause, followed by Dieulafoy's lesion, tumors, and non-steroidal anti-inflammatory drug-induced ulcers.

Diagnosis

Second-Look Endoscopy

Bleeding lesions may be overlooked in the first upper gastrointestinal endoscopy and colonoscopy if the endoscopic technician lacks the required skill and experience, and if the test is performed 48 h after the onset of gastrointestinal bleeding. Intermittent hemorrhage, anemia, dehydration, weakening of vascular lesions due to sedation, difficulty in securing visibility due to blood or insufficient bowel preparation, and failure of the ampulla of Vater observation could result in a failure of diagnosis or a misdiagnosis. However, secondary upper endoscopy and colonoscopy have been shown to have low diagnostic yield and to not be cost-effective. Therefore, they should be selectively performed in cases of OGIB [3].

Small-Bowel Capsule Endoscopy

Small-bowel capsule endoscopy is highly useful as the first diagnostic tool for OGIB, according to the recent Korean and international guidelines [2–4]. The diagnosis yield of capsule endoscopy in patients with OGIB is usually 50–60% [6], and is higher (48 vs. 78%) when performed within 48 h after bleeding [1]. In addition, capsule endoscopy is also recommended as the first diagnostic tool for iron deficiency anemia [2]. Therefore, capsule endoscopy may be preferentially performed after upper endoscopy and colonoscopy in hemodynamically stable patients with acute or chronic gastrointestinal bleeding.

Small-Bowel Enteroscopy

Small-bowel enteroscopy is an invasive method used for both diagnosis and treatment that com-plements the disadvantages of capsule endoscopy. It includes double- or single-balloon small-bowel endoscopy and spiral enteroscopy [7]. It is difficult to simultaneously perform small-intestine capsule endoscopy and double-balloon endoscopy in patients with OGIB.

In cases of OGIB, it is recommended to perform capsule endoscopy before small-bowel enteroscopy for making a diagnosis [2–4].

Radiographic Examination

Computed Tomography (CT) Enterography

CT enterography has been used to diagnose small-bowel tumors as well as small-intestinal mucosal lesions including angiodysplasia, which are difficult to diagnose using conventional radiologic examinations [5, 8]. CT enterography may be helpful in the diagnosis of OGIB. Furthermore, it could be useful especially in the presence of suspicion of intestinal obstruction due to Crohn's disease. It can be performed as a primary test for OGIB.

According to the 2015 guidelines of the American College of Gastroenterology, CT angiography in patients with OGIB can diagnose and localize mucosal lesions in small-bowel tumors when capsule endoscopy is negative in patients suspected of having small-bowel bleeding. CT enterography is recommended because of its high sensitivity and role in guiding small-bowel endoscopy [4].

CT Angiography

According to the 2015 American Society of Gastroenterology guidelines, traditional angiography for acute gastrointestinal bleeding should be performed in hemodynamically unstable patients. In hemodynamically stable patients, CT angiography should be performed to determine the location of bleeding and for subsequent treatment [4]. CT angiography is the preferred method for rapid gastrointestinal bleeding [4].

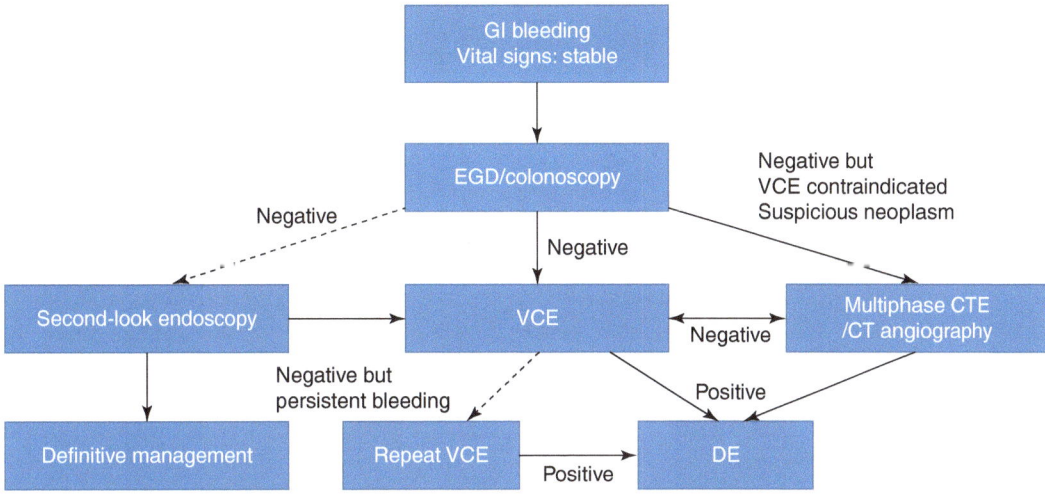

Fig. 1 Diagnosis and treatment algorithm for obscure gastrointestinal bleeding. *GI* gastrointestinal, *EGD* esophagogastroduodenoscopy, *VCE* video capsule endoscopy, *CTE* computed tomography enterography, *DE* deep enteroscopy

Summary

The algorithm for the diagnosis and treatment of acute or chronic bleeding in hemodynamically stable patients is shown in Fig. 1. Upper endoscopy and colonoscopy should first be performed. If the result is negative, second-look endoscopy and capsule endoscopy should be followed. If capsule endoscopy is not possible or a small-bowel tumor is suspected, CT enterography and CT angiography could be performed. If the cause of small-bowel bleeding is not found, a secondary capsule endoscopy can be performed if there is persistent bleeding or a double-balloon or single-balloon endoscopy can be performed when the results of capsule endoscopy or CT enterography and CT angiography are positive.

References

1. Singh A, Baptista V, Stoicov C, Cave DR. Evaluation of small bowel bleeding. Curr Opin Gastroenterol. 2013;29:119–24.

2. Shim KN, Moon JS, Chang DK, et al. Guideline for capsule endoscopy: obscure gastrointestinal bleeding. Clin Endosc. 2013;46:45–53.

3. Pennazio M, Spada C, Eliakim R, et al. Small-bowel capsule endoscopy and device-assisted enteroscopy for diagnosis and treatment of small-bowel disorders: European society of gastrointestinal endoscopy (ESGE) clinical guideline. Endoscopy. 2015;47:352–76.

4. Gerson LB, Fidler JL, Cave DR, Leighton JA. ACG clinical guideline: diagnosis and management of small bowel bleeding. Am J Gastroenterol. 2015;110:1265–87.

5. ASGE Standards of Practice Committee, Gurudu SR, Bruining DH, Acosta RD, Eloubeidi MA, Faulx AL, Khashab MA, Kothari S, Lightdale JR, Muthusamy VR, Yang J, JM DW. The role of endoscopy in the management of suspected small-bowel bleeding. Gastrointest Endosc. 2017;85:22–31.

6. ASGE Standards of Practice Committee, Fisher L, Lee Krinsky M, et al. The role of endoscopy in the management of obscure GI bleeding. Gastrointest Endosc. 2010;72:471–9.

7. Elena RM, Riccardo U, Rossella C, Bizzotto A, Domenico G, Guido C. Current status of device-assisted enteroscopy: technical matters, indication, limits and complications. World J Gastrointest Endosc. 2012;4:453–61.

8. Liu K, Kaffes AJ. Review article: the diagnosis and investigation of obscure gastrointestinal bleeding. Aliment Pharmacol Ther. 2011;34:416–23.

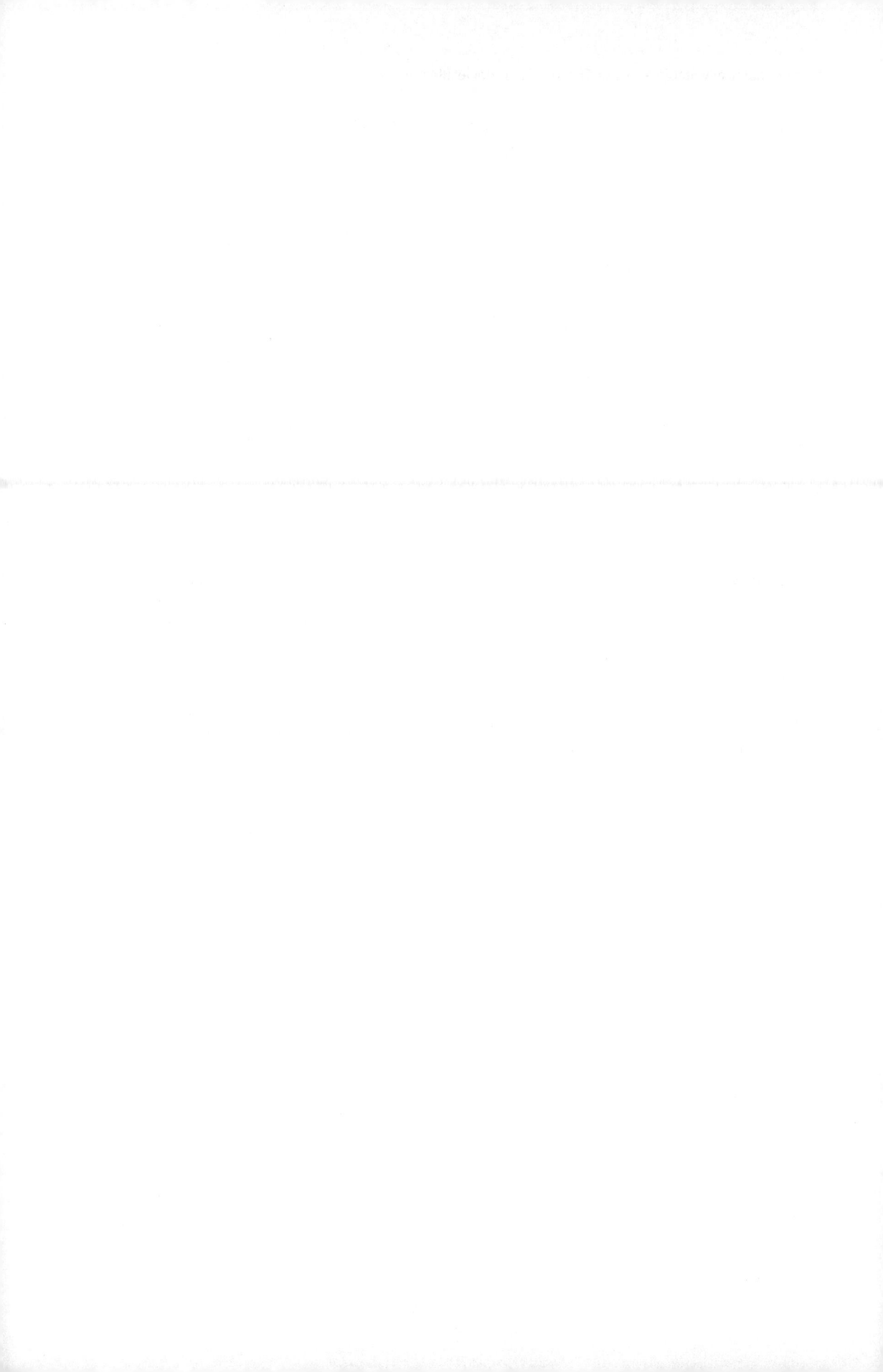

Vascular Diseases of the Small Intestine

Junseok Park and Jin-Oh Kim

Key Points
1. In principle, the treatment of acute mesenteric infarction is surgery.
2. The most common cause of small-bowel bleeding is angioectasia.
3. Diverse symptoms can be caused by inflammatory changes resulting from various causes.

Vascular Anatomy and Physiology of the Small Intestine

The duodenum is located at the branch of the celiac artery, and the jejunum and ileum receive blood supply from the superior mesenteric artery [1]. After the ligament of Treitz, the arteries that supply blood to the small intestine run arch-like in the peritoneum, with small branches extending into the serosa and the proper muscles, and further extending to the villus in the form of arterioles. The arteries supplying blood to the duodenum form collateral circulations connected to adjacent arteries. The venous flow in the small intestine leads to the portal vein through the superior mesenteric vein.

About 10–15% of the cardiac output is supplied to the small intestine [2]. Changes in blood pressure within the normal range do not affect perfusion; however, severe hypotension causes a sudden drop in perfusion. This leads to a functional closure of the arterioles, especially in the mucous membranes. An increase in portal venous pressure may lead to an increase in small-bowel venous pressure.

The clinical features of small-intestinal vascular disorders are highly diverse [3]. Symptoms may be absent or various symptoms such as abdominal pain, nausea, vomiting, diarrhea, bleeding, and weight loss may occur. Perfusion disorders directly result from occlusion of the blood vessels, and secondary changes including inflammation can cause symptoms.

Ischemic Disorders

The ileocecal region is the most vulnerable region to ischemia because this area is supplied by the longest segment of the superior mesenteric artery. About half of the cases are caused by occlusion due to atheroma, thrombosis, embolism, or inflammatory changes. The risk factors are age >50 years, heart failure, arrhythmia, recent myocardial infarction, hypovolemia, hypotension, and sepsis. Symptoms occur when the cross-sectional area of the blood vessel is reduced to about two-third or when blood flow is reduced to about 50–80% [4]. Further, ischemia appears

J. Park · J.-O. Kim (✉)
Soonchunhyang University Hospital, Seoul, Korea
e-mail: junspark@schmc.ac.kr; jokim@schmc.ac.kr

© Springer Nature Singapore Pte Ltd. 2022
H. J. Chun et al. (eds.), *Small Intestine Disease*, https://doi.org/10.1007/978-981-16-7239-2_35

more frequently in female patients, those with severe sclerosis of the aorta or coronary artery sclerosis, and those with diabetes. A chronic splanchnic syndrome is characterized by abdominal pain, weight loss, and diarrhea that occur after meals, presumably caused by intestinal ischemia that is not more severe than infarction. Venous obstruction induces 5–15% of all mesenteric ischemia; however, it is difficult to immediately diagnose and its mortality rate reaches 20–50% [5]. Most commonly, venous flow is disturbed owing to pressure externally derived from intestinal tract abnormalities, including hernias, abdominal lymph nodes, and appendicitis. Oral contraceptive medication or abnormalities of prothrombin and protein C produce blood clots that can disrupt the flow. Portal vein thrombosis caused by cirrhosis or liver tumors may also be affected.

The pressure in the superior mesenteric artery is the same as that in the aorta, and the portal pressure is one-tenth of that. The blood vessels located between them are sensitive to amine compounds associated with blood pressure control and contribute to maintaining blood pressure even in hypotensive conditions. Left ventricular failure, aortic valve closure, and shock may cause intestinal ischemia without marked vascular occlusion. In addition, increased blood viscosity due to blood concentration or erythropoiesis may be caused by small blood clots in disseminated intravascular coagulation.

Under ischemia, the small intestine develops edema and changes its color tone from purple to green [6]. The necrosis of the mucous membrane is covered by mucus, fibrin, and blood cells. Hemorrhage occurs in the submucosal layer and may be seen as a nodule. If the degree of ischemia is severe, it may lead to damage to the deep muscular layer. Persistent ischemic injury of the small intestine may lead to ulcerative bleeding or stenosis of the mucosa.

Computed tomography with contrast enhancement is effective in identifying small-bowel abnormalities [7]. It is possible to determine the degree of damage and the occlusion of blood vessel, as well as to diagnose bleeding, by checking the extravasation of the contrast agent. Magnetic resonance imaging and ultrasonography may also be helpful in the diagnosis of small-bowel vascular diseases.

Prompt treatment of acute small-intestinal ischemia improves the prognosis [7]. In principle, the treatment of obstruction of the superior mesenteric artery is reperfusion through surgical treatment. Excision of the intestinal tract with ischemic injury should be simultaneously considered. Depending on the cause, vasodilators and thrombolytic agents can be used, but only if the patient does not have peritonitis. This is because the use of medicines may cause unexpected contraction of blood vessels. Radiologic interventions may be helpful for the reperfusion of blood vessels (Fig. 1).

Portal Hypertensive Enteropathy

In addition to cirrhosis, thrombotic diseases such as splenic vein thrombosis and Budd–Chiari syndrome cause elevated portal pressure that influences the gastrointestinal vasculature. The small-intestinal mucosa is characterized by edema, redness, enlargement of small vessels, varicose veins, and bleeding [8].

Although the efficacy of drug therapy for small-bowel lesions caused by portal hypertension has not been clarified, treatment with beta-blockers, somatostatin derivatives, and thalidomide has been reported. If hemorrhage occurs, endoscopic hemostasis, radiologic intervention, or surgery may be considered. For small-bowel varices, more active treatment should be considered, such as coil embolization, transjugular intrahepatic portosystemic shunt, and endoscopic injection of a sclerotic agent.

Vasculitis

Inflammation can develop in blood vessels and surrounding tissues in various immune diseases including systemic sclerosis, rheumatoid arthritis, Henoch-Schönlein purpura, and allergic granulomatous vasculitis [6]. Chronic ischemia or acute occlusion may also occur in the peritoneum. It is

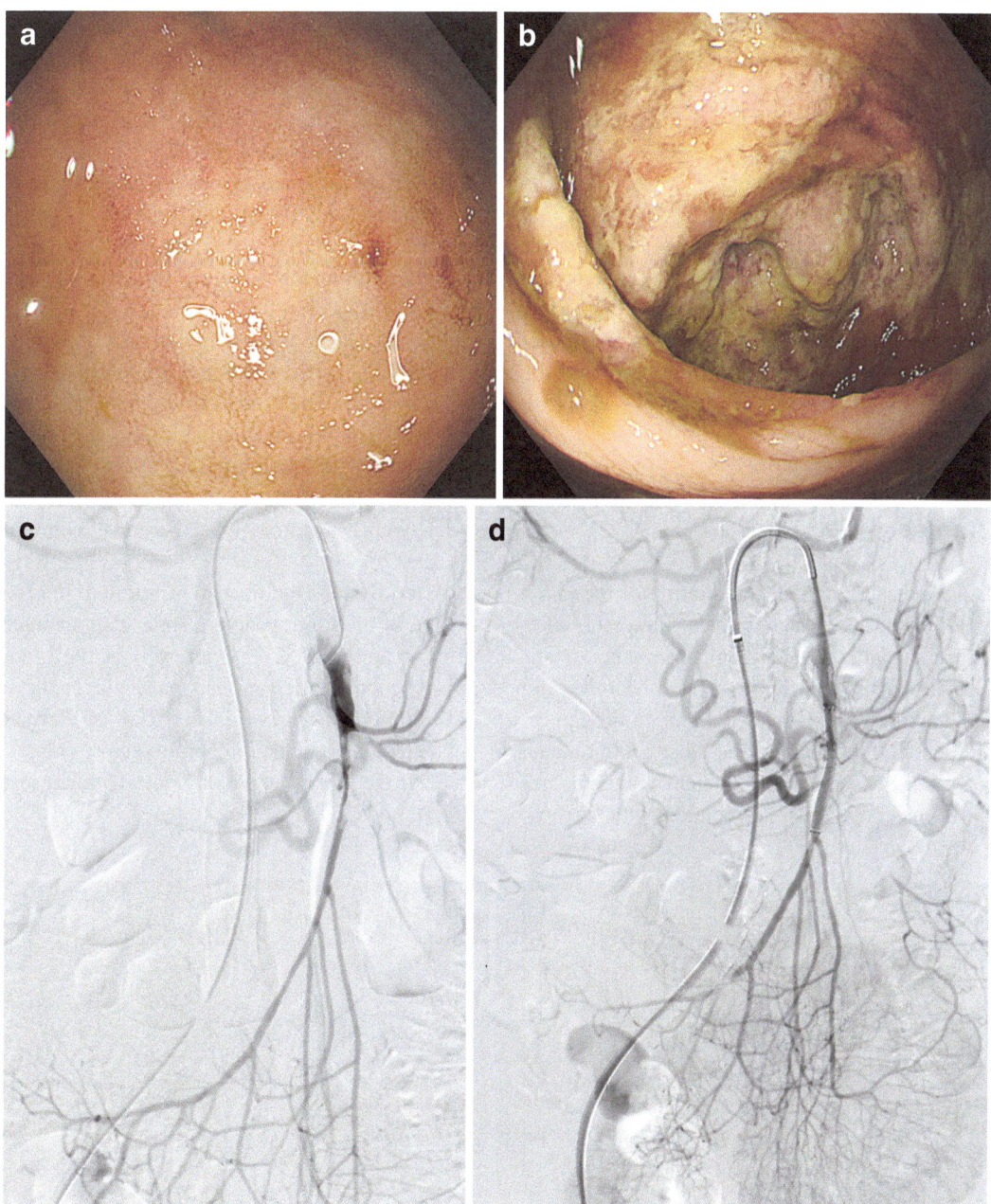

Fig. 1 Treatment with radiologic intervention of superior mesenteric artery occlusion due to a thrombus. (**a**, **b**) Endoscopic features—erosions and ulcers developed in the ileocecal area. (**c**) Angiography—intraluminal throm-bus is observed in the superior mesenteric artery. (**d**) Radiologic intervention—reperfusion is achieved after stent insertion

often difficult to confirm the diagnosis through histologic examination alone. Extraintestinal symptoms and serological findings should be considered together. If severe complications such as bleeding, perforation, or infarction are present, surgical treatment may be necessary.

Thromboangiitis Obliterans

Thromboangiitis obliterans, also known as Buerger's disease, rarely invades the distal branch of the superior mesenteric artery and causes localized intestinal ischemia. It can invade the small intestine and the large intestine, usually accompanied by claudication of the limb. The blood vessels of the submucosa and serosa are occluded by thrombi, accompanied by the proliferation of vascular endothelial cells and mesenteric fibrosis. Compared with other vasculitis conditions, the collagenous layer of the vascular endothelium is preserved.

Angioectasia

Angioectasia refers to the dilation of blood vessels without cellular dysplasia. In vessels of the intestinal mucosa and submucosa, smooth muscle disappears and the inner wall becomes thinner, increasing in diameter and turning into a serpentine form. This is the most common cause of small-bowel bleeding in elderly patients aged >50 years. It is also associated with cirrhosis, chronic kidney disease, and heart valve disease. It manifests as red spots of a few millimeters in size and with a pale halo [9]. It is more common in the jejunum than in the ileum, and more often occurs in multiple forms (Fig. 2).

When the submucosal vein is dilated, it can be observed in the form of a blue nodule, which is called phlebectasia. Although the covering mucosa is thin, the bleeding tendency is relatively low (Fig. 2).

Telangiectasia is vasodilation secondary to systemic disease or syndrome. In contrast to the expansion of blood vessels throughout the intestinal wall, simple vasodilation is mainly confined to mucosal or submucosal blood vessels. Hereditary hemorrhagic telangiectasia (Rendu Osler–Weber syndrome) is the most common disease.

Arteriovenous malformation refers to the formation of an arteriovenous fistula without intervening capillaries. The inner wall of the blood vessel becomes thick and the muscle layer shows proliferation. It appears in the form of elevated pulsatile lesions with peripheral vascular enlargement. If the size is large, surgical treatment may be required (Fig. 3).

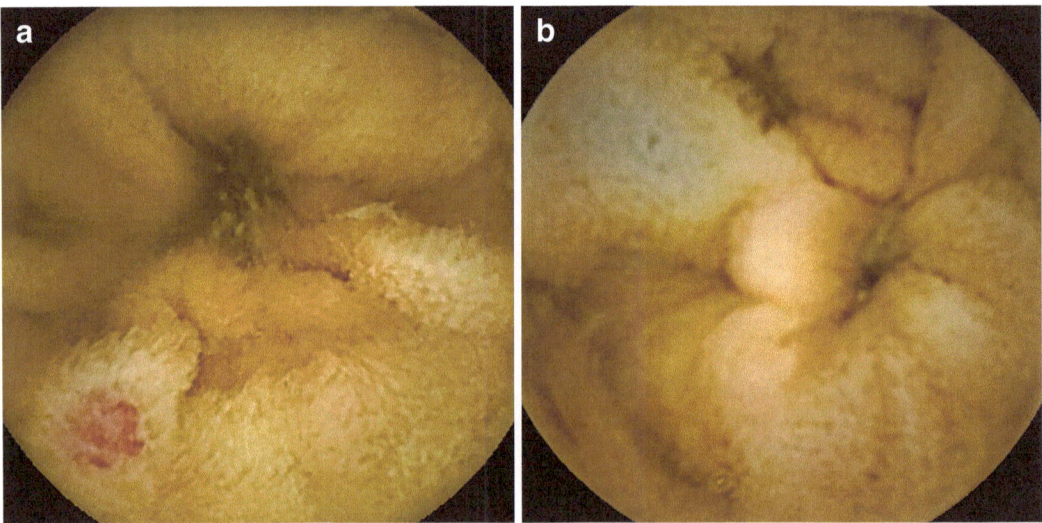

Fig. 2 Vascular dilations discovered with capsule endoscopy. (**a**) Capsule endoscopy—angioectasia. (**b**) Capsule endoscopy—blue-colored venous dilation

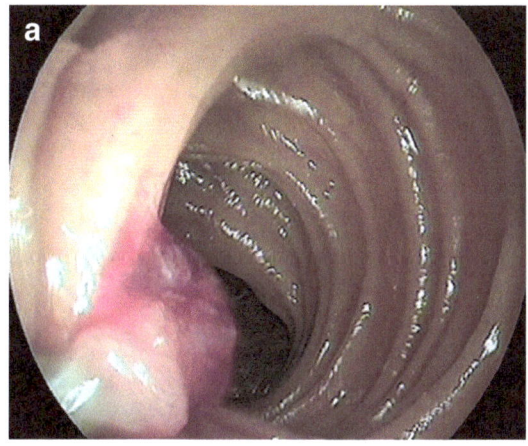
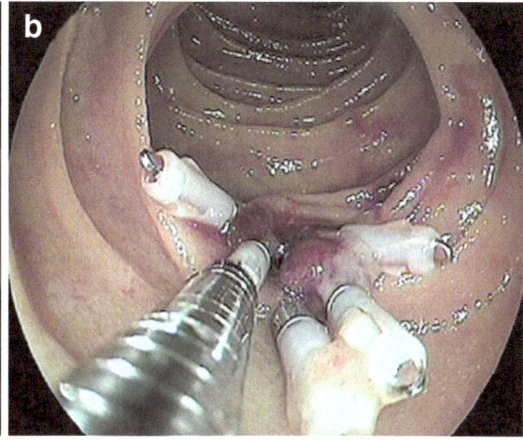
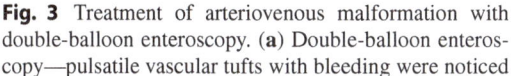

Fig. 3 Treatment of arteriovenous malformation with double-balloon enteroscopy. (**a**) Double-balloon enteroscopy—pulsatile vascular tufts with bleeding were noticed on the ileal mucosa. (**b**) Double-balloon enteroscopy—hemostasis was performed by clipping

Hemangioma

Hemangioma is a neoplasm of proliferating blood vessels and is rarely malignant. It accounts for 7–10% of small-bowel benign tumors. Gastrointestinal bleeding, anemia, obstruction, and platelet sequestration can occur. It grossly appears as a small, red polypoid lesion. Histologically, it is divided into the capillary, cavernous, and mixed types [7].

Suppurative granuloma can also develop in the intestinal mucosa. Lobular proliferation of capillaries is stimulated by external irritation or hormones and has been shown as red polyps with inflammatory changes covered with exudates. Blue rubber bleb nevus syndrome and other diseases that cause cavernous hemangiomas can result in gastrointestinal complications. These usually occur in the small intestine and on the left side of the colon. They may vary in size and shape and may be accompanied by bleeding.

Summary

The small intestine beyond the duodenum receives blood supply from the superior mesenteric artery, and venous return occurs through the portal vein. The blood vessels of the small intes-tine are well equipped with a physiological adaptation mechanism that prevents ischemic injury. Ischemic injury of the small intestine can manifest as various clinical symptoms. Ulceration or stenosis can develop in chronic cases. Damage of the blood vessels can occur in various immune diseases and may extend to the surrounding area. Ectasia of the blood vessels may be secondary to other diseases, and bleeding may occur. Increased portal pressure due to cirrhosis can cause small-bowel varices. Malignancies are rare; however, some neoplastic diseases such as hemangiomas result from the proliferation of blood vessels.

References

1. Reiner L, Platt R, Rodriguez FL, Jimenez FA. Injection studies on the mesenteric arterial circulation. II. Intestinal infarction. Gastroenterology. 1960;39:747–57.
2. Lundgren O, Svanvik J. Mucosal hemodynamics in the small intestine of the cat during reduced perfusion pressure. Acta Physiol Scand. 1973;88:551–63.
3. Gore RM, Thakrar KH, Mehta UK, Berlin J, Yaghmai V, Newmark GM. Imaging in intestinal ischemic disorders. Clin Gastroenterol Hepatol. 2008;6:849–58.
4. Wilson C, Gupta R, Gilmour DG, Imrie CW. Acute superior mesenteric ischaemia. Br J Surg. 1987;74:279–81.
5. Schoots IG, Koffeman GI, Legemate DA, Levi M, van Gulik TM. Systematic review of survival after acute

mesenteric ischaemia according to disease aetiology. Br J Surg. 2004;91:17–27.

6. Noffsinger AE. Morson and Dawson's gastrointestinal pathology. 5th ed. Malden: Blackwell; 2013.

7. Filippone A, Cianci R, Milano A, Valeriano S, Di Mizio V, Storto ML. Obscure gastrointestinal bleeding and small bowel pathology: comparison between wireless capsule endoscopy and multidetector-row CT enteroclysis. Abdom Imaging. 2008;33:398–406.

8. Jeon SR, Kim JO. Capsule endoscopy for portal hypertensive enteropathy. Gastroenterol Res Pract. 2016;2016:8501394.

9. Lee BI. Clinical gastrointestinal endoscopy: a comprehensive atlas. New York, NY: Springer; 2014.

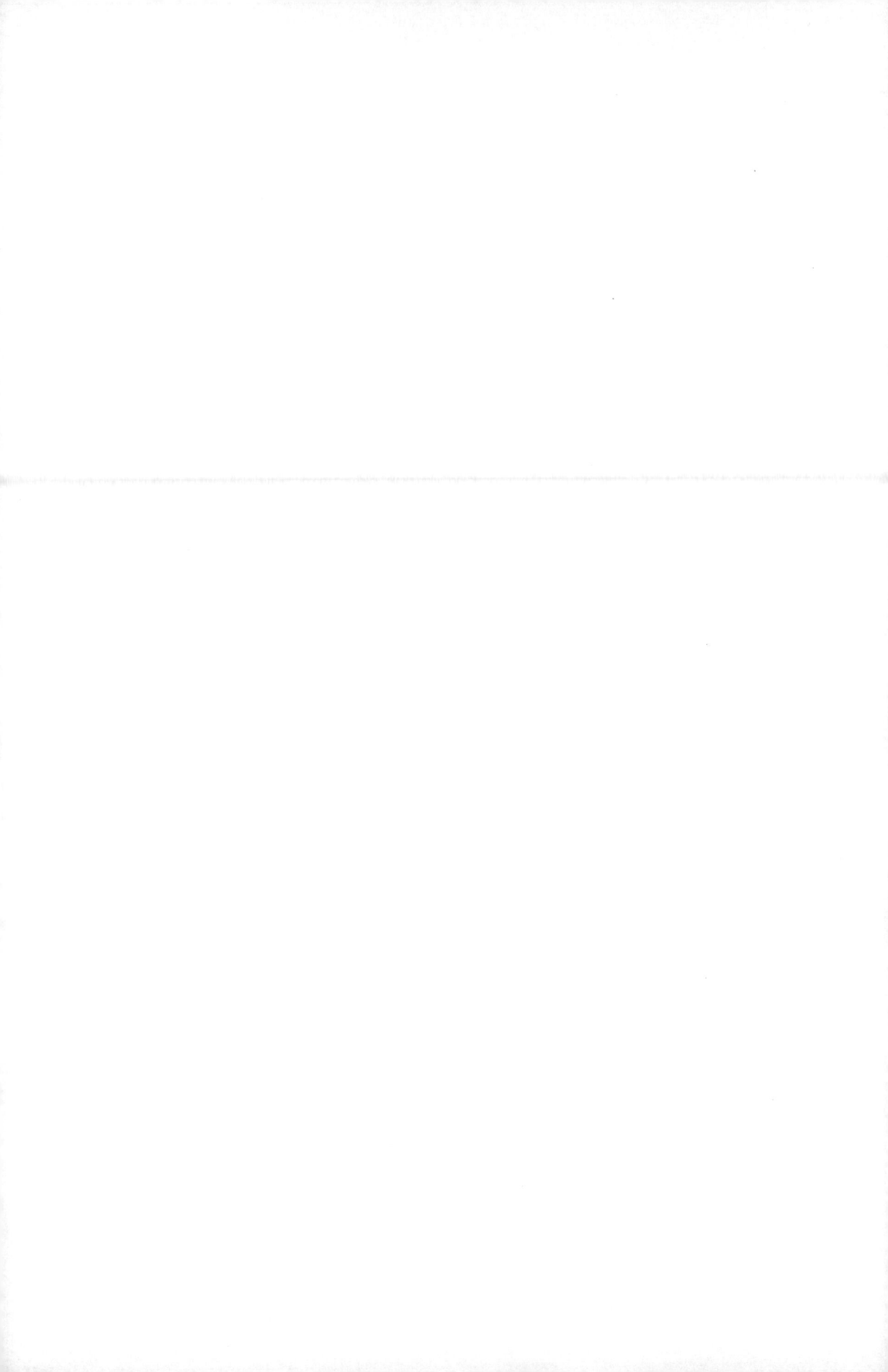

Diagnostic Criteria for Crohn's Disease

Sung Chul Park and Yoon Tae Jeen

Key Points
- Diagnostic criteria for Crohn's disease (CD) : No definite diagnostic gold standard currently exists. Therefore, the diagnosis is based on the comprehensive evaluation of clinical, endoscopic, histological, surgical, imaging, and laboratory findings.
- Diagnostic method for CD: Primarily, ileocolonoscopy and biopsy are recommended. Capsule endoscopy can be considered if small-bowel CD is clinically suspected but there are no specific findings in colonoscopy or imaging studies.

Crohn's disease (CD) is a heterogeneous disease with diverse phenotypes in terms of age of onset, lesion location, and disease pattern. No single gold standard method for diagnosing CD presently exists; thus, the diagnosis is based on the comprehensive evaluation of clinical, endoscopic, histological, surgical, imaging, and laboratory findings [1, 2]. As no definite criteria for diagnosing CD have been established, the diagnosis is still difficult. The differential diagnoses include acute infectious enterocolitis, irritable bowel syndrome, ulcerative colitis (UC), intestinal tuberculosis, and intestinal Behcet's disease. This chapter will describe the diagnostic criteria for CD.

Medical History Taking and Physical Examination

Among the various symptoms of CD, abdominal pain, diarrhea, and weight loss are the most common. CD should be suspected if such symptoms are noted, especially in patients in their teens up to the late 20s. Medical history taking for the diagnosis of CD must include the onset of symptoms, recent travel history, food intolerance, drug history including the use of antibiotics and nonsteroidal anti-inflammatory drugs (NSAIDs), and appendectomy history, while paying attention to the risk factors of CD such as smoking, family history, and recent infectious enterocolitis. Furthermore, nighttime symptoms; extraintestinal symptoms involving the mouth, skin, eye, or joints; and perianal lesions (anal fissures, anal fistulas, and perianal abscesses) must be evaluated.

S. C. Park
Division of Gastroenterology and Hepatology, Department of Internal Medicine, Kangwon National University School of Medicine, Chuncheon, Kangwon-do, South Korea

Y. T. Jeen (✉)
Division of Gastroenterology and Hepatology, Department of Internal Medicine, Korea University Anam Hospital, Korea University College of Medicine, Seoul, Seongbuk-gu, South Korea
e-mail: ytjeen@korea.ac.kr

© Springer Nature Singapore Pte Ltd. 2022
H. J. Chun et al. (eds.), *Small Intestine Disease*, https://doi.org/10.1007/978-981-16-7239-2_36

Physical examination should include the assessment of general appearance; measurement of blood pressure, body temperature, and pulse rate; examination of the abdomen (tenderness, distention, and mass); perineal and oral inspection; digital rectal examination; and calculation of body mass index.

Laboratory Tests

Basic laboratory tests include C-reactive protein levels and complete blood count. Further, inflammatory markers such as fecal calprotectin and erythrocyte sedimentation rate (ESR) can also be measured. Such tests can help identify acute or chronic inflammatory reaction, anemia, dehydration, malnutrition, and malabsorption. A fecal calprotectin test can help determine the need for an endoscopic evaluation, which is especially useful in pediatric patients. To distinguish CD from infectious enterocolitis, microbiological tests including *Clostridium difficile* toxin assay are recommended. Moreover, if there is a history of travel, stool analysis may be performed. Serum anti-*Saccharomyces cerevisiae* antibody is positive in 35–50% of patients with CD, but in only <1% of patients with UC;

thus, it can be used as a diagnostic tool together with perinuclear anti-neutrophil cytoplasmic autoantibody, which is commonly positive in 11–84% of patients with UC. Further, interferon-gamma release assay can be considered to differentiate CD from intestinal tuberculosis [3]. Currently, no genetic testing is available for diagnosing CD.

Endoscopy

When CD is suspected, ileocolonoscopy and biopsy are primarily recommended. The characteristic endoscopic findings of CD include longitudinal ulcers parallel to the longitudinal direction of the gastrointestinal (GI) tract, a cobblestone-like appearance, discontinuous multiple aphthous ulcerations, asymmetrical inflammation, and skipped lesions. Moreover, fissures, fistulas, and strictures may be found.

If CD is clinically suspected but no characteristic findings are found in ileocolonoscopy and radiological tests such as small-bowel follow-through, computed tomography (CT), or magnetic resonance imaging (MRI), capsule endoscopy can be helpful in the diagnosis (Fig. 1) [4]. Capsule endoscopy is a sensitive tool used

Fig. 1 Diagnostic process in patients with suspected small-bowel Crohn's disease

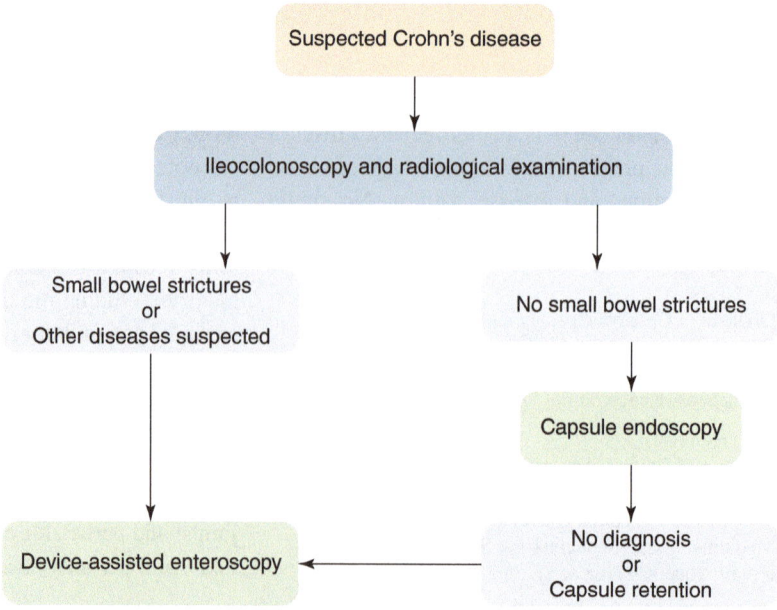

for detecting small-bowel mucosal abnormalities. It can help assess the extent of small-bowel involvement of CD and the degree of damage. The diagnostic yield of capsule endoscopy in small-bowel CD is superior to that of small-bowel follow-through or CT. Furthermore, capsule endoscopy has a high negative predictive value in excluding a diagnosis of small-bowel CD. However, owing to its low specificity in detecting small-bowel CD, a clear definition of CD-related lesions is needed. Mucosal breaks and erosions in the small bowel can be found in up to 10% of healthy individuals without CD, and it is difficult to distinguish CD-related lesions from NSAID-related lesions; thus, it recommended to perform capsule endoscopy after the discontinuation of NSAIDs for at least 1 month [5]. The contraindications of capsule endoscopy include intestinal obstruction, strictures, and dysphagia. Small-bowel imaging or patency capsule endoscopy is recommended before capsule endoscopy, to evaluate small-bowel strictures that may cause capsule retention.

As device-assisted enteroscopy procedures such as single-balloon or double-balloon enteroscopy are invasive and difficult to perform, they are only recommended when histological confirmation or endoscopic therapies, such as dilation of the stricture site, withdrawal of a retained capsule, and hemostasis, are needed.

Esophagogastroduodenoscopy is recommended when upper GI symptoms are present; however, whether it should be recommended as a routine test in adults is still controversial.

Radiology

To identify the location and extent of small-bowel involvement of CD, radiological tests should be considered regardless of colonoscopic findings. Topographic evaluations, such as CT enterography or magnetic resonance enterography, and abdominal ultrasound are complementary methods to endoscopy and therefore could be helpful in identifying complications, such as strictures, fistulas, and abscess, while differentiating inflammatory from fibrotic strictures.

Histopathology

To obtain an accurate diagnosis of CD, it is recommended to obtain more than two tissue samples from each of the five segments (terminal ileum, ascending colon, transverse colon, sigmoid colon, and rectum) and to acquire samples from lesions as well as normal sites [6]. Clinical information such as patient age, disease duration, and type and duration of treatment should be provided to the pathologists in addition to tissue samples.

Focal or patchy chronic inflammation (infiltration of lymphocytes and plasma cells), focal (segmental or discontinuous) crypt architectural abnormalities, granuloma in the lamina propria that is not adjacent to the crypt damage, and mucin preservation in active parts are histological findings commonly observed in CD. Although non-caseating granuloma is a characteristic histological finding, it is neither pathognomonic nor sensitive. When the diagnosis is difficult, the existence of granuloma, focally enhanced gastritis, or focal active gastritis in the gastric specimens may be helpful.

Diagnostic Criteria

Although there is no gold standard method for diagnosing CD, some guidelines have suggested diagnostic criteria. The criteria for diagnosing CD recommended by the World Health Organization are shown in Table 1 [4]. The diagnostic criteria published in Japan include three major criteria (A: longitudinal ulcer, B: cobblestone-like appearance, and C: non-caseating epithelial cell granuloma) and three minor criteria (a: irregularly shaped and/or quasi-circular ulcers, or aphthous ulcerations appearing extensively in the GI tract; b: characteristic perianal lesions; and c: characteristic gastric and/or

Table 1 World Health Organization diagnostic criteria for Crohn's disease [4]

	Clinical findings	Radiological tests	Endoscopy	Biopsy	Resected specimen
Discontinuous or segmental lesions		+	+		+
Cobblestone appearance or longitudinal ulcer		+	+		+
Transmural inflammation	+	+		+	+
Non-caseating granuloma				+	+
Fissures and fistulas	+	+			+
Perianal disorders	+				

duodenal lesions) [7]. CD is definitively diagnosed when A or B, C with a or b, or all three minor criteria are met. Otherwise, the diagnosis can only be suspected.

Conclusions

No gold standard method for diagnosing CD presently exists. Therefore, the diagnosis should be based on thorough history taking and careful physical examination with appropriate laboratory tests, in addition to a comprehensive evaluation of endoscopic, radiological, and histological findings. To identify the location and extent of small-bowel involvement of CD, diagnostic tests in the small bowel should be considered. For patients with suspected small-bowel CD with no specific findings in colonoscopy and radiological tests, capsule endoscopy is recommended, and device-assisted enteroscopy may be considered if histologic confirmation or endoscopic therapies for stricture, capsule retention, and bleeding are required.

References

1. Shim KN, Jeon SR, Jang HJ, Kim J, Lim YJ, Kim KO, Song HJ, Lee HS, Park JJ, Kim JH, Chun J, Park SJ, Yang DH, Min YW, Keum B, Lee BI. Quality indicators for small bowel capsule endoscopy. Clin Endosc. 2017;50:148–60. https://doi.org/10.5946/ce.2017.030.

2. Ye BD, Jang BI, Jeen YT, Lee KM, Kim JS, Yang SK. Diagnostic guideline of Crohn's disease. Korean J Gastroenterol. 2009;53:161–76.

3. Kim YS, Kim YH, Lee KM, Kim JS, Park YS. Diagnostic guideline of intestinal tuberculosis. Korean J Gastroenterol. 2009;53:177–86.

4. Bernstein CN, Eliakim A, Fedail S, Fried M, Gearry R, Goh KL, Hamid S, Khan AG, Khalif I, Ng SC, Ouyang Q, Rey JF, Sood A, Steinwurz F, Watermeyer G, LeMair A. World gastroenterology organisation global guidelines inflammatory bowel disease: update august 2015. J Clin Gastroenterol. 2016;50:803–18. https://doi.org/10.1097/mcg.0000000000000660.

5. Pennazio M, Spada C, Eliakim R, Keuchel M, May A, Mulder CJ, Rondonotti E, Adler SN, Albert J, Baltes P, Barbaro F, Cellier C, Charton JP, Delvaux M, Despott EJ, Domagk D, Klein A, McAlindon M, Rosa B, Rowse G, Sanders DS, Saurin JC, Sidhu R, Dumonceau JM, Hassan C, Gralnek IM. Small-bowel capsule endoscopy and device-assisted enteroscopy for diagnosis and treatment of small-bowel disorders: European Society of Gastrointestinal Endoscopy (ESGE) Clinical Guideline. Endoscopy. 2015;47:352–76. https://doi.org/10.1055/s-0034-1391855.

6. Gomollon F, Dignass A, Annese V, Tilg H, Van Assche G, Lindsay JO, Peyrin-Biroulet L, Cullen GJ, Daperno M, Kucharzik T, Rieder F, Almer S, Armuzzi A, Harbord M, Langhorst J, Sans M, Chowers Y, Fiorino G, Juillerat P, Mantzaris GJ, Rizzello F, Vavricka S, Gionchetti P. 3rd European evidence-based consensus on the diagnosis and management of Crohn's disease 2016: part 1: diagnosis and medical management. J Crohn's Colitis. 2017;11:3–25. https://doi.org/10.1093/ecco-jcc/jjw168.

7. Ueno F, Matsui T, Matsumoto T, Matsuoka K, Watanabe M, Hibi T. Evidence-based clinical practice guidelines for Crohn's disease, integrated with formal consensus of experts in Japan. J Gastroenterol. 2013;48:31–72. https://doi.org/10.1007/s00535-012-0673-1.

Clinical Features of Small Bowel Crohn's Disease

Chang Soo Eun

Key Points

- Approximately 70% of patients with Crohn's disease have an affected small bowel, and approximately a third of patients with Crohn's disease have exclusive small intestine involvement.
- Small-bowel Crohn's disease is difficult to diagnose and treat due to its non-specific symptoms and anatomical location. Especially when the proximal small intestine is involved, the risk of stricture, surgery, or recurrence is increased.
- It is essential to differentiate small-bowel Crohn's disease from other inflammatory disorders affecting the small intestine, in particular intestinal tuberculosis and NSAID-induced enteropathy.
- Small-bowel adenocarcinoma with poor prognosis may develop in the presence of small-bowel Crohn's disease, and should be suspected in patients with symptom recurrence after long-term remission and small-bowel stricture unresponsive to medical treatment.

Crohn's disease is one of the inflammatory bowel diseases of unclear etiology. The inflammation can involve the entire gastrointestinal tract from the oral cavity to the anus. The condition develops at a young age and shows chronic progression by repeated improvement and deterioration. Crohn's disease may lead to severe complications such as perforation, stricture, fistula, and abscess formation. About one-third of patients with Crohn's disease have only the small intestine affected, while another one-third of patients involve both the small bowel and colon. Crohn's disease patients affecting the small intestine show different clinical features and undergo different diagnostic modalities and have prognoses different from those of patients with the colonic disease. It can be based on the anatomical and physiologic differences between the small intestine and the colon. Additionally, the small intestine is not easily accessible by endoscopy, thereby presenting challenges to disease diagnosis in the early stages. Small-bowel Crohn's disease is known to be difficult to differentiate from other infectious diseases such as intestinal tuberculosis and drug-induced enteropathy. In addition, it has been reported to have a high risk of complications such as stricture and recurrence. This chapter briefly reviews the incidence of small-bowel Crohn's disease and its clinical features.

C. S. Eun (✉)
Department of Gastroenterology, Hanyang University College of Medicine, Seoul, South Korea
e-mail: cseun@hanyang.ac.kr

© Springer Nature Singapore Pte Ltd. 2022
H. J. Chun et al. (eds.), *Small Intestine Disease*, https://doi.org/10.1007/978-981-16-7239-2_37

Incidence of Small-Bowel Crohn's Disease

Although Crohn's disease can affect any part of the gastrointestinal tract, the exact incidence of small-bowel Crohn's disease remains unclear and underestimated in many studies. The most common area affected by Crohn's disease is the terminal ileum and colon simultaneously, but it may involve only the small intestine, especially in younger patients. Population-based epidemiologic studies have reported that over 50% of Western patients with Crohn's disease, and 77–87.7% of Asian patients have an affected small intestine at the time of diagnosis [1].

In general, about 70% of patients with Crohn's disease have an affected small intestine, and the most common site involved is the distal ileum. The Montreal classification of Crohn's disease defines L1 as cases with an affected area in only the small intestine including the terminal ileum, L2 as cases where the affected area is within the colon only, and L3 as cases where both the small intestine and colon are affected. The involved area in Crohn's disease varies significantly among Western and Asian patients. It indicates that L1, L2, and L3 are distributed in similar proportions in Western patients. On the contrary, in Asian patients, L3 is most commonly reported. In Korean studies, L3 was the most common with an incidence of 53–71%, followed by L1 with an incidence of 21–32%, and L2 with an incidence of 7–14% [2].

It has been reported that approximately one-third of patients with Crohn's disease have only small intestine involvement. However, when the small intestine is exclusively affected, diagnosis and treatment are often difficult due to non-specific symptoms and the anatomical location of the small intestine. Most patients with small-bowel Crohn's patients have terminal ileum involvement, which enables observation of the affected mucosa and biopsy by ileo-colonoscopy. However, in some patients with small bowel Crohn's disease, the terminal ileum is not affected, and therefore, diagnosis is challenging. Accordingly, ileo-colonoscopy cannot exclude Crohn's disease even if the terminal ileum appears normal. If there is clinical suspicion of the disease, especially in the case of anemia, weight loss, abdominal pain, diarrhea, and extra-intestinal symptoms, a thorough examination of the entire small intestine is required. Several studies using capsule endoscopy have demonstrated that small bowel involvement in patients with Crohn's disease is more common than it was in the past.

Clinical Features of Small-Bowel Crohn's Disease

The clinical manifestations of small-bowel Crohn's disease are vague and variable, depending on the location of the affected area, intensity of inflammation, and intestinal and extra-intestinal complications. Abdominal pain is the most common and persistent symptom, which can occur as an intermittent colic and may be persistent and severe pain resulting from inflammation, abscess, or stricture. In some patients, mild symptoms may persist for a long time resulting in delayed diagnosis. They may manifest as a form of small-bowel obstruction exacerbated by non-digestible vegetables or fruits. Additionally, they may be accompanied by intermittent colic, nausea, and vomiting, resulting from the fibrosis associated with small-bowel inflammation in patients with no clinical symptoms for long periods. Sometimes, acute right lower abdominal pain can cause a misdiagnosis of appendicitis. In patients with active small-bowel inflammation, abdominal pain accompanies nausea, diarrhea, weight loss, fever, and malnutrition. In particular, weight loss, malnutrition, and growth failure can be severe problems in pediatric patients.

Patients with small-bowel Crohn's disease often present with non-specific symptoms, so it is essential to differentiate it from other small bowel inflammatory diseases, which cause various symptoms such as abdominal pain, diarrhea, hemorrhage, iron deficiency anemia, malabsorption, and weight loss. These include infectious diseases such as intestinal tuberculosis, NSAID-induced enteropathy, ischemic small bowel diseases, radiation-induced enteritis, Behcet's enteritis, and lymphoproliferative disorders [3].

The prevalence of intestinal tuberculosis is particularly high in Korea, so it is crucial to differentiate between small-bowel Crohn's disease and intestinal tuberculosis. Empirical anti-tuberculous therapy may be helpful in differential diagnosis. The clinical findings favoring Crohn's disease include a longer duration of symptoms, medical history of appendectomy, diarrhea, hematochezia, weight loss, perianal lesions, and extra-intestinal symptoms. On the contrary, clinical findings suggesting intestinal tuberculosis include fever, night sweat, and medical history of pulmonary tuberculosis.

Small-bowel Crohn's disease, especially that involving the proximal small intestine, often increases the risk of complications or recurrence. In a retrospective study of 108 patients with Crohn's disease, the incidence of small bowel involvement was studied with capsule endoscopy. This study revealed that more than half of the patients had jejunal involvement, which increased the risk of clinical relapses [4]. Other studies have also shown an increased risk of stricture or multiple abdominal operations in patients with Crohn's disease with jejunal involvement. The incidence of jejunal involvement in patients with Crohn's disease may vary in different populations. In a Korean study with 1403 patients with Crohn's disease, the authors found a higher rate of jejunal involvement compared to that of Western patients. Additionally, the risk of surgery or hospitalization was increased in Korean patients with Crohn's disease and jejunal involvement [5].

The most common problem encountered in patients with small-bowel Crohn's disease is the occurrence of strictures, which can cause several bowel resections, leading to an intestinal failure (short bowel syndrome) and malnutrition. The causes of intestinal fibrosis have not yet been elucidated, but many studies have been focused on the role of interleukin-17, Th17 immune responses, the renin-angiotensin system, and intestinal microbiota [6]. In patients with small-bowel Crohn's disease, risk factors for intestinal strictures remain unknown, and there is no effective anti-fibrotic treatment. Therefore, current treatment is planned based on the location, length, and number of strictures.

Conversely, a rare complication in patients with small-bowel Crohn's disease is small-bowel adenocarcinoma, which has a poor prognosis and can be preoperatively diagnosed only in a small number of patients. Diagnosis is often delayed due to a lack of specific symptoms distinguishing it from small bowel strictures, lack of proper screening method, and the very low prevalence. Three meta-analyses on small-bowel cancer incidence in Crohn's disease reported standardized incidence ratios of 27.1–33.2. In a prospective observational study with 8222 patients with small-bowel Crohn's patients, the incidence rate of small bowel cancer was 0.235 per 1000 patient-years. Small-bowel cancer in patients with Crohn's disease develops at a younger age and mainly in the ileum in contrast to sporadic small-bowel cancer. The possibility of small-bowel cancer should be suspected in cases of symptom recurrence after long-term remission and small-bowel stricture unresponsive to medical treatment in patients with small-bowel Crohn's disease [7].

Conclusion

Approximately 70% of patients with Crohn's disease have small intestine involvement at the time of diagnosis, and approximately a third of patients with Crohn's disease exclusively involve the small intestine. Small-bowel Crohn's disease is harder to diagnose and treat due to its non-specific symptoms and anatomical location than colonic disease and increases the risk of stricture, surgery, or recurrence. Recently, the advancement of small-bowel imaging and endoscopic techniques has improved the ability to diagnose and treat small-bowel Crohn's disease. However, future study is necessary to understand the occurrence and progression of small-bowel Crohn's disease and establish early diagnostic markers and a more definitive treatment strategy.

References

1. Yang DH, Keum B, Jeen YT. Capsule endoscopy for Crohn's disease: current status of diagnosis and management. Gastroenterol Res Pract. 2016;2016:8236367.
2. Lee JM, Lee KM. Crohn's disease in Korea: past, present, and future. Korean J Intern Med. 2014;29:558–70.
3. Leighton JA, Pasha SF. Inflammatory disorders of the small bowel. Gastrointest Endosc Clin N Am. 2017;27:63–77.
4. Flamant M, Trang C, Maillard O, et al. The prevalence and outcome of jejunal lesions visualized by small bowel capsule endoscopy in Crohn's disease. Inflamm Bowel Dis. 2013;19:1390–6.
5. Park SK, Yang SK, Park SH, et al. Long-term prognosis of the jejunal involvement of Crohn's disease. J Clin Gastroenterol. 2013;47:400–8.
6. Fong SC, Irving PM. Distinct management issues with Crohn's disease of the small intestine. Curr Opin Gastroenterol. 2015;31:92–7.
7. Cahill C, Gordon PH, Petrucci A, Boutros M. Small bowel adenocarcinoma and Crohn's disease: any further ahead than 50 years ago? World J Gastroenterol. 2014;20:11486–95.

Indication of Small Bowel Evaluation in Crohn's Disease

Byong Duk Ye

Key Points
- In cases of clinically suspected Crohn's disease without the presence of lesions supporting the diagnosis of Crohn's disease through colonoscopy, evaluation of the small intestine is indicated. Even if a diagnosis of Crohn's disease was already established based on clinical features, colonoscopy with biopsy and blood tests, etc., examination of the small bowel should be performed to evaluate the small bowel lesions.
- In established Crohn's disease, a small bowel evaluation is required in the following conditions: (1) a change in clinical status with a suspected change of small intestinal lesions, (2) evaluation of small bowel mucosal healing, (3) evaluation of postoperative recurrence, and (4) endoscopic treatment for small bowel lesions.

B. D. Ye (✉)
Department of Gastroenterology and Inflammatory Bowel Disease Center, Asan Medical Center, University of Ulsan College of Medicine, Seoul, South Korea
e-mail: bdye@amc.seoul.kr

Initial Diagnosis of Crohn's Disease

Crohn's disease can involve the entire gastrointestinal tract from the mouth to the anus. The ileum and colon are the most commonly affected areas. Therefore, to diagnose Crohn's disease, the standard procedure is colonoscopic evaluation of the colon and terminal ileum together with biopsy [1, 2]. However, Crohn's disease can involve only the small intestine and not the colon. According to previous Western reports, approximately 30% of patients with Crohn's disease had lesions limited to the small intestine [3], and a Korean population-based epidemiologic study reported that 24.9% of patients with Crohn's disease had small intestinal lesions only [4]. When Crohn's disease is clinically suspected but no lesions are observed through colonoscopy, evaluation of the small intestine is necessary [1]. However, even with symptoms such as chronic abdominal pain and diarrhea, the diagnostic yield of the small-bowel examination for Crohn's disease is decreased if inflammatory biomarkers such as C-reactive protein, erythrocyte sedimentation rate, and fecal calprotectin are not elevated [5].

Even if a diagnosis of Crohn's disease was already established based on clinical features, colonoscopy with biopsy, and blood tests, evaluation of the presence, location, extent, and severity of small bowel lesions is required at the time of diagnosis of Crohn's disease [1, 2]. That is, evaluation of the small intestine should be performed at the time of diagnosis of Crohn's

© Springer Nature Singapore Pte Ltd. 2022
H. J. Chun et al. (eds.), *Small Intestine Disease*, https://doi.org/10.1007/978-981-16-7239-2_38

disease for phenotyping, prognostication, and therapeutic planning.

For imaging of the small bowel, barium small-bowel follow-through or enteroclysis, CT (computed tomography) enterography or enteroclysis, MR (magnetic resonance) enterography or enteroclysis, and small bowel sonography can be used. Small bowel endoscopies include push enteroscopy, enteroscopy with sonde or the rope-way method, capsule endoscopy, and device-assisted enteroscopy [6]. Currently, the most commonly used endoscopic evaluation methods are capsule endoscopy and device-assisted enteroscopy. Compared with that of radiologic imaging tests, small intestine endoscopy has the advantage of enabling direct observation of the intestinal lumen and mucosa. Conversely, radiologic imaging methods such as CT enterography, MR enterography, and small bowel sonography have the advantage of evaluating transmural inflammation of the intestinal tract and extraluminal organs. In cases of suspected Crohn's disease, the choice of small bowel evaluation depends on the individual clinical manifestations of each patient. In general, colonoscopy and small bowel radiologic imaging tests are performed first; then, small bowel capsule endoscopy is performed if Crohn's disease cannot be diagnosed by colonoscopy and radiologic imaging test [1–3, 7, 8]. However, the risk of capsule retention should be considered; if patients have symptoms suggesting intestinal obstruction, a patency capsule or small bowel radiologic imaging tests should be performed before capsule endoscopy [3, 8]. Device-assisted enteroscopy is performed when a diagnosis cannot be made by other tests such as colonoscopy, small bowel imaging, and small bowel capsule endoscopy; a definitive diagnosis is required through biopsy of small bowel lesions [9].

Evaluation of Small Bowel Lesions for Established Crohn's Disease

If patients with Crohn's disease show a change in clinical status during the course of the disease such as elevation of disease activity index and suspected intra-abdominal complications, bowel lesions should be evaluated by colonoscopy or small bowel imaging, depending on the patient's condition. When the cause of clinical deterioration cannot be evaluated through colonoscopy or small intestine imaging, small bowel capsule endoscopy could be helpful through visualizing the small bowel mucosa [5].

Recently, the therapeutic goal of Crohn's disease has evolved to aim to achieve mucosal healing, not only clinical remission. Therefore, it is needed to monitor the mucosal status of the small intestine as well as the colon, evaluate the response to treatment, and evaluate mucosal healing regularly [10]. Although MR imaging, CT imaging, and ultrasonography are widely used to evaluate the small bowel, small bowel capsule endoscopy has the advantage of direct visualization of the small intestinal mucosa. However, because the rate of capsule retention in established Crohn's disease has been reported to be as high as 13.2%, patency capsule or small bowel radiologic imaging tests should be considered before capsule endoscopy [1].

Colonoscopy is primarily used for the evaluation of postoperative recurrence of Crohn's disease. However, for evaluating recurrence in the proximal small bowel that cannot be reached by colonoscopy, small intestine examinations are required [7].

Device-assisted enteroscopy is indicated when therapeutic procedures are required for small bowel lesions of Crohn's disease, such as hemostasis, dilatation of stricture, and foreign body removal [9].

References

1. Ye BD, Jang BI, Jeen YT, et al. Diagnostic guideline of Crohn's disease. Korean J Gastroenterol. 2009;53:161–76.
2. Gomollon F, Dignass A, Annese V, et al. 3rd European evidence-based consensus on the diagnosis and management of Crohn's disease 2016: part 1: diagnosis and medical management. J Crohns Colitis. 2017;11:3–25.
3. Lichtenstein GR, Loftus EV, Isaacs KL, et al. ACG clinical guideline: Management of Crohn's disease in adults. Am J Gastroenterol. 2018;113:481–517.

4. Park SH, Kim YJ, Rhee KH, et al. A 30-year trend analysis in the epidemiology of inflammatory bowel disease in the Songpa-Kangdong District of Seoul, Korea in 1986-2015. J Crohns Colitis. 2019;13:1410–7.

5. Enns RA, Hookey L, Armstrong D, et al. Clinical practice guidelines for the use of video capsule endoscopy. Gastroenterology. 2017;152:497–514.

6. Kim J. Training in endoscopy: enteroscopy. Clin Endosc. 2017;50:328–33.

7. Carter D, Eliakim R. Current role of endoscopy in inflammatory bowel disease diagnosis and management. Curr Opin Gastroenterol. 2014;30:370–7.

8. Park SK, Ye BD, Kim KO, et al. Guidelines for video capsule endoscopy: emphasis on Crohn's disease. Clin Endosc. 2015;48:128–35.

9. Kim M, Jang HJ. The role of small bowel endoscopy in small bowel Crohn's disease: when and how? Intest Res. 2016;14:211–7.

10. Peyrin-Biroulet L, Sandborn W, Sands BE, et al. Selecting therapeutic targets in inflammatory bowel disease (STRIDE): determining therapeutic goals for treat-to-target. Am J Gastroenterol. 2015;110:1324–38.

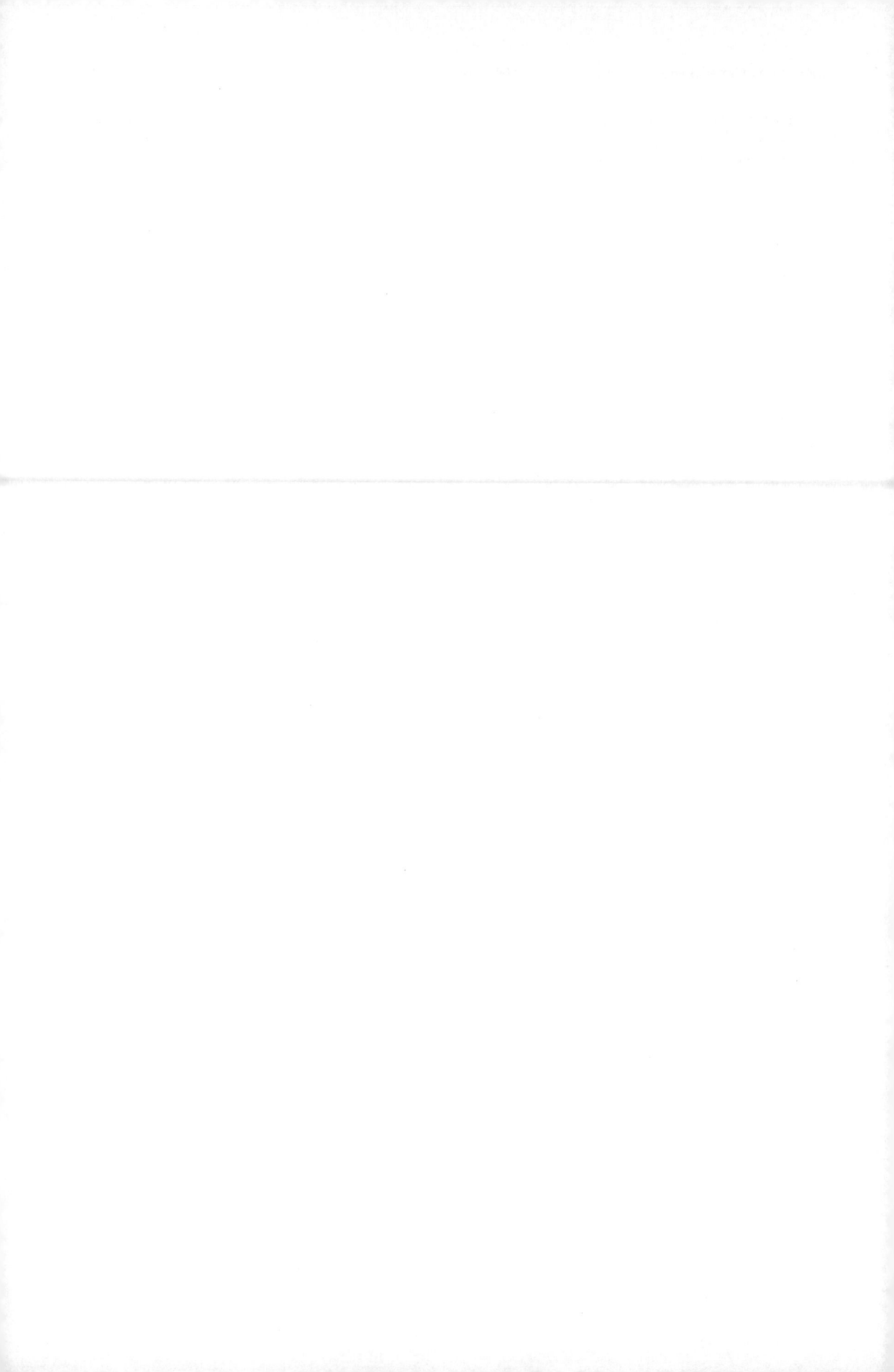

Part X

Usefulness of the Diagnostic Studies to Evaluated Small Bowel Involvement of Crohn's Disease

Radiologic Examination: Small-Bowel Follow-Through, Computed Tomography Enterography, and Magnetic Resonance Enterography

Dae Bum Kim and Kang-Moon Lee

Key Points

1. *Accuracy of radiologic examinations for evaluating small-bowel involvement in Crohn's disease*
   (a) Sensitivity: computed tomography (CT) enterography = magnetic resonance (MR) enterography > small bowel follow-through
   (b) Specificity: CT enterography = MR enterography > small bowel follow-through
2. *Advantages and limitations of each radiologic examination*
   (a) Small bowel follow-through
      (i) Advantages: relatively easy to perform, no intravenous contrast agent required, can demonstrate fine mucosal change
      (ii) Limitations: long examination time, radiation exposure, difficult to interpret
   (b) CT enterography
      (i) Advantages: short scan time, high sensitivity and specificity, can diagnose extraintestinal manifestations
      (ii) Limitations: risk of adverse effects of radiation exposure and intravenous contrast injections
   (c) MR enterography
      (i) Advantages: radiation free, high sensitivity and specificity, excellent soft-tissue contrast
      (ii) Limitations: expensive, time consuming, image quality can decrease because of movement or gas

D. B. Kim · K.-M. Lee (✉)
Department of Internal Medicine, St. Vincent's Hospital, College of Medicine, The Catholic University of Korea, Seoul, Korea
e-mail: drmaloman@catholic.ac.kr

Introduction

Crohn's disease is a chronic disease characterized by non-specific granulomatous inflammation that can occur anywhere in the gastrointestinal tract from the mouth to the anus. The small bowel is the most commonly involved site, with a simultaneous invasion of the small bowel and colon in 45–55% of the patients and invasion of the small bowel alone in 30–40% of the patients [1]. In addition, more than one-third of patients with Crohn's disease have complications, such as a stricture or fistula, at the time of diagnosis, which are often difficult to diagnose without a radiologic examination. Although small bowel follow-through (SBFT) has traditionally been used for small-bowel imaging in Crohn's disease, recent

© Springer Nature Singapore Pte Ltd. 2022
H. J. Chun et al. (eds.), *Small Intestine Disease*, https://doi.org/10.1007/978-981-16-7239-2_39

advances in imaging modalities have enabled faster and more accurate screening of the small bowel on combined computed tomography (CT) or magnetic resonance (MR) imaging (MRI). This chapter will review the usefulness of radiologic examinations in diagnosing and evaluating small-bowel involvement in Crohn's disease.

SBFT

Fluoroscopic evaluation of the small bowel provides images of the small intestinal mucosa by fluoroscopically observing that a contrast agent, such as barium or Gastrografin, travels with the peristaltic movement of the small intestine (Fig. 1). Although the frequency of use of fluoroscopic imaging has decreased because of recent developments in capsule endoscopy, CT, and MRI, fluoroscopic imaging is still important in the evaluation of the small intestine, which is difficult to access endoscopically. The two most commonly used fluoroscopic examinations are SBFT and small-bowel enteroclysis (performed

using a catheter). SBFT is easy to perform, does not require intubation or sedation, and causes less discomfort in the patient. In addition, it has the advantage of low radiation exposure. However, it has the disadvantages of long examination time, insufficient expansion of the mucosal folds, and less double-contrast effect. Enteroclysis has the advantages of sufficient expansion of the mucosal folds, excellent double-contrast effect, and short examination time owing to the rapid administration of the contrast agent; however, it is difficult to perform and has a relatively large radiation exposure. In a study comparing the two tests in Crohn's disease, SBFT was found to be safer, more comfortable for the patient, and superior in diagnosing fistulas and gastroduodenal lesions [2]. In a previous study assessing the sensitivity and specificity of SBFT, capsule endoscopy, and CT enterography in diagnosing small bowel Crohn's disease, the sensitivity, specificity, and accuracy of SBFT were 41–80%, 73–100%, and 63–90%, respectively. Although the sensitivity was lower than that of capsule endoscopy, the specificity or accuracy was not significantly dif-

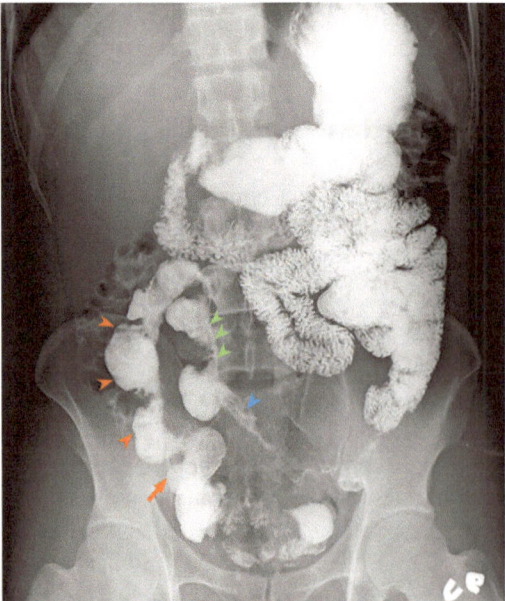

➤ Pseudosacculation on the anti-mesenteric border
➤ Shortening and linear ulcers on the mesenteric border
➤ Mucosal nodularity

Fig. 1 Small bowel follow-through image showing multiple, segmental mucosal thickening from the proximal ileum to the distal ileum and pseudosacculation at the antimesenteric border

ferent. However, both sensitivity and specificity tended to be slightly lower than those of CT enterography [3].

SBFT can easily examine the entire small bowel and is relatively inexpensive; however, it has the disadvantages of long examination time, insufficient information about the small bowel wall and surrounding structures, and difficult image analysis because of overlapping of the small intestine. Therefore, it has recently been replaced by CT and MRI. However, it is still a useful method in cases with difficulty in evaluating fine mucosal changes, contraindication to capsule endoscopy, and a high risk of adverse effects of intravenous contrast agents.

CT Enterography

CT enterography is a test in which a CT scan is performed after the oral administration of a large amount of contrast medium, similar to SBFT and administration of a drug that pauses or decreases small-bowel peristalsis. CT scan can minimize imaging errors due to motion and intestinal peristalsis through rapid image acquisition. In particular, on CT enterography, changes in the small intestinal mucosa and thickening of the small bowel wall can be observed better than on conventional CT. Thus, it is a useful radiologic examination for small-bowel involvement of Crohn's disease (Fig. 2). In addition, CT enterography is useful for diagnosing obstructions, penetrating disease, and extraintestinal manifestations. Since Raptopoulos et al. first reported CT enterography as a method for examining the extent and severity of Crohn's disease in 1997, it has been actively used in clinical practice [4]. Although there are limitations in assessing fine mucosal changes, small ulcers, and ulcer shapes, a recent meta-analysis on the accuracy of CT enterography for small bowel involvement demonstrated sensitivity and specificity of 86% and 84%, respectively [5].

As CT is relatively easy to perform and has high sensitivity and specificity, it can be used as the primary test to confirm small bowel involvement of Crohn's disease. Although it has been

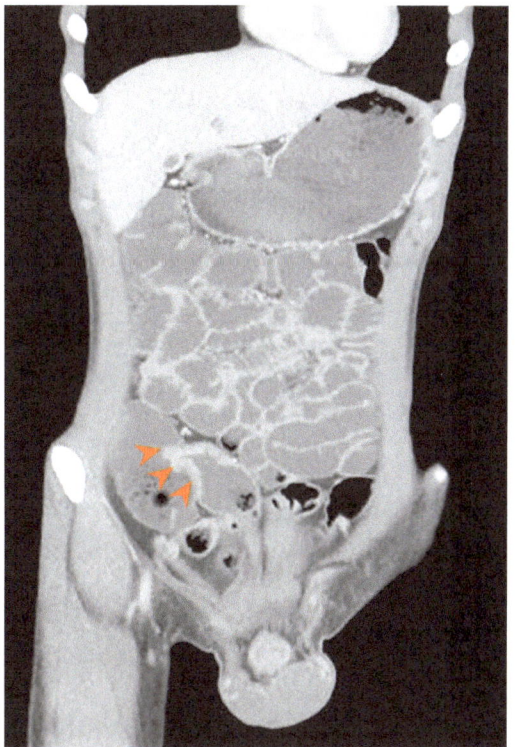

Fig. 2 Computed tomography enterography image showing multiple mucosal thickening in the proximal and distal ileum

established as an important radiologic examination for confirming small-bowel involvement of Crohn's disease, the associated radiation exposure is a drawback. Patients with Crohn's disease are often young and can be susceptible to the effects of radiation. In recent studies, small-dose multidetector CT using low current or low voltage alone, or their combination, was demonstrated to reduce radiation exposure without reducing the diagnostic accuracy [6]. However, excessive reduction in radiation dose warrants caution because it can reduce the image quality and diagnostic accuracy.

MR Enterography

In the past, MR enterography was not frequently used because of the lack of adequate contrast agents, severe image quality deterioration due to breathing or intestinal movement, and long

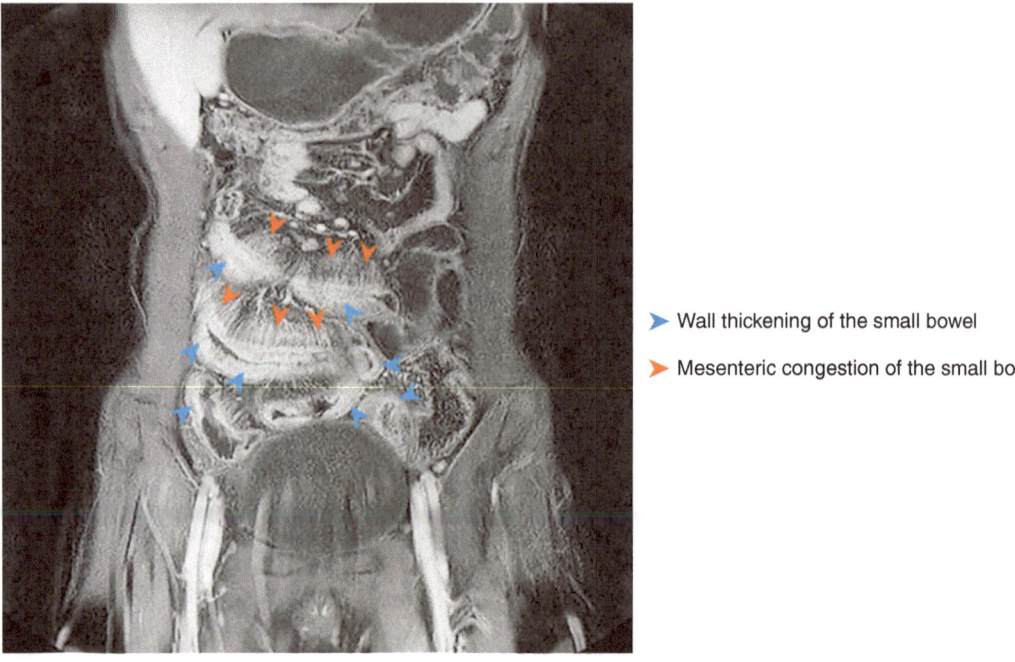

> Wall thickening of the small bowel

> Mesenteric congestion of the small bowel

Fig. 3 Magnetic resonance enterography image showing multiple bowel wall thickening and mesenteric vessel engorgement in the distal jejunum, ileum, and proximal colon

examination time; however, rapid imaging acquisition techniques and the introduction of various gastrointestinal contrast agents have overcome most of the aforementioned limitations. MR enterography can be used to distinguish between active inflammation and stricture caused by fibrosis because of the excellent soft-tissue contrast obtained using the difference in water contents (Fig. 3). In addition, as there is no risk of radiation exposure, it can be useful as an imaging technique to complement the limitations of CT enterography. In recent studies, the sensitivity and specificity of MR enterography for detecting small-bowel involvement of Crohn's disease were 88% and 81%, respectively, which are not significantly different from those of capsule endoscopy and are superior to those of SBFT [5, 7]. In addition, there is no difference in accuracy between CT and MR enterography in evaluating small-bowel involvement in Crohn's disease; however, MR enterography has the advantage of no radiation exposure. Therefore, it is the preferred method for pediatric and young patients with

Crohn's disease. Other advantages include good soft-tissue resolution, availability of quantitative techniques (e.g., diffusion-weighted imaging), and less frequent adverse effects of intravenous contrast agents. However, the disadvantages are long examination time, high cost, reduced image quality due to intestinal peristalsis or gas, and low negative predictive value. Therefore, even when negative findings are observed on MR enterography, the possibility of small-bowel involvement in Crohn's disease and complications such as strictures and fistulas should be considered [8].

Conclusion

A radiologic examination is effective and useful for the diagnosis and evaluation of small bowel involvement in Crohn's disease. Table 1 shows the advantages and disadvantages of each radiologic examination. The appropriate modality should be selected based on the individual patient's situation and the purpose of the test.

Table 1 Advantages and limitations of radiologic examination for evaluating small-bowel involvement in Crohn's disease

Radiologic examination	Advantages	Limitations
Small bowel follow-through	• Easy to perform • Cheap • Can demonstrate fine mucosal changes • No intravenous contrast agents required	• Long examination time • Radiation exposure • Difficult to interpret • Lack of information about the surrounding structures
Computed tomography enterography	• Short scan time • High sensitivity and specificity • Can diagnose extraintestinal manifestations	• Radiation exposure • Risk of intravenous contrast agent-associated adverse effects • Limited to the evaluation of fine mucosal change
Magnetic resonance enterography	• Excellent soft-tissue contrast • Radiation free • High sensitivity and specificity • Relatively less contrast agent-associated adverse effects	• Time-consuming • Expensive • Decreased image quality because of motion or gas

References

1. Farmer RG, Hawk WA, Turnbull RB Jr. Clinical patterns in Crohn's disease: a statistical study of 615 cases. Gastroenterology. 1975;68:627–35.
2. Bernstein CN, Boult IF, Greenberg HM, van der Putten W, Duffy G, Grahame GR. A prospective randomized comparison between small bowel enteroclysis and small bowel follow-through in Crohn's disease. Gastroenterology. 1997,113.390–8.
3. Solem CA, Loftus EV Jr, Fletcher JG, et al. Small-bowel imaging in Crohn's disease: a prospective, blinded, 4-way comparison trial. Gastrointest Endosc. 2008;68:255–66.
4. Raptopoulos V, Schwartz RK, McNicholas MM, Movson J, Pearlman J, Joffe N. Multiplanar helical CT enterography in patients with Crohn's disease. AJR Am J Roentgenol. 1997;169:1545–50.
5. Qiu Y, Mao R, Chen BL, et al. Systematic review with meta-analysis: magnetic resonance enterography vs. computed tomography enterography for evaluating disease activity in small bowel Crohn's disease. Aliment Pharmacol Ther. 2014;40:134–46.
6. Kambadakone AR, Prakash P, Hahn PF, Sahani DV. Low-dose CT examinations in Crohn's disease: impact on image quality, diagnostic performance, and radiation dose. AJR Am J Roentgenol. 2010;195:78–88.
7. Lee SS, Kim AY, Yang SK, et al. Crohn disease of the small bowel: comparison of CT enterography, MR enterography, and small-bowel follow-through as diagnostic techniques. Radiology. 2009;251:751–61.
8. Jensen MD, Kjeldsen J, Rafaelsen SR, Nathan T. Diagnostic accuracies of MR enterography and CT enterography in symptomatic Crohn's disease. Scand J Gastroenterol. 2011;46:1449–57.

Effectiveness of Endoscopic Examinations for the Detection of Small Bowel Crohn's Disease: Capsule Endoscopy and Device-Assisted Enteroscopy

Hyun-Soo Kim

Introduction

Capsule endoscopy and device-assisted enteroscopy are considered the most effective methods for diagnosing small bowel Crohn's disease, with a diagnosis rate of 40–60%. Capsule endoscopy enables direct observation of the small intestinal mucosa and is very useful for diagnosing superficial or small lesions without causing any pain or radiation effect (Table 1) [1]. Device-assisted enteroscopy aids in the histological diagnosis of diseases associated with the small intestinal mucosa and in the treatment of stenosis or hemorrhage.

Capsule Endoscopy

Capsule endoscopy is more effective in diagnosing small bowel Crohn's disease than abdominal computed tomography or small bowel barium study and has a diagnostic effect similar to that of magnetic resonance imaging [2]. Considering the poor prognosis of Crohn's disease with extensive small intestinal involvement or Crohn's disease of the upper small bowel, diagnosing these diseases via capsule endoscopy is important for treatment decision-making. Furthermore, capsule

H.-S. Kim (✉)
Department of Gastroenterology, Chonnam National University Hospital, Chonnam National University Medical School, Gwangju, South Korea
e-mail: dshskim@jnu.ac.kr

endoscopy plays an exceptional role in the diagnosis of proximal small intestine lesions compared with other imaging studies.

Suspected Crohn's Disease

Colonoscopy is preferred for diagnosis if Crohn's disease is suspected (i.e., abdominal pain, chronic diarrhea, weight loss, growth disturbance). Nonetheless, capsule endoscopy can be performed in patients without any colonoscopic abnormalities, symptoms of small intestinal obstruction, or stenosis. The diagnostic sensitivity and specificity of capsule endoscopy are 91–100% and 91–92%, respectively; while the specificity of capsule endoscopy is low, its sensitivity is high [3]. Additionally, the negative predictive value is high; thus, in case of negative findings on colonoscopy and capsule endoscopy, we can rule out 96% of Crohn's disease. Endoscopic findings include edema, loss of villi, erosion, erythema, aphthous ulcer, and stenosis (Fig. 1). Nonspecific ulcers and erosions are also found in 14% of normal individuals [4]. These lesions are similar to the nonsteroidal anti-inflammatory drug (NSAID)-induced enteropathy, tuberculosis, Behcet's disease, lymphoma, small bowel ischemia, and radiation enteritis and are hence difficult to distinguish. As NSAIDs may cause lesions similar to those of Crohn's disease in the small intestine, it is preferable to stop taking NSAIDs until 1 month

© Springer Nature Singapore Pte Ltd. 2022
H. J. Chun et al. (eds.), *Small Intestine Disease*, https://doi.org/10.1007/978-981-16-7239-2_40

Table 1 Wireless capsule endoscopy

Advantages	Disadvantages
Sensitivity to identifying mucosal abnormalities	Specificity and positive predictive value not known
Useful when other imaging modalities are negative	Cost
Easy to administer	Requires experienced gastroenterologist to review
Nonionizing radiation	Capsule retention
No sedation required	Nontherapeutic, no biopsy possible

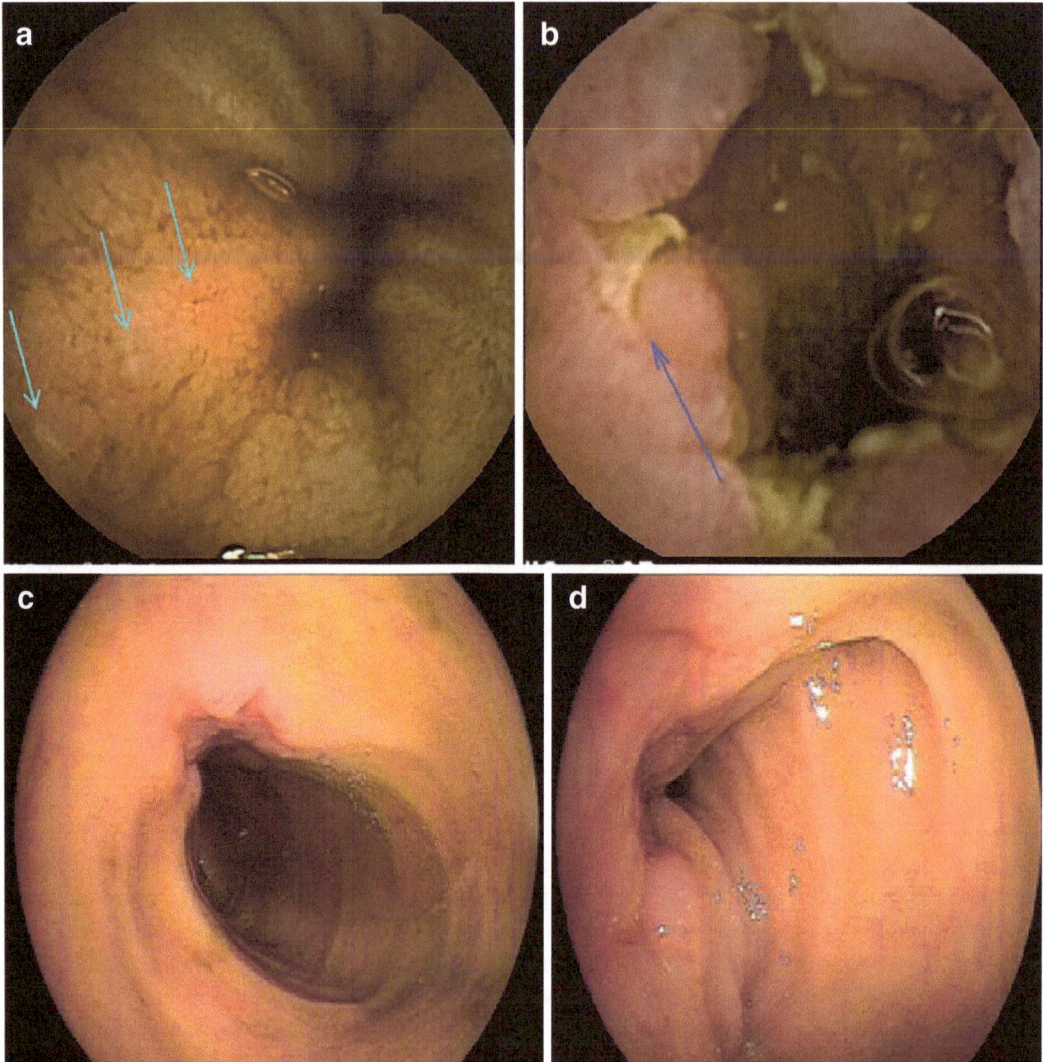

Fig. 1 Findings of capsule endoscopy (**a**, **b**) and enteroscopy (**c**, **d**). (**a**) Longitudinally arranged erosions; (**b**) multiple ulcers; (**c**) ulcer; (**d**) ulcer and stricture

Table 2 Lewis score

	Number	Extent	Descriptors
Villous appearance (worst-affected tertile) Ulcer (worst-affected tertile)	Normal—0 Edematous—1 None—0 Single—3 2–7—5 ≥8—10	≤10%—8 11–50%—12 >50%—20 ≤10%—5 11–50%—10 >50%—15	Single—1 Patchy—14 Diffuse—17 <1/4—9 1/4–1/2—12 ≥1/2—18 (percentage of the frame occupied by the largest ulcer)
Stenosis (whole study)	None—0 Single—14 Multiple—20	Non-ulcerated—2 Ulcerated—24	Traverse—7 Not traverse—10

Table 3 Capsule endoscopy Crohn's disease activity index (Niv score)

A. Inflammation score
0 = None
1 = Edema/hyperemia/denudation (mild to moderate)
2 = Edema/hyperemia/denudation (severe)
3 = Bleeding, exudate, aphthae, erosion, ulcer <0.5 cm
4 = Ulcer 0.5–2 cm, pseudopolyp
5 = Large ulcer >2 cm

B. Extent of disease score
0 = No disease
1 = Focal disease (1 segment)
2 = Patchy disease (2–3 segments)
3 = Diffuse disease (>3 segments)

C. Stricture score
0 = None
1 = Single—passed
2 = Multiple—passed
3 = Obstruction (non-passage)

CECDAI = proximal (A1 × B1 + C1) + distal (A2 × B2 + C2)

before the examination. Recent guidelines have recommended the use of Lewis score or Capsule Endoscopy Crohn's Disease Activity Index (CECDAI) to objectify the degree of inflammation in small bowel diseases (Tables 2 and 3) [5]. A Lewis score <135 may indicate normal or nonsignificant inflammation; between 135 and 790, mild inflammation; and >790, moderate or severe inflammation. CECDAI of 3.8 and 5.9 had been shown to be consistent with Lewis scores of 135 and 790, respectively, although the correlation with fecal calprotectin was more consistent with the Lewis score than with CECDAI [5].

Confirmed Crohn's Disease

The roles of capsule endoscopy are as follows:

1. Phenotype, location, and prognosis of lesion
2. Mucosal healing test for therapeutic purpose
3. Postoperative recurrence examination
4. Evaluations of discrepancies in clinical symptoms, blood test, and endoscopic findings

When the disease is confirmed as Crohn's disease, capsule endoscopy is required for the detection of invasion range and activity. Jejunum involvement is associated with the severity of Crohn's disease, increasing the risk of recurrence and hospitalization as well as steroid and immunosuppressant use. Recent studies have reported an increased incidence of biological agent use when the upper small bowel is invaded [6]. Mucosal healing not only is a goal of treatment for Crohn's disease but also an important indicator of treatment response. Assessment indicators should be relatively objective, with the Lewis score or CECDAI being used. Despite clinical improvement, mucosal healing can be observed on capsule endoscopy only in approximately 15–40% of patients [7]. Therefore, capsule endoscopy is important for treatment evaluation. Colonoscopy can diagnose postoperative recurrence in Crohn's disease in 25% of patients; in contrast, capsule endoscopy can diagnose postoperative recurrence in 62% of patients [6]. Capsule endoscopy can be performed for the evaluation of postoperative recurrence if no abnormality is found on colonoscopy. Ulcerative colitis and Crohn's disease are difficult to differentiate by imaging tests in approximately 10–15% of cases, and additional capsule endoscopy may be diagnosed as Crohn's disease [8]. Capsule endoscopy can be performed to diagnose unexplained iron deficiency anemia or detect an intestinal bleeding site.

Among the disadvantages of capsule endoscopy is that the capsule may be retained in the small intestine. If the capsule remains in the small intestine for more than 14 days, as identified on plain abdominal radiograph, capsule retention is suspected. The capsule retention rate in suspected and confirmed Crohn's disease has been reported to be 0–5.4% and 0–13.2%, respectively [2]. Patency capsules and computerized images can be used to predict residual stenosis in order to prevent or reduce capsule retention.

Device-Assisted Enteroscopy

Compared with other forms of endoscopy, device-assisted enteroscopy is very invasive and requires a longer time to complete. Nevertheless, device-assisted enteroscopy is very useful for diagnosing small bowel diseases. If other imaging studies are negative, approximately 40% of additional diagnosis is possible with device-assisted enteroscopy [9]. If Crohn's disease is suspected, the diagnostic yield of small intestinal enteroscopy is 22–70%, and complications can occur in approximately 1% of cases [4]. A recent meta-analysis reported that the diagnostic yield of enteroscopy for the presence of inflammatory lesions in the small intestine is 16%, which is comparable to that of capsule endoscopy (18%). Hence, the primary examination should be capsule endoscopy, which is an easier test than enteroscopy in patients without stenosis [4]. Nevertheless, enteroscopy plays an exceptional role in the treatment of hemorrhage and stenosis and has the advantage of the performance of biopsy for the diagnosis of Crohn's disease. Approximately 60–80% of anastomotic stenosis or stenosis measuring <5 cm without severe inflammation can be treated through endoscopy,

and there is a risk of perforations in approximately 9%; therefore, caution should be exercised when severe inflammation is present or steroids are used [4].

Summary and Conclusion

Crohn's disease involves the small intestine in more than 50% of cases, and examining this disease is fraught with several difficulties. If colonoscopy is negative, capsule endoscopy may be performed in patients with suspected Crohn's disease. Device-assisted enteroscopy can be used when histological diagnosis or treatment for complications such as hemorrhage and stenosis is needed.

References

1. Morris M, Chu DI. Imaging for inflammatory bowel disease. Surg Clin N Am. 2015;95:1143–58.
2. Park SK, Ye BD, Kim KO, et al. Guidelines for video capsule endoscopy: emphasis on Crohn's disease. Clin Endosc. 2015;48:128–35.
3. Enns RA, Hookey L, Amstrong D, et al. Clinical practice guideline for the use of video capsule endoscopy. Gastroenterology. 2017;152:497–514.
4. Kim M, Jang HJ. The role of small bowel endoscopy in small bowel Crohn's disease: when or how? Intest Res. 2016;14:211–7.
5. Rosa B, Pinho R, Ferro SM, et al. Endoscopic score for evaluation of Crohn's disease activity at small bowel capsule endoscopy: general principles and current applications. GE Port Gastroenterol. 2016;23:36–41.
6. Rosa B, Cotter J. Current clinical indications for small bowel capsule endoscopy. Acta Medica Port. 2015;28:632–9.
7. Koylov U, Yung DE, Engel T, et al. Diagnostic yield of capsule endoscopy versus magnetic resonance enterography and small bowel contrast ultrasound in the evaluation of small bowel Crohn's disease: systemic review and meta-analysis. Dig Liver Dis. 2017;49:854–63.
8. Kypylov U, Ben-Horin S, Seidman EG, Elikaim R. Video capsule endoscopy of small bowel for monitoring of Crohn's disease. Inlamm Bowel Dis. 2015;21:2726–35.
9. Tun GSZ, Ratehalli D, Sander DS, et al. Clinical utility of double-balloon enteroscopy in suspected Crohn's disease: a single-centre experience. Eur J Gastroenterol Hepatol. 2016;28:820–5.

Non-steroidal Anti-inflammatory Drug Enteropathy

Seong-Eun Kim

Key Points
- The incidence of non-steroidal anti-inflammatory drug (NSAID) enteropathy is increasing, as are its serious clinical complications.
- The pathogenic mechanism of NSAID enteropathy is suggested to be as follows:
  - Local mucosal damage—"three-hit hypothesis" (mitochondrial damage; increased mucosal permeability; and interactions among bile, gut microbiota, and enterohepatic circulation);
  - Systemic effects—decrease in prostaglandin (inhibition of cyclooxygenase [COX]-1 and that of COX-2 are both important).
- The main complications are iron deficiency anemia, protein-losing enteropathy, and diaphragm-like strictures.
- The most important factor for the diagnosis of NSAID enteropathy is a detailed history of NSAID intake.
- There are no standard treatments at present; however, selective COX-2 inhibitors, mucosal protective agents (e.g., rebamipide), antibiotics, and probiotics are reported to be useful.

Non-steroidal anti-inflammatory drugs (NSAIDs) are a class of medications used as anti-inflammatory, analgesic, and anti-thrombotic agents. They are commonly prescribed in a wide range of diseases, including arthritis, cardiovascular disease, and cerebrovascular disease. However, they have the drawback of occasionally causing gastrointestinal (GI) complications, such as ulcers, bleeding, and perforation.

Previous studies have focused on NSAID-induced complications in the upper GI tract, as well as the effects of gastric acid suppressants in preventing and treating these diseases. NSAID enteropathy, in contrast, has not been well documented because its clinical symptoms are non-specific and difficult to diagnose. Recent advances in endoscopy have led to the development of capsular endoscopy and balloon-assisted small-bowel enteroscopy, which have made the diagnostic approach to small-intestinal diseases easier. Additionally, the interest in small-intestinal diseases induced by NSAIDs has increased the reported incidence of NSAID enteropathy.

S.-E. Kim (✉)
Department of Internal Medicine, Ewha Womans University College of Medicine, Seoul, South Korea
e-mail: kimse@ewha.ac.kr

© Springer Nature Singapore Pte Ltd. 2022
H. J. Chun et al. (eds.), *Small Intestine Disease*, https://doi.org/10.1007/978-981-16-7239-2_41

In this chapter, we will review current knowledge on NSAID enteropathy.

Epidemiology

Upper GI complications secondary to NSAIDs, such as bleeding and perforation, have decreased. However, complications in the small intestine and colon are increasing. The ratio of upper to lower NSAID-related GI events decreased from 4.1 in 1996 to 1.4 in 2005 [1]. In a recent large-scale clinical study, 40% of severe GI complications induced by NSAIDs were lower GI complications [2]. This suggests that NSAID-induced mucosal damage may be as common and serious in the small intestine as in the stomach and duodenum.

NSAID enteropathy can occur in 53–80% of healthy individuals who have used NSAIDs for a short period. Between 50 and 70% of chronic users (>3 months of use) are reported to be affected [3].

Aspirin has been considered less likely to damage the small intestine than other NSAIDs. However, when a small dose of aspirin was administered to healthy subjects for 2 weeks, the incidence of enteropathy, including in a mild form, significantly increased in comparison to a control group [4].

Pathogenesis

Various hypotheses have been suggested to explain the mechanism of NSAID enteropathy. However, none has been well-validated (Fig. 1).

The "three-hit hypothesis" posits that NSAIDs have a direct toxic effect on intestinal cells. First, phospholipids in the cell membrane on the mucosal surface are directly damaged by the drugs, resulting in mitochondrial damage in the cell. Second, mitochondrial damage leads to a decrease in intracellular energy production, followed by calcium efflux and the generation of free radicals. As a result, the intercellular junction is damaged and mucosal permeability increased. Third, intestinal luminal contents like bile, proteolytic enzymes, gut flora and its byproducts, and toxins enter the cells through the damaged barrier, leading to inflammation [5, 6].

The systemic effects of NSAIDs are associated with a reduction in prostaglandin (PG). PG plays an important role in intestinal blood flow and mucus production, and inhibition of PG synthesis may cause GI mucosal damage. COX-1, which is one of two predominant COX isozymes, plays an important role in PG formation and the maintenance of GI mucosal homeostasis. In the past, only COX-1 inhibition was believed to be associated with mucosal damage; however, recent animal studies have shown that inhibition of COX-2 can also lead to damage of the mucosa in the small intestine. It has been suggested that COX-2 products have an important role in maintaining small bowel integrity [6, 7].

Among the previously mentioned pathophysiologic factors involved in the COX-independent mechanism, enterohepatic circulation, gut microbiota, and bile are thought to have very important roles in the development of NSAID enteropathy. When NSAIDs are excreted into bile ducts from hepatocytes, they are deconjugated by bacterial β-glucuronidase in the small intestine and re-enter the enterohepatic circulation through the intestinal epithelial cells. Repeated enterohepatic circulation of NSAIDs, and the toxic effects of bile, may cause local damage to the mucosa. The gut microbiota may have an important role in the pathogenesis of NSAID enteropathy as a source of pathogens, and not only (as mentioned previously) as a β-glucuronidase producer. There is evidence of gut microbiota involvement in the pathogenesis of NSAID enteropathy. In germ-free mice, the small-intestinal mucosa was not damaged by NSAID administration. However, colonization with gram-negative bacteria caused mucosal damage in the small intestine. Antibiotic treatment targeting the gram-negative bacteria reduced the incidence of NSAID enteropathy. Lipopolysaccharides from gram-negative bacteria have been shown to activate the Toll-like receptors of macrophages in the lamina propria. In this way, they stimulate the innate immune system, recruit inflammatory cells, and cause mucosal damage in the small intestine. Prolonged

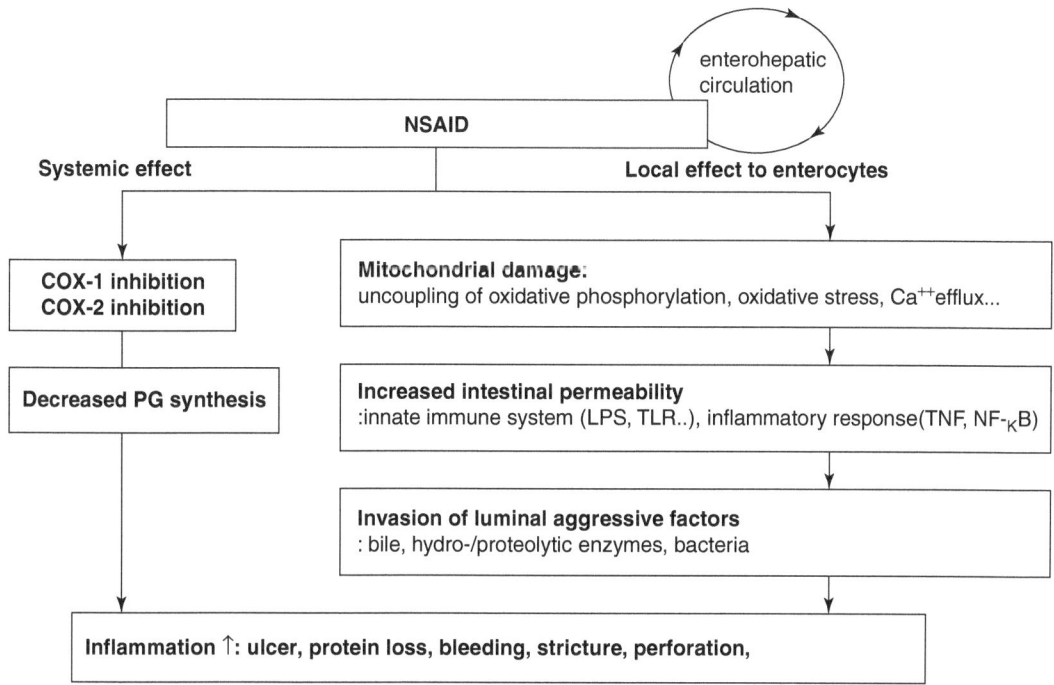

Fig. 1 The pathogenesis of non-steroidal anti-inflammatory drug (NSAID) enteropathy. The figure summarizes the main suggested mechanisms that NSAID may lead to small intestinal inflammation [13]

use of proton pump inhibitors (PPIs) may exacerbate NSAID enteropathy by weakening stomach acidity, altering the gut environment, and causing dysbiosis of the gut microbiota [6, 8].

Because aspirin is rapidly absorbed in the stomach and duodenum and does not enter the enterohepatic circulation, lesions caused by aspirin are typically localized in the stomach and duodenum. However, enteric-coated aspirin, which has been developed to reduce gastric mucosal damage, is mainly soluble in the small intestine and enters the enterohepatic circulation, giving rise to mucosal damage in the distal area of the small intestine. One study showed that 16.7% of users of non-coated aspirin developed small-intestinal ulcers, versus 56.3% of users of enteric-coated aspirin [4, 6].

Clinical Manifestations

The symptoms of NSAID enteropathy, unlike those of NSAID gastropathy, are usually non-specific and present in various ways.

Manifestations include dyspepsia, constipation, diarrhea, abdominal pain, occult blood, hypoalbuminemia, malabsorption, iron deficiency anemia, and protein-losing enteropathy. Severe life-threatening complications like hemorrhage, intestinal obstruction due to stenosis, and perforation are rare but possible. Other rare manifestations of NSAID enteropathy include diverticulitis, diverticular bleeding, and malabsorption of vitamin B12 or bile acid [3, 6].

Iron Deficiency Anemia

Unexplained iron deficiency anemia manifests in 30–40% of cases of obscure GI bleeding. NSAID enteropathy, along with angiodysplasia, is a common cause of unexplained GI bleeding.

Protein-Losing Enteropathy

Protein-losing enteropathy is a rare manifestation. However, when a patient taking NSAIDs for a prolonged period shows hypoalbuminemia (albumin < 3.0 g/dL) of unknown cause, malnutrition, and micronutrient deficiencies, protein-losing enteropathy should be suspected. Hypoalbuminemia has been reported in approximately 10% of patients with rheumatoid arthritis taking NSAIDs. Measurement of alpha-1-antitrypsin clearance in suspected cases may aid the diagnosis. In studies using isotopes, protein loss in these patients was mainly observed in the distal ileum [6].

Small Bowel Stricture

The diaphragm-like stricture is a rare but pathognomonic finding suggesting long-term use of NSAIDs. It is more common in the ileum than jejunum and was observed in approximately 2% of chronic NSAID users in a capsule endoscopy study. It is usually caused by fibrosis originating from mucosal or submucosal inflammation. This leads to the development of multiple concentric membranes or mucosal webs, resulting in stenosis and occlusion with progressive narrowing of the lumen. Because the muscle layer is usually well preserved, perforation rarely occurs unless serious inflammation is present. These characteristics suggest that balloon dilation or needle knife electro-incision may be more suitable than surgery for treating NSAID-induced isolated stenosis. Surgery is recommended if lesions are extensive and multiple, refractory to endoscopic therapy, and need to be differentiated from malignancy.

High-Risk Groups

Prevention and treatment regimens for NSAID enteropathy have not been established. Therefore, an important aspect of clinical practice may be the identification of those at high risk of NSAID enteropathy, and avoidance or careful monitoring of NSAID use in this group. Thus far, high-risk individuals have been identified as those aged 70 years or older, using a combination of antithrombotic agents, having two or more chronic dis-

eases, having polymorphisms such as CYP2C9, and using specific NSAIDs (diclofenac and oxicam agents such as meloxicam, ampiroxicam, and loxocam). No studies have examined whether ulcers and erosions or diaphragm-like lesions are more common in patients with certain clinical characteristics.

Animal studies have reported that concomitant administration of a PPI to prevent NSAID gastropathy instead causes gut dysbiosis, further exacerbating small-intestinal mucosal lesions. However, the clinical relevance of this finding remains unclear [3, 6].

Diagnosis

History-Taking

The most important step in diagnosing NSAID enteropathy is taking a detailed history of NSAID use. NSAIDs are often prescribed for long periods to patients who are not aware that they are taking NSAIDs. Therefore, if the cause of a lesion is unclear, NSAID use should always be suspected and investigated. Small-intestinal mucosal damage may occur in 53–80% of healthy adults with only short-term NSAID use. It is not known how long it takes for damaged mucosa to recover after NSAIDs are discontinued. However, lesions have been reported to persist for 18 months or longer [3]. Care should also be taken to rule out the possibility of Crohn's disease, even in patients who have taken NSAIDs.

Capsule Endoscopy and Device-Assisted Enteroscopy

Capsule endoscopy and device-assisted enteroscopy are the most suitable diagnostic methods because they are able to confirm disease severity and the location of mucosal lesions. Capsule endoscopy should be considered first because it is a non-invasive test that does not cause pain. Because diaphragm-like stenosis is one of the most common causes of capsule retention, it is recommended that patency capsule endoscopy be performed before capsule endoscopy in at-risk patients. The ability of NSAID ulcers to cause capsule retention is less widely recognized, but one study reported that radiography identified small mucosal defects in only 17% of patients with small bowel stenosis caused by NSAIDs [9]. The findings of capsule endoscopy can be divided into five categories: petechiae, reddened folds, denuded areas of villus loss, mucosal breaks (including erosions and ulcers), and presence of blood without a visualized lesion [10]. Device-assisted enteroscopy may also reveal discrete ulcers, red spots, and large and small erosions.

Isotopic Tests

Chromium-51-labeled EDTA (^{51}Cr EDTA) or 111-indium (In)-labeled leukocyte scanning may be used to indirectly assess the severity of inflammatory damage by measuring the permeability of the small intestine. However, these tests have limited clinical applications due to their high costs.

Fecal Calprotectin

Fecal calprotectin can be used as a marker of inflammation in the small intestine, as well as to evaluate disease severity. However, its specificity is low. The range of significant values is similar to that of inflammatory bowel disease, infectious colitis, and colorectal cancer.

Computed Tomography (CT) and Magnetic Resonance (MR) Enterography

Computed tomography (CT) and magnetic resonance (MR) enterography are more useful for diagnosing stenosis than conventional CT; however, it is important to have a complete understanding of the patient's clinical history to improve the diagnostic yield for NSAID enteropathy. NSAID-induced stenoses are shorter in length, symmetrical, and more numerous than stenoses associated with Crohn's disease, and they typically spare the terminal ileum.

Treatment and Prevention

The most effective way to prevent NSAID enteropathy is to stop NSAID use. However, there are many clinical situations in which these drugs cannot be avoided. Thus, effective preventive medicines that can be used in combination with NSAIDs are needed. Unfortunately, there are no clinically proven drugs or preventive strategies for NSAID enteropathy. Medications for preventing NSAID gastropathy, such as H2 blockers and PPIs, do not prevent NSAID enteropathy.

Selective COX-2 Inhibitors

Selective COX-2 inhibitors have been reported to lower the incidence of GI ulcers and bleeding, and reduce the risk of small-intestinal complications compared with conventional NSAIDs. The risk of mucosal injury in the small intestine was lower in patients treated with celecoxib for 2 weeks than in those treated with a combination of naproxen and omeprazole for the same period. However, selective COX-2 inhibitors may not provide complete protection against injury to the small intestine. When a selective COX-2 inhibitor was administered for 3 months, there was no significant difference in the risk of small-intestinal damage from NSAIDs [2].

Mucoprotective Agents

Misoprostol, a synthetic PG analog, was expected to have a protective effect on NSAID enteropathy. However, conflicting results have been reported. In addition, the misoprostol may cause adverse effects such as nausea, dyspepsia, abdominal pain, and diarrhea, and patient compliance may be low [11].

Rebamipide is known to protect the GI mucosa by increasing mucus and PG production, eliminating reactive oxygen species, and inhibiting myeloperoxidase activity. It is safe for long-term administration because it has few adverse effects. A study using capsule endoscopy showed that rebamipide was effective in the treatment of NSAID gastroenteropathy in healthy adults. Its prophylactic effect has been confirmed, even when it is used on a short-term basis in combination with diclofenac. However, a preventive effect has not yet been demonstrated in large clinical studies, and studies of its therapeutic effects are lacking. Irsogladine and geranylgeranylacetone have also been proposed as candidate prophylactic agents for NSAID enteropathy.

Manipulation of the Gut Microbiota

Treating NSAID enteropathy through manipulation of the gut microbiota is based on evidence of an association between changes in the composition of the microbiota and disease development. It has been reported that the combination of an NSAID and metronidazole, the latter of which targets anaerobic bacteria, reduces the incidence of NSAID enteropathy. An evaluation using capsule endoscopy found that delayed-release rifaximin was associated with a significant short-term decrease in the incidence of the disease [12]. Use the probiotics *Lactobacillus acidophilus* and *Bifidobacterium adolescentis* have also shown potential therapeutic and prophylactic effects against NSAID enteropathy. VSL#3, a probiotic mixture consisting of eight bacterial strains, is also expected to prevent indomethacin-induced mucosal damage in the small intestine [3].

Others

The PPI lansoprazole has been reported to increase the production of heme oxygenase-1, which is expected to have a therapeutic effect in NSAID enteropathy. However, because there are conflicting reports, further studies are still needed. In patients with rheumatoid arthritis, the combination of an NSAID and sulfasalazine reduced intestinal inflammation and bleeding. This suggests that sulfasalazine is a possible prophylactic agent against NSAID enteropathy.

New NSAIDs currently under investigation include NO- and H2S-releasing NSAIDs. NO and H2S protect the mucosa by increasing mucosal blood flow and inhibiting the adhesion of leukocytes to the vascular endothelium.

NSAIDs with a phosphatidylcholine base are also being studied. These may prevent the penetration of mucosal surfaces by acids, bile, and other toxic substances.

Conclusion

NSAID enteropathy is as common and severe as NSAID-related complications in the upper GI tract. Various pathogenic mechanisms have been proposed; however, further studies are needed. The clinical manifestations of NSAID enteropathy are usually non-specific. Therefore, it is important to identify high-risk patients and observe them carefully. Once long-term NSAID use has caused progression to severe complications (e.g., diaphragm-like stricture), the disease cannot be treated by simple cessation of NSAID use. Advances in small-intestinal endoscopy and imaging studies have made it easier to diagnose NSAID enteropathy. However, taking a detailed history is still important for diagnosing the disease in a timely manner. Currently, there are no standard treatments or effective methods for preventing NSAID enteropathy. Although selective COX-2 inhibitors, various mucoprotective agents, antibiotics, and probiotics have been proposed as therapeutic and prophylactic agents, treatment and prevention strategies that can be applied in clinical practice are still needed.

References

1. Lanas A, García-Rodríguez LA, Polo-Tomás M, et al. Time trends and impact of upper and lower gastrointestinal bleeding and perforation in clinical practice. Am J Gastroenterol. 2009;104:1633–41.

2. Laine L, Curtis SP, Langman M, et al. Lower gastrointestinal events in a double-blind trial of the cyclo-oxygenase-2 selective inhibitor etoricoxib and the traditional nonsteroidal anti-inflammatory drug diclofenac. Gastroenterology. 2008;135:1517–25.
3. Srinivasan A, De Cruz P. A practical approach to the clinical management of NSAID enteropathy. Scand J Gastroenterol. 2017;52(9):941–7.
4. Endo H, Sakai E, Kato T, et al. Small bowel injury in low-dose aspirin users. J Gastroenterol. 2015;50(4):378–86.
5. Bjarnason I, Hayllar J, MacPherson AJ, Russell AS. Side effects of nonsteroidal anti-inflammatory drugs on the small and large intestine in humans. Gastroenterology. 1993;104:1832–47.
6. Shin SJ, Noh CK, Lim SG, et al. Non-steroidal anti-inflammatory drug-induced enteropathy. Intest Res. 2017;15(4):446–55.
7. Sigthorsson G, Simpson RJ, Walley M, et al. COX-1 and 2, intestinal integrity, and pathogenesis of non-steroidal antiinflammatory drug enteropathy in mice. Gastroenterology. 2002;122:1913–23.
8. Wallace JL. NSAID gastropathy and enteropathy: distinct pathogenesis likely necessitates distinct prevention strategies. Br J Pharmacol. 2012;165(1):67–74.
9. Matsumoto T, Esaki M, Kurahara K, et al. Double-contrast barium enteroclysis as a patency tool for nonsteroidal anti-inflammatory drug-induced enteropathy. Dig Dis Sci. 2011;56:3247–53.
10. Maiden L, Thjodleifsson B, Theodors A, et al. A quantitative analysis of NSAID-induced small bowel pathology by capsule enteroscopy. Gastroenterology. 2005;128:1172–8.
11. Watanabe T, Sugimori S, Kameda N, et al. Small bowel injury by low-dose enteric-coated aspirin and treatment with misoprostol: a pilot study. Clin Gastroenterol Hepatol. 2008;6:1279–82.
12. Scarpignato C, Dolak W, Lanas A, et al. Rifaximin reduces number and severity of intestinal lesions associated with use of non-steroidal anti-inflammatory drugs in humans. Gastroenterology. 2017;152:980–2.
13. Matsui H, Shimokawa O, Kaneko T, et al. The pathophysiology of non-steroidal anti-inflammatory drug (NSAID)-induced mucosal injuries in stomach and small intestine. J Clin Biochem Nutr. 2011;48(2):107–11.

Small Intestinal Tuberculosis

Jaeyoung Chun

Key Points

1. Small intestinal tuberculosis predominantly involves the terminal ileum around the ileocecal valve, requiring a differential diagnosis of Crohn's disease.
2. Chest X-ray is essential for the diagnosis but can be negative in patients with suspected small intestinal tuberculosis.
3. Histopathologic examinations, acid-fast bacilli smear and culture, and a polymerase chain reaction (PCR) of the intestinal tissue from the endoscopic biopsy specimen are required to confirm small intestinal tuberculosis despite the low diagnostic sensitivity. Screening for latent tuberculosis using interferon-gamma releasing assay tests can also be used in patients with suspected small intestinal tuberculosis.
4. A 6-month standard therapy is recommended for the treatment of small intestinal tuberculosis, similar to that of pulmonary tuberculosis. A follow-up endoscopy between 2 and 3 months after therapy initiation is helpful to determine the treatment response.

J. Chun (✉)
Gangnam Severance Hospital, Yonsei University College of Medicine, Seoul, South Korea

Epidemiology and Routes of Infection

Tuberculosis mainly involves the lungs but can develop in all extrapulmonary organs. In Korea, extrapulmonary tuberculosis accounts for approximately 15% of incident tuberculosis and its incidence among tuberculosis cases has been reported to have increased since 2001 [1]. Among extrapulmonary tuberculosis, intestinal tuberculosis (1–3% of incident tuberculosis) is less common than tuberculous lymphadenitis, urogenital tuberculosis, tuberculous osteomyelitis, miliary tuberculosis, and tuberculous meningoencephalitis. The risk factors for intestinal tuberculosis involve human immunodeficiency virus infection, an immunocompromised state, malignancy (especially malignant lymphoma), and immunosuppressive therapy such as steroids and tumor necrosis factor inhibitors. Intestinal tuberculosis is mostly caused by *Mycobacterium tuberculosis*; however, *M. bovis* can also induce intestinal tuberculosis in some cases.

The presentation of intestinal tuberculosis has been previously considered to be highly associated with active pulmonary tuberculosis. However, for many patients, there is no evidence of pulmonary tuberculosis at the time of diagnosis of intestinal tuberculosis. Recent evidence has shown that tuberculosis infection is mainly caused due to the direct invasion of mycobacteria (derived from infected food or sputum inserted into the oral cavity) in the intestinal mucosa.

Intestinal tuberculosis can also develop through direct invasion of tuberculosis in the surrounding organs or via a hematogenous spread of miliary tuberculosis [2].

Clinical Manifestations

In general, intestinal tuberculosis symptoms are nonspecific. Esophageal tuberculosis is very rare and requires the exclusion of esophageal cancer as a differential diagnosis in some cases. Endoscopic findings of gastroduodenal tuberculosis are similar to those of peptic ulcer diseases. Patients with gastroduodenal tuberculosis occasionally have complicated pyloric stricture, which requires the exclusion of adenocarcinoma as a differential diagnosis. Colonic tuberculosis accounts for 10% of intestinal tuberculosis cases and requires the exclusion of colon cancer. Anorectal tuberculosis leads to anorectal bleeding and fistula; therefore, anorectal cancer or perianal Crohn's disease should also be excluded.

Intestinal tuberculosis can occur in any part of the gastrointestinal tract; however, intestinal tuberculosis generally involves both the terminal ileum and cecum around the ileocecal valve and accounts for more than 75% of all intestinal tuberculosis cases. Patients with intestinal tuberculosis involving the ileocecal area present with abdominal pain, a palpable mass in the right iliac fossa, altered bowel habits, hematochezia, fever, and weight loss, making it difficult to distinguish from Crohn's disease in many cases. Intestinal tuberculosis has also been reported to mimic cancer, amebic colitis, enteric fever, or *Yersinia enterocolitica* infection [3].

Diagnosis

Small intestinal tuberculosis is diagnosed by physicians' decisions using a comprehensive approach including subjective symptoms, endoscopic and histopathologic findings of biopsy specimens, acid-fast bacilli (AFB) smear and culture, and radiological examinations. PCR of the intestinal tissue from an endoscopic biopsy specimen and screening for latent tuberculosis using the tuberculin skin test (TST) or the interferon-gamma releasing assay (IGRA) test can be used in the diagnosis of small intestinal tuberculosis.

Endoscopic Findings

Generally, small intestinal tuberculosis shows ileocecal-predominant involvement with a segmental distribution similar to Crohn's disease observed on ileocolonoscopy. Ileocolonoscopic findings can be used to confirm the presence of small intestinal tuberculosis at as far as the terminal ileum; however, inflammation in the small intestine should be evaluated using enteroscopy or small bowel capsule endoscopy in rare cases of small intestinal tuberculosis without ileocecal inflammation.

On the endoscopic findings of small intestinal tuberculosis, small lesions appear as aphthous or round ulcers. Large lesions appear to be irregularly shaped-geographic ulcers. Characteristic circumferential ulcers surrounding the intestinal lumen distinguish small intestinal tuberculosis from Crohn's disease (Fig. 1). Another characteristic of small intestinal tuberculosis is a patulous ileocecal valve that results from chronic inflammation. In general, the ulcer base is shallow and flat, and the mucosa at the peri-ulcer margins appears normal. Stricture can develop as a complication or progress due to fibrotic scarring during the healing phase.

Radiologic Findings

In Korea, the incidence of active pulmonary tuberculosis ranges from 27 to 67% among intestinal tuberculosis cases, which is relatively high compared to other countries, and inactive pulmonary tuberculosis accounts for 8–14% of those with intestinal tuberculosis. Therefore, chest X-ray should be performed to evaluate the presence of concomitant pulmonary tuberculosis in patients with suspected small intestinal tuberculosis.

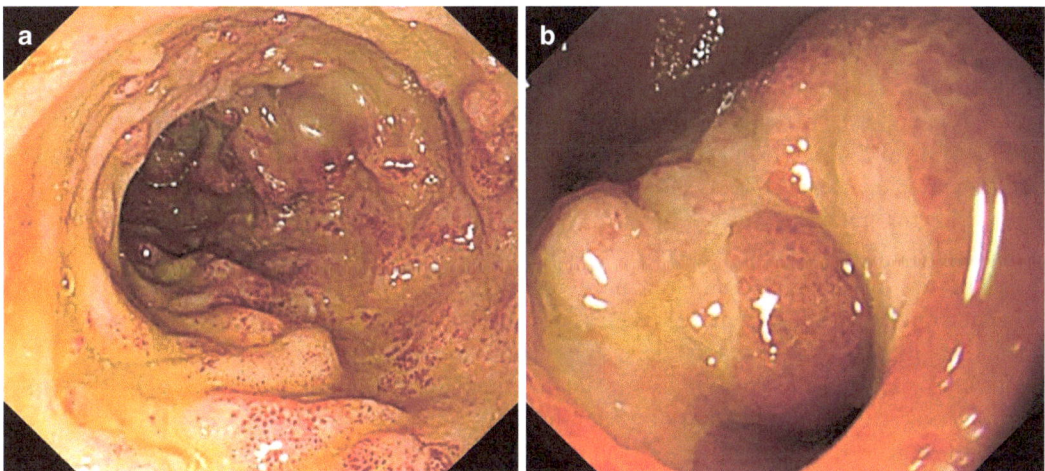

Fig. 1 Small intestinal tuberculosis identified using balloon-assisted enteroscopy. (**a**) Diffuse hyperemic erosions and (**b**) A typical circumferential ulcer encircling the intestinal lumen with stricture is observed on the distal ileum

Small bowel series that show longitudinal ulcers on the mesenteric border and pseudosacculation on the anti-mesenteric border suggest typical findings of small intestinal Crohn's disease and can help rule out small intestinal tuberculosis [4].

On computed tomography (CT) enterography, the most common abnormality of small intestinal tuberculosis is a symmetrical concentric mural thickening and homogenous mural enhancement with short-segment strictures [5]. Magnetic resonance (MR) enterography depicts mural thickening with multifocal stricture, lymphadenopathy, ascites, and peritoneal enhancement for diagnosing small intestinal tuberculosis with a relatively high degree of accuracy [6].

Histopathologic Findings

Histopathologic evaluations, AFB smear and culture, and PCR of the intestinal mucosa from a colonoscopic or enteroscopic biopsy specimen can be used for the diagnosis of small intestinal tuberculosis. Multiple biopsy specimens should be obtained from the ulcer base and margins to improve diagnostic sensitivity. The greater the number of biopsy specimens, the better the diagnostic sensitivity. It is recommended to obtain more than 3 pieces of endoscopic biopsy,

although the optimal number of biopsy specimens required to detect small intestinal tuberculosis remains to be determined [4]. Small intestinal tuberculosis can be confirmed if the AFB smear of the intestinal tissue is positive or chronic granulomatous inflammation with caseation necrosis is noted on histologic examinations of the intestinal mucosa. However, the sensitivity of typical histologic findings from a biopsy specimen is less than 30% in patients with small intestinal tuberculosis. Histologic findings comprising a large number and size of granulomas or histiocytic aggregates also suggest small intestinal tuberculosis.

Intestinal tissue PCR can detect the presence of mycobacteria with high specificity; however, the low sensitivity of PCR limits its usefulness as a confirmative diagnostic tool to distinguish Crohn's disease in patients with suspected small intestinal tuberculosis. Therefore, PCR can be used as an adjunctive method for diagnosing patients with suspected small intestinal tuberculosis.

Small intestinal tuberculosis is confirmed through intestinal tissue AFB culture. Minimally, 3–4 biopsies should be performed during an enteroscopic or an ileocolonoscopic procedure for intestinal tissue AFB culture. Sensitivity for the detection of mycobacteria is low and has been reported to range from 21 to 55% [7].

Skin Test

TST detects delayed-type hypersensitivity to mycobacterial antigens present in a purified protein derivative (PPD), which is a result of skin infiltration of monocytes and T and B lymphocytes. This infiltration is initiated by memory T cells localized in the skin that recognize proteins included in the intradermally administered PPD. Interpretation of TST depends on measurement (in millimeters) of the induration, history of tuberculosis infection, and risk of progression to disease if infected. An induration of 15 mm or more (10 mm or more in high-prevalent countries) is considered positive in individuals with no known risk factors for tuberculosis. Even when not infected with *M. tuberculosis*, a false-positive TST may result from infection with non-tuberculosis mycobacteria and previous BCG vaccination. Due to a lack of studies regarding the usefulness of TST for diagnosing small intestinal tuberculosis, diagnosis cannot be confirmed through positive TST alone.

Interferon-Gamma Releasing Assay

IGRA is a test measuring serum interferon-gamma (IFN-γ) levels secreted from T lymphocytes (QuantiFERON®-TB Gold) or IFN-γ-releasing T lymphocytes directly (T SPOT-TB®) that are stimulated by mycobacteria-specific antigens. Considering that mycobacteria-specific antigens used for IGRA tests are rarely shared by BCG or non-tuberculous mycobacteria, the specificity of IGRA for tuberculosis is higher than that of TST. In a recent meta-analysis, the sensitivity and specificity of IGRA were 81% and 85%, respectively, and the sensitivity of T SPOT-TB was higher than that of QuantiFERON-TB Gold [8].

Treatment

Treatment for intestinal tuberculosis is the same as that for pulmonary tuberculosis and tuberculous peritonitis. A previous random- ized clinical trial showed no significant difference in complete remission and relapse rates between 6- and 9-month regimens in patients with intestinal tuberculosis [9]. Therefore, the standard treatment for intestinal tuberculosis is a 6-month regimen similar to the treatment of pulmonary tuberculosis [1]. The dosage and adverse events of anti-tuberculosis medications as a first-line standard regimen are shown in Table 1.

Isoniazid has the most potent bactericidal effect on the proliferation of mycobacteria and is a critical therapeutic agent in the early phase of anti-tuberculosis therapy. Isoniazid can induce pyridoxine (vitamin B_6) deficiency, leading to peripheral neuropathy. Therefore, pyridoxine (10–50 mg per day) should be administered with isoniazid to prevent the complication of peripheral neuropathy.

Rifamycin which includes rifampin and rifabutin is an important therapeutic agent against intestinal tuberculosis due to its potent bactericidal effects on mycobacteria. Rifampin, the most commonly used rifamycin, can induce orange discoloration of urine due to its color. Rifampin, a potent inducer of cytochrome P450, decreases blood concentrations of various drugs including anti-arrhythmic agents, such as quinidine and phenytoin, warfarin, oral contraceptives, steroids, insulin, and oral hypoglycemic agents such as sulfonylurea. It is, therefore, necessary to double the dose of warfarin and steroids for patients who take rifampin.

Optic neuropathy is the most serious complication of ethambutol. It occurs 2 months after starting ethambutol in most cases. Visual disturbance slowly improves after stopping ethambutol, but it is permanent in some cases. High-dose ethambutol (25 mg/kg/day) or renal insufficiency increases the risk of optic neuropathy. Ethambutol is not recommended for patients with difficulty in assessing the presence of visual disturbance.

Among the anti-tuberculosis medications, pyrazinamide is the most bactericidal agent against mycobacteria located in early inflammatory lesions with caseation necrosis. Therefore, the therapeutic effect of pyrazinamide is high in the early phase of treatment, and its use is recom-

Table 1 Dosage and adverse events of anti-tuberculosis medications [1]

Drugs	Dose (maximum)	Dosage	Major adverse events
Isoniazid	5 mg/kg (300 mg)	Once a day, before meals 300 mg	Hepatotoxicity, peripheral neuropathy, and skin hypersensitivity
Rifampin	10 mg/kg (600 mg)	Once a day, before meals 450 mg (<50 kg) 600 mg	Hepatotoxicity, flu-like syndrome, skin hypersensitivity, thrombocytopenia, gastrointestinal disturbance, and orange discolorat on of body fluids
Rifabutin	5 mg/kg (300 mg)	Once a day, before or after meals 300 mg	Hepatotoxicity and neutropenia
Ethambutol	15–20 mg/kg (1600 mg)	Once a day, before or after meals	Optic neuropathy
Pyrazinamide	20–30 mg/kg (2000 mg)	Once a day, before or after meals 1000 mg (<50 kg) 1500 mg (50–70 kg) 2000 mg (≥70 kg)	Hepatotoxicity, arthralgia, and gastrointestinal disturbance

mended in the first 2 months of the anti-tuberculosis therapy. Major adverse events include hepatotoxicity and arthralgia. Arthralgia occurs in approximately 40% of pyrazinamide users and can be treated with symptomatic treatment using nonsteroidal anti-inflammatory medication. Pyrazinoic acid, a metabolite of pyrazinamide, inhibits renal excretion of uric acid leading to hyperuricemia but rarely induces an acute gouty attack.

Patients with small intestinal tuberculosis clinically respond to the standard combination regimen of isoniazid, rifampin, ethambutol, and pyrazinamide within 2 weeks after the start of medication; however, abdominal masses and small intestinal strictures improve more slowly. One literature review reported endoscopic improvement of small intestinal tuberculosis in 93% of patients 3 months after starting antituberculotic medications. Therefore, a follow-up endoscopic assessment 2–3 months after starting medication may be useful for evaluating the therapeutic response in patients with small intestinal tuberculosis. Most patients with small intestinal tuberculosis are usually cured with medical treatment; however, surgical treatment may be required for patients with complications such as intestinal obstruction, perforation, and bleeding.

References

1. Joint Committee for the Revision of Korean Guidelines for Tuberculosis. Korean guidelines for tuberculosis. 3rd ed; 2017. p. 1–232.
2. Charles F, Haines CLS. Infectious enteritis and proctocolitis. In: Mark Feldman LSF, Brandt LJ, editors. Sleisenger and Fordtran's gastrointestinal and liver disease. 10th ed. Philadelphia: Saunders; 2016. p. 1926–7.
3. Donoghue HD, Holton J. Intestinal tuberculosis. Curr Opin Infect Dis. 2009;22:490–6.
4. Kim YS, Kim YH, Lee KM, et al. Diagnostic guideline of intestinal tuberculosis. Korean J Gastroenterol. 2009;53:177–86.
5. Kalra N, Agrawal P, Mittal V, et al. Spectrum of imaging findings on MDCT enterography in patients with small bowel tuberculosis. Clin Radiol. 2014;69:315–22.
6. Krishna S, Kalra N, Singh P, et al. Small-bowel tuberculosis: a comparative study of MR enterography and small-bowel follow-through. AJR Am J Roentgenol. 2016;207:571–7.
7. Yonal O, Hamzaoglu HO. What is the most accurate method for the diagnosis of intestinal tuberculosis? Turk J Gastroenterol. 2010;21:91–6.
8. Ng SC, Hirai HW, Tsoi KK, et al. Systematic review with meta-analysis: accuracy of interferon-gamma releasing assay and anti-Saccharomyces cerevisiae antibody in differentiating intestinal tuberculosis from Crohn's disease in Asians. J Gastroenterol Hepatol. 2014;29:1664–70.
9. Park SH, Yang SK, Yang DH, et al. Prospective randomized trial of six-month versus nine-month therapy for intestinal tuberculosis. Antimicrob Agents Chemother. 2009;53:4167–71.

Cryptogenic Multifocal Ulcerous Stenosing Enteritis

Jae Jun Park

Key Points

Cryptogenic multifocal ulcerous stenosing enteritis (CMUSE) is a chronic disease of the small intestine characterized by multiple superficial ulcers, stenosis, and recurrent partial intestinal obstruction.

No confirmatory tests are available to definitively diagnose CMUSE, and diagnosis is established based on medical history, clinical features, laboratory tests, imaging studies, small bowel endoscopy, and histopathological examination.

Steroids constitute first-line therapy in patients with CMUSE; however, varying response rates are reported in the available literature, and surgery is required in a significant number of patients.

Cryptogenic multifocal ulcerous stenosing enteritis (CMUSE) is a rare chronic disease characterized by multiple shallow ulcerations and stenosis of the small intestine with recurrent partial or complete intestinal obstruction. This condition was first described by Debray et al. in 1964 [1]. Although the exact etiopathogenetic contributors to CMUSE remain unclear, it is presumed that immunological mechanisms play a causal role, primarily because some patients respond to steroid therapy. A recent study has reported that mutation of the *PLA2G4A* gene on chromosome 1 is involved in the development of CMUSE [2].

Clinical Characteristics

CMUSE typically manifests with chronic and recurrent partial small-intestinal atresia secondary to multiple areas of intestinal stenosis. Abdominal pain secondary to small intestinal obstruction is the most common clinical symptom (observed in 60–70% of patients) [3, 4]. Approximately 25–50% of patients present with chronic iron deficiency anemia secondary to potential small intestinal bleeding. Notably, anemia may precede the diagnosis of CMUSE by several years [3, 4]. Diarrhea, malabsorption, hematochezia, or fever are relatively rare in patients with CMUSE. Reportedly, the time interval between symptom onset and diagnosis of CMUSE is approximately 50 months, which suggests that early diagnosis of this condition is difficult [3]. Extraintestinal manifestations occur in 15–40% of patients and often include peripheral neuropathy, aphthous stomatitis, Sicca syndrome, multiple arthralgia, Raynaud's phenomenon, arterial hypertension, and subclavian vein thrombosis [3, 5].

J. J. Park (✉)
Yonsei University, Seoul, South Korea

© Springer Nature Singapore Pte Ltd. 2022   227
H. J. Chun et al. (eds.), *Small Intestine Disease*, https://doi.org/10.1007/978-981-16-7239-2_43

Diagnosis

CMUSE is diagnosed based on the patient's medical history, clinical features, serological testing, radiological examination, small bowel endoscopy, and histopathological examination. No specific serological testing is available to confirm the diagnosis of CMUSE. Anemia is commonly detected in patients, and the mean serum hemoglobin level at the time of diagnosis is reported to be 10–11 g/dL. Laboratory tests such as estimation of the white blood cell count or serum C-reactive protein levels, which reflect a systemic inflammatory response, are usually within the reference range; only 10–15% of patients show mildly elevated levels of the aforementioned parameters [3, 4].

Histopathological findings in a resected surgical specimen are characterized by multiple superficial ulcerations and stenosis confined to the mucosa or submucosa. In a few segments, stenosis is accompanied by ulceration with thickening secondary to submucosal fibrosis associated with the ulcer [4]. Some patients may also show chronic cryptitis, pyloric gland metaplasia, and lymphocytic infiltration. No inflammatory involvement of the small intestinal segments is observed between the ulcers, and giant cell granulomas, transmural inflammation, and/or fistulas are not usually identified in patients with CMUSE. These findings are similar to those observed on imaging or endoscopic examination [4].

A study in which abdominal computed tomography (CT) and CT/magnetic resonance enterography were performed in 20 patients with CMUSE reported that 17 patients (85%) showed only ileal stenosis, 2 patients (10%) showed only jejunal stenosis, and 1 patient (5%) showed both ileal and jejunal stenosis (Fig. 1) [4]. The stenosed segment was short (mean length 10 mm), high-grade obstruction was rare (10%), and most patients (90%) showed no or only low-grade obstruction [4].

Endoscopic findings following balloon-assisted enteroscopy or capsule endoscopy performed in all patients revealed multiple small bowel ulcers with various features, such as a relatively well-demarcated margin and a linear, round, irregular, or geographic shape [4, 6]. Some ulcers showed a circular alignment, and the intervening mucosa between ulcers appeared normal. Most patients showed multiple areas of stenoses, although only short segments were stenosed, and some segments showed accompanying ulcers (Fig. 2) [4]

A multicenter study performed in Korea reported the use of various imaging and endoscopic modalities, including small bowel series, balloon-assisted enteroscopy, CT enterography, and capsule endoscopy to diagnose CMUSE [3]. Notably, CMUSE is a condition involving small bowel stenosis; therefore, capsule retention may occur during capsule endoscopy, and utmost caution is warranted. Perlemuter et al. summarized the clinicopathological features of CMUSE (Table 1), and to date, several studies have used these guidelines to diagnose CMUSE [5].

Crohn's disease must first be excluded when considering the differential diagnosis of CMUSE. Unlike CMUSE, Crohn's disease involves transmural inflammation causing complications such as fistulas, abscesses, and perforation and may invade other small intestine or large intestines. Moreover, Crohn's disease is usually associated with elevated serum levels of inflammatory

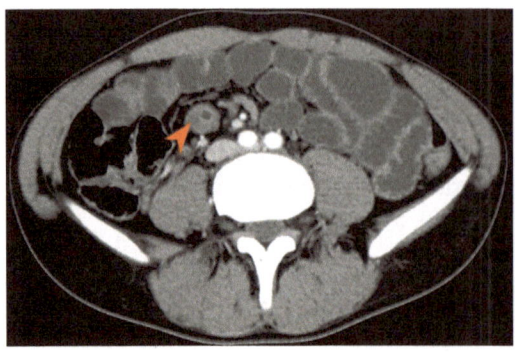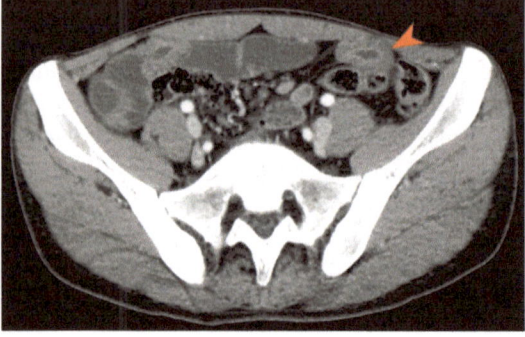

Fig. 1 CT enterography findings in patients with CMUSE. CMUSE: Cryptogenic multifocal ulcerous stenosing enteritis, CT: computed tomography. Jejunal and ileal stenosis

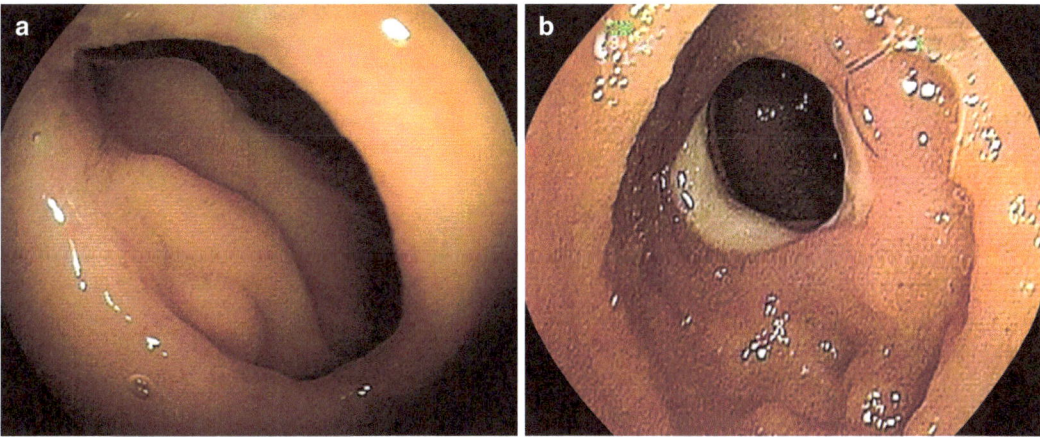

Fig. 2 Endoscopic findings in a patient with CMUSE. (**a**) Short-segment fibrotic stenosis of the distal ileum. (**b**) Annular ulcer of the ileum. CMUSE: Cryptogenic multifocal ulcerous stenosing enteritis

Table 1 Clinicopathological features of CMUSE [5]

1.	Unexplained small intestinal strictures observed in adolescents and middle-aged patients
2.	Superficial ulceration of the mucosa and submucosa
3.	Chronic or relapsing clinical course, even after surgery
4.	No biological signs of systemic inflammatory reaction
5.	Favorable response to systemic corticosteroids

CMUSE Cryptogenic multifocal ulcerous stenosing enteritis

Table 2 Comparison of CMUSE vs. Crohn's disease - characteristics of CMUSE [7]

1.	Absence of clinical or laboratory features of an inflammatory syndrome
2.	Absence of a small intestinal transmural inflammatory process or ulceration
3.	Absence of histopathological evidence of small intestinal granulomatous inflammation with giant cells
4.	Absence of small intestinal fistula formation despite recurrent chronic disease
5.	Absence of disease in other parts of the gastrointestinal tract (i.e., stomach or colon)
6.	Absence of most extraintestinal features of Crohn's disease (e.g., cutaneous manifestations)

CMUSE Cryptogenic multifocal ulcerous stenosing enteritis

markers (Table 2) [7]. It should be remembered that all conditions associated with multiple ulcers and stenosis of the small intestine should be considered in the differential diagnosis of CMUSE, including drug-induced enteropathy (particularly nonsteroidal anti-inflammatory drug enteropathy), tuberculosis, intestinal Behcet's disease, lymphoma, eosinophilic enteritis, infectious enteritis (*Campylobacter, Yersinia* infections), gastrin-secreting tumors (Zollinger–Ellison syndrome), traumatic injury (endoscopy related, seat-belt damage), and ischemic bowel damage (collagen vascular disease, and/or vasculitis) [8].

Matsumoto et al. proposed chronic nonspecific multiple ulcers of the small intestine (CNSU), an enteropathy similar to CMUSE [9]. They reported that a *SLCO2A1* gene mutation could serve as an etiopathogenetic contributor to CNSU. They reported a chronic enteropathy associated with the *SLCO2A1* gene, which was diagnosed in patients with the *SLCO2A1* gene mutation among patients with clinical manifestations of CNSU [10]. Considering that both conditions involve idiopathic chronic small bowel ulcers, it is reasonable to conclude that both diseases are similar. However,

CNSU differs from CMUSE with regard to the following characteristics: All patients present with anemia, a significant number of patients show low serum protein levels, abdominal pain is relatively rare (13%), and stenosis is not included in the diagnostic criteria used for CNSU. Future studies are warranted to conclusively establish whether CNSU and CMUSE represent different presentations of the same disease.

Treatment

The pathogenesis of CMUSE remains unclear; therefore, optimal treatment based on the etiopathogenesis is unknown. Steroids are considered first-line medical therapy for CMUSE [5]. To date, the standard dose of steroids required to treat CMUSE has not been established. Previous studies have reported favorable outcomes with prednisone administered at an initial dose of 30–50 mg with gradual dose reduction following response to treatment [5]. A significant number of patients receiving steroid therapy develop steroid dependence and many require repeat courses of steroids [5]. Although previous studies in the literature have reported a favorable treatment response to steroids in patients with CMUSE, and this part has also been included in Table 1, Korean multicenter studies have reported a relatively low response rate (25%) [3]. Small-sized case studies have reported that oral administration of 5-aminosalicylic acid, azathioprine, and methotrexate is ineffective [5].

A significant number of patients with CMUSE are required to undergo surgical treatment owing to multiple fibrotic stenoses. Reportedly, the rate of surgery in patients with CMUS is 65–83% [3–5]. However, recent technological advances in small bowel endoscopy have enabled endoscopic access to strictures located even deep within the small bowel, and enteroscopy-guided balloon dilation is an effective alternative to surgical treatment in patients with CMUSE with relatively short-segment stenosis. However, a careful approach is warranted because patients with CMUSE present with multiple stenoses. Although intestinal obstruction is the most common cause necessitating surgical treatment in patients with CMUSE, surgery is occasionally performed to treat bleeding and/or perforation [3]. A Korean study reported that 33% of patients with CMUSE received medical treatment, 33% underwent surgery, and 33% received both medical and surgical treatment [3].

Reportedly, the median time until recurrence was 2.6–5.6 years after improvement with medical or surgical treatment [3, 4], the clinical recurrence rate was 25–70% [3–5], and the reoperation rate was 25% [3]. The long-term prognosis of CMUSE remains unclear, and the recurrence rate is reportedly higher in men than in women [3].

Conclusion

CMUSE is a chronic disease of the small intestine characterized by multiple superficial ulcerations, stenosis, and recurrent partial intestinal obstruction. Although CMUSE is rare, it should be considered in the differential diagnosis in patients presenting with these clinical features. Recently, technological advances in genetic analysis techniques have led to the identification of genes associated with the development of CMUSE, and it is expected that the etiopathogenesis of this condition will become clearer in the near future. To date, reports describing CMUSE in the available literature include only small-sized studies. Large-scale multinational studies are warranted in the future to gain a deeper understanding of this condition. Moreover, regarding the definition of CMUSE, similar diseases have been proposed according to the region and country, thus further discussions and agreements related to this issue are needed in the future.

References

1. Debray C, Besancon F, Hardouin JP, et al. Cryptogenic plurifocal ulcerative stenosing enteritis. Arch Mal Appar Dig Mal Nutr. 1964;53:193–206.
2. Brooke MA, Longhurst HJ, Plagnol V, et al. Cryptogenic multifocal ulcerating stenosing enteritis associated with homozygous deletion mutations in cytosolic phospholipase A2-alpha. Gut 2014;63:96–104.
3. Chung SH, Park SU, Cheon JH, et al. Clinical characteristics and treatment outcomes of cryptogenic multifocal ulcerous stenosing enteritis in Korea. Dig Dis Sci. 2015;60:2740–5.
4. Hwang J, Kim JS, Kim AY, et al. Cryptogenic multifocal ulcerous stenosing enteritis: Radiologic features and clinical behavior. World J Gastroenterol. 2017;23:4615–23.
5. Perlemuter G, Guillevin L, Legman P, et al. Cryptogenetic multifocal ulcerous stenosing enteritis: an atypical type of vasculitis or a disease mimicking vasculitis. Gut 2001;48:333–8.
6. Chang DK, Kim JJ, Choi H, et al. Double balloon endoscopy in small intestinal Crohn's disease and other inflammatory diseases such as cryptogenic multifocal ulcerous stenosing enteritis (CMUSE). Gastrointest Endosc. 2007;66:S96–8.
7. Freeman HJ. Multifocal stenosing ulceration of the small intestine. World J Gastroenterol 2009;15:4883–5.
8. Freeman HJ. Small intestinal multifocal stenosing ulceration. Dig Dis Sci. 2015;60:2568–70.
9. Matsumoto T, Iida M, Matsui T, et al. Chronic nonspecific multiple ulcers of the small intestine: a proposal of the entity from Japanese gastroenterologists to Western enteroscopists. Gastrointest Endosc. 2007;66:S99–107.
10. Umeno J, Hisamatsu T, Esaki M, et al. A hereditary enteropathy caused by mutations in the SLCO2A1 gene, encoding a prostaglandin transporter. PLoS Genet. 2015;11:e1005581.

Peutz–Jeghers syndrome

Soo Jung Park and Jung Min Kim

Prevalence and Related Genes

PJS has an estimated prevalence of 1:5000 to 1:25,000 births [1], and may manifest with various clinical features. One family member may exhibit pigmentation, while the other family member may have pigmentation and polyps. PJS can be diagnosed by identifying mutations in *STK11 (serine/threonine-protein kinase 11; LKB1)* through genetic testing. The *STK11* gene is located on chromosome 19p13.3 and is known to suppress AMP activator protein kinase

S. J. Park (✉) · J. M. Kim
Department of Internal Medicine and Institute of Gastroenterology, Yonsei University College of Medicine, Seoul, South Korea
e-mail: sjpark@yuhs.ac

(AMPK) and the mTOR signaling pathway. However, the precise mechanism of action of *STK11* is unknown.

Clinical Features

PJS can be diagnosed when positive family history, hyperpigmentation, small intestinal polyps, or more than two of these clinical features are exhibited [2, 3]. Hyperpigmentation occurs as spots on the mucous membranes of the lips, mouth, eyes, and ball, and may rarely occur on the fingers, toes, palms, soles of the feet, or intestinal mucosa. It is very rare that the disease becomes malignant and it may disappear in adolescence. The unique characteristic of the hamartomatous polyps caused by PJS is that the cellular components are normal, but the polyp structure is distorted [2].

Therefore, endoscopy cannot distinguish the polyps, but PJS can be diagnosed through histological confirmation. Polyps usually appear in the small bowel of patients aged 11–13 years. Double-balloon enteroscopy, capsule endoscopy, and magnetic resonance (MR) enterography may be helpful in the diagnosis of small intestinal polyps (Figs. 1, 2). Before 30 years of age, approximately 50% of the patients show symptoms of anemia, gastrointestinal bleeding, abdominal pain, intussusception, or ileus [4–5]. Intussusception is usually seen in the small bowel [6], but the association between intussusception and the *STK11* mutation is unclear [7] (Fig. 3).

© Springer Nature Singapore Pte Ltd. 2022
H. J. Chun et al. (eds.), *Small Intestine Disease*, https://doi.org/10.1007/978-981-16-7239-2_44

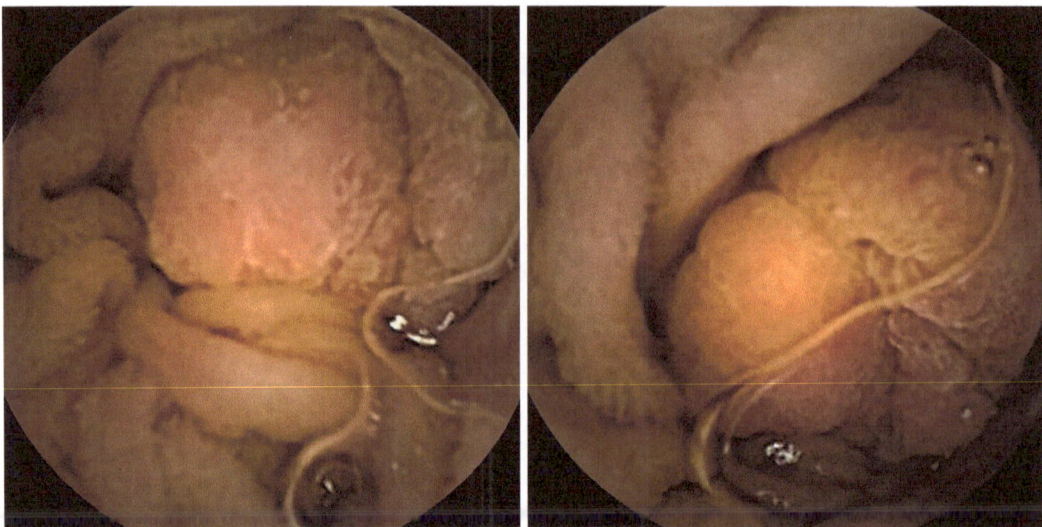

Fig. 1 Hamartomatous polyps in capsule endoscopy

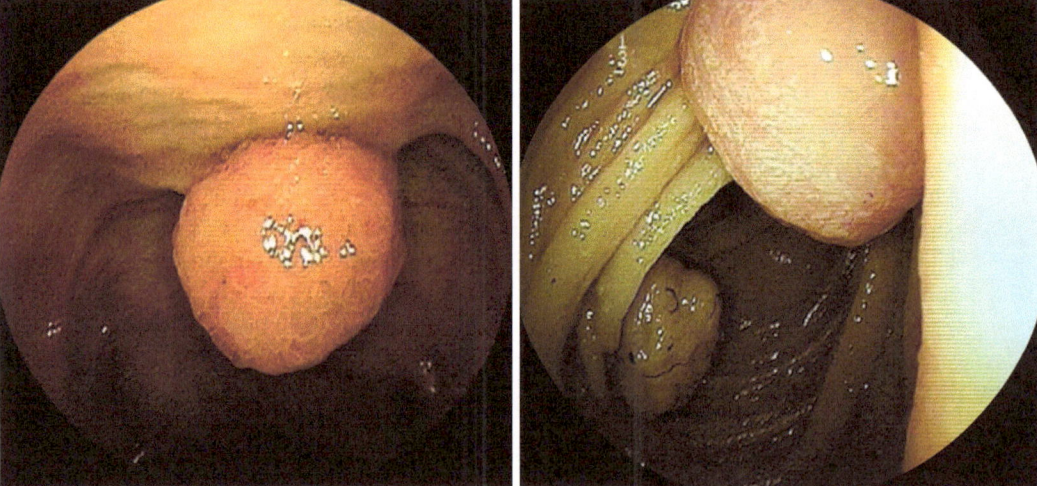

Fig. 2 Hamartomatous polyps in double-balloon endoscopy

Extraintestinal Tumor

PJS is associated with the development of extraintestinal tumors as well as breast cancer, lung cancer, pancreatic cancer, uterine cancer, and ovarian cancer due to a specific gene mutation. Therefore, screening for multiple polyps of the gastrointestinal tract as well as screening for cancer are required regularly [8].

Testicular screening in males is required every year until 12 years of age. If an abnormality of the testis is reported, testicular ultrasound should

be performed. Women should complete a breast self-examination every month from the age of 18 years; a breast cancer screening should be performed every year between the ages of 25 and 50 years. Pap smears and liquid cytology should be performed every 3 years after 25 years of age. At 8 years of age, the first esophagogastroduodenoscopy and colonoscopy are necessary. If polyps are observed, they should be examined regularly every 3 years until 50 years of age. If polyps are not observed, the patients should be examined annually until 18 years of age and every 3 years between 18 and 50 years of age.

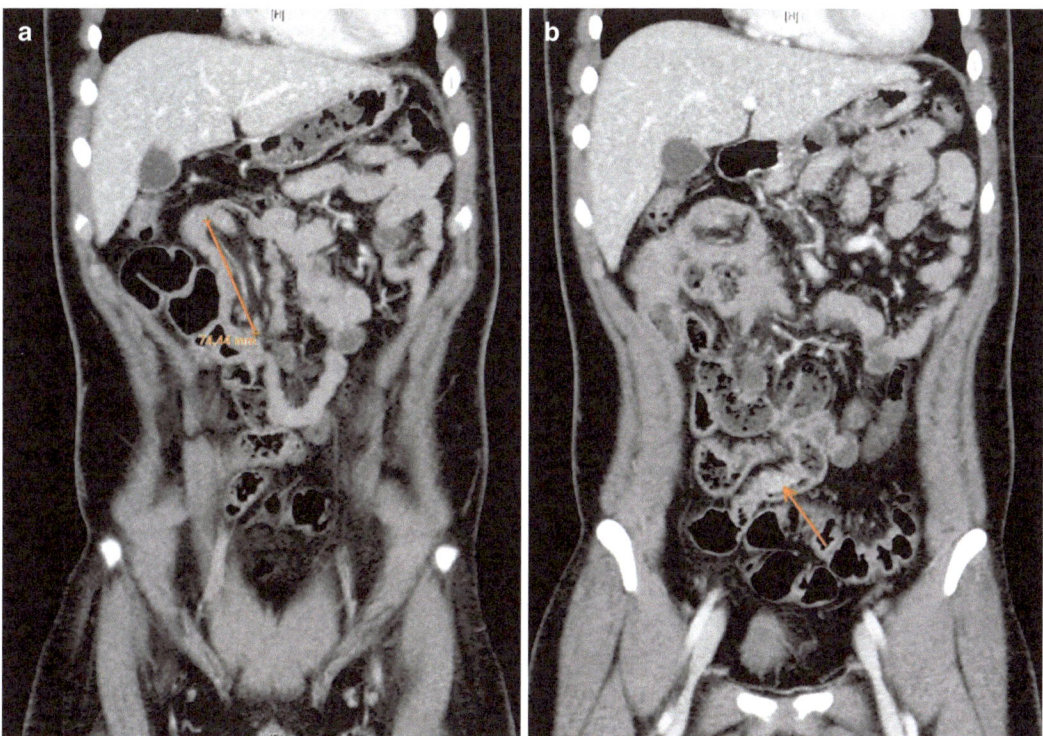

Fig. 3 Small bowel intussusception in abdominal computed tomography. (**a**) Intussusception is noted to be at least 15 cm in length in the small bowel (arrow). (**b**) Multiple polyps are observed in the small bowel

Summary

PJS is inherited through an autosomal dominant *STK11 (LKB1)* gene mutation that may result in hyperpigmentation and hamartomatous polyps. Before 30 years of age, approximately 50% of patients experience anemia, gastrointestinal bleeding, abdominal pain, intussusception, or ileus. Regular cancer screening is needed because it is associated with the development of breast cancer, lung cancer, pancreatic cancer, uterine cancer, and ovarian cancer as well as gastrointestinal and extraintestinal malignancy.

References

1. Giardiello FM, Trimbath JD. PeutzeJeghers syndrome and management recommendations. Clin Gastroenterol Hepatol. 2006;4:408e15.

2. Chen HM, Fang JY. Genetics of the hamartomatous polyposis syndromes. A molecular review. Int J Color Dis. 2009;24:865–74.

3. Noel RJ, Werlin SL. Peutz-Jeghers syndrome. Are "shaggy" villi part of the pathology? Gastrointest Endosc. 2008;68:1004–5.

4. Schreibman IR, Baker M, Amos C, McGarrity TJ. The hamartomatous polyposis syndromes: a clinical and molecular review. Am J Gastroenterol. 2005;100:476–90.

5. Gammon A, Jasperson K, Kohlmann W, Burt RW. Hamartomatous polyposis syndromes. Best Pract Res Clin Gastroenterol. 2009;23:219–31.

6. Hinds R, Philp C, Hyer W, Fell JM. Complications of childhood Peutz-Jeghers syndrome: implications for pediatric screening. J Pediatr Gastroenterol Nutr. 2004;39:219–20.

7. Hearle N, Schumacher V, Menko FH, et al. STK11 status and intussusception risk in Peutz-Jeghers syndrome. J Med Genet. 2006;43:e41.

8. Beggs AD, Latchford AR, Vasen HF, Moslein G, Alonso A, Arctz S. Peutz Jeghers syndrome: a systematic review and recommendations for management. Gut. 2010;59:975–86.

Small Bowel Adenocarcinoma

Jun Lee

Key Points
1. Small bowel adenocarcinoma is a rare malignant tumor with a poor prognosis.
2. Recent advances in small bowel enteroscopy and radiologic imaging have enabled early diagnosis.
3. The treatment of small bowel adenocarcinoma requires extensive local excision, with regional lymph node resection (>8–10 lymph nodes) if surgery is possible, and systemic chemotherapy if surgery is not possible.

Small bowel adenocarcinoma is difficult to diagnose as there are no specific symptoms and accessing the small intestine using a conventional endoscope is challenging. Recently, both capsule endoscopy and balloon-assisted enteroscopy have been used clinically, and radiographical developments have made it easier to diagnose small bowel disease. Moreover, genetic studies have revealed molecular pathogenesis, and improved surgery and systemic chemotherapy have led to increased interest in small bowel adenocarcinoma. In this article, we discuss the latest developments and treatment of small intestinal adenocarcinoma.

Epidemiology

Small bowel cancer is a rare malignancy, comprising approximately 5% of all gastrointestinal malignancies, and is most frequently diagnosed as carcinoid tumor (44%), adenocarcinoma (33%), lymphoma (15%), and gastrointestinal stromal tumors or sarcoma (8%) [1]. The annual incidence of small bowel adenocarcinoma is 7.3 cases per million persons [2]. The incidence is high among individuals of African ethnicity, whereas it is relatively low in individuals of Asian ethnicity, including Korean individuals [3]. The most common site of occurrence is the duodenum, followed by the jejunum and the ileum.

Etiology and Pathogenesis

The etiology of small bowel adenocarcinoma is unclear; however, hereditary familial syndrome and Crohn's disease are the main risk factors. In one meta-analysis, small bowel cancer was reported to be 27.1 times more common in individuals with Crohn's disease than in general population [4]. Other risk factors include alcohol consumption, cigarette smoking, and red meat or refined carbohydrate consumption. The con-

J. Lee (✉)
Department of Internal Medicine, College of Medicine, Chosun University, Gwangju, South Korea
e-mail: leejun@chosun.ac.kr

sumption of coffee, fish, fruits, and vegetables is helpful for prevention [5].

In the molecular biology of small bowel adenocarcinoma, KRAS mutation, loss of 18q, and loss of p53 occur in a similar manner to colorectal cancer. However, APC mutations are very rare, unlike in colorectal cancer. In a recent large-scale gene analysis, small bowel adenocarcinoma has been shown to be significantly different from gastric and colorectal cancer, and small bowel adenocarcinoma is considered to be an independent molecular biological cancer [6].

Clinical Features and Diagnosis

The average age at the time of diagnosis is approximately 66 years, and this disease is common among elderly people [2]. Clinical symptoms vary according to the anatomic location. Adenocarcinoma arising in the duodenum is asymptomatic in approximately 50% of patients, while adenocarcinomas in the jejunum and ileum produce a variety of nonspecific symptoms [7]. The most common symptoms are abdominal pain and nausea, vomiting, and weight loss, and GI bleeding may occur. The small intestine is a relatively narrow, very long organ that occupies most of the abdominal cavity. Therefore, if there is no significant obstruction, conventional abdominal computed tomography (CT) (Fig. 1) is limited in terms of diagnosis. Recently, new radiographic techniques such as CT enterography, CT enteroclysis, and magnetic resonance enteroclysis have been shown to have higher sensitivity and specificity than conventional radiologic techniques [8]. Capsule endoscopy can be directly visualized in the small intestine with a high-resolution image, and balloon-assisted enteroscopy (Fig. 2) allows direct diagnosis of lesions and simultaneous biopsy. Serum tumor markers are not appropriate as diagnostic tools but are useful for evaluating recurrence and prognosis.

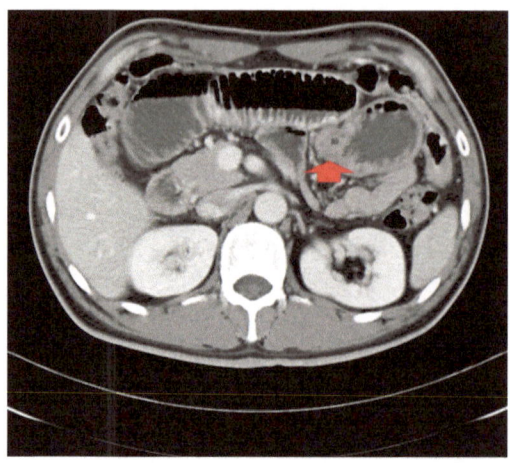

Fig. 1 Abdominal CT scan. An irregular thickness and stenosis is seen in the jejunum (arrow) and abnormal dilatation of lumen is revealed at the proximal part

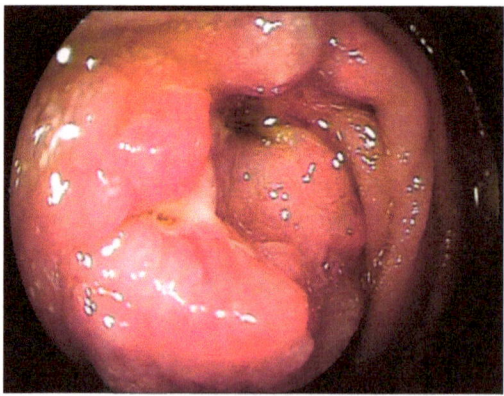

Fig. 2 Double-balloon enteroscopy. An encircled and elevated mass (approximately 4 cm in size) with an irregular margin is seen in the jejunum

Prognosis

The 5-year overall survival rate is between 14% and 33%, which indicates a poor prognosis. Tumor stage at the time of diagnosis is the most important prognostic factor. Other factors include being male, of older age, the duodenal location, invasive margins, and lymph node invasion. Additionally, when only a small number of lymph

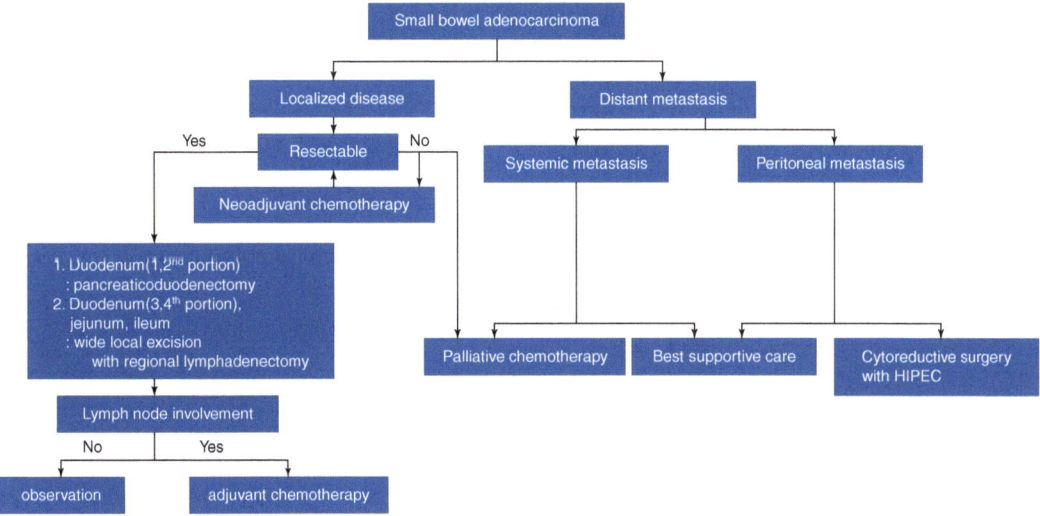

Fig. 3 Therapeutic algorithm for small bowel adenocarcinoma. HIPEC, hyperthermic intraperitoneal chemotherapy. Data adapted from Raghav K, Overman, M. Nat Rev. Clin Oncol. 2013;10(9):534–44

nodes have been surgically removed, this has been associated with a poor prognosis. Therefore, a minimum of 8–10 lymph nodes should be excised during surgery [2].

Treatment

The standard treatment for localized small bowel adenocarcinomas is surgical resection. The surgical procedure depends on the location; pancreaticoduodenectomy is performed for tumors located in the more proximal part of the second portion of the duodenum and wide local excision with regional lymph node dissection is performed for tumors located in the distal part of the second portion of the duodenum. Adjuvant therapy choices for patients with resected, non-metastatic small bowel adenocarcinomas depend on the disease stage. Despite limited data, it is reasonable to consider the role of adjuvant fluoropyrimidine-based chemotherapy for patients with stage III disease (patients with positive lymph nodes). The current management for metastatic small bowel adenocarcinomas involves a combination treatment with fluoropyrimidine and oxaliplatin (FOLFOX

or CAPEOX), with a reported therapeutic 45%–50% response rate, a disease control rate of 80%–90%, and a median overall survival of 15–20 months [9]. Approximately 20%–50% of patients with metastatic small bowel adenocarcinoma have peritoneal metastasis. Patients with peritoneal metastasis have a relatively low response to chemotherapy. Recently, treatment of small bowel adenocarcinoma with peritoneal metastasis using cytoreductive surgery with hyperthermic intraperitoneal chemotherapy has been reported to have resulted in a median disease-free survival rate of 10–12 months and a median overall survival time of 16–47 months [10]. In addition, many studies on target therapy and immune therapy to increase survival time are being undertaken. The treatment of small bowel adenocarcinoma is summarized in Fig. 3 [11].

Conclusion

Small bowel adenocarcinoma is a rare, malignant tumor with a poor prognosis. Recently, advances in diagnostic techniques and equipment have made it possible to perform a rapid diagnosis. The standard treatment for localized small bowel adenocarcinoma is wide local excision with regional lymph node dissection. Despite limited data, palliative chemotherapy should be considered for metastatic small adenocarcinomas and cytoreductive surgery with hyperthermic intraperitoneal chemotherapy should be considered if there is peritoneal metastasis.

References

1. Siegel RL, Miller KD, Jemal A. Cancer statistics, 2016. CA Cancer J Clin. 2016;66(1):7–30.
2. Overman MJ, Hu CY, Wolff RA, Chang GJ. Prognostic value of lymph node evaluation in small bowel adenocarcinoma: analysis of the surveillance, epidemiology, and end results database. Cancer. 2010;116(23):5374–82.
3. Goodman MT, Matsuno RK, Shvetsov YB. Racial and ethnic variation in the incidence of small-bowel cancer subtypes in the United States, 1995-2008. Dis Colon Rectum. 2013;56(4):441–8.
4. Jess T, Gamborg M, Matzen P, Munkholm P, Sorensen TI. Increased risk of intestinal cancer in Crohn's disease: a meta-analysis of population-based cohort studies. Am J Gastroenterol. 2005;100(12):2724–9.
5. Aparicio T, Zaanan A, Svrcek M, et al. Small bowel adenocarcinoma: epidemiology, risk factors, diagnosis and treatment. Digestive and Liver Dis. 2014;46(2):97–104.
6. Schrock AB, Devoe CE, McWilliams R, et al. Genomic Profiling of Small-Bowel Adenocarcinoma. JAMA Oncol. 2017;3(11):1546–53.
7. Sakae H, Kanzaki H, Nasu J, et al. The characteristics and outcomes of small bowel adenocarcinoma: a multicentre retrospective observational study. Br J Cancer. 2017;117(11):1607–13.
8. Pilleul F, Penigaud M, Milot L, Saurin JC, Chayvialle JA, Valette PJ. Possible small-bowel neoplasms: contrast-enhanced and water-enhanced multidetector CT enteroclysis. Radiology. 2006;241(3):796–801.
9. Xiang XJ, Liu YW, Zhang L, et al. A phase II study of modified FOLFOX as first-line chemotherapy in advanced small bowel adenocarcinoma. Anti-Cancer Drugs. 2012;23(5):561–6.
10. Elias D, Glehen O, Pocard M, et al. A comparative study of complete cytoreductive surgery plus intraperitoneal chemotherapy to treat peritoneal dissemination from colon, rectum, small bowel, and nonpseudomyxoma appendix. Ann Surg. 2010;251(5):896–901.
11. Raghav K, Overman MJ. Small bowel adenocarcinomas--existing evidence and evolving paradigms. Nat Rev Clin Oncol. 2013;10(9):534–44.

Small Bowel Lymphoma

Hyun Jin Kim

Key Points
- The most common site of primary small bowel lymphoma is the ileum, especially the terminal ileum. Approximately 50% cases involve single lesions in the small intestine, whereas the remaining 50% cases involve multiple lesions in the small and large intestines.
- The most common pathologic type of small bowel lymphoma is diffuse large B-cell lymphoma, followed by follicular lymphoma, Burkitt's lymphoma, and mantle cell lymphoma. Cases of mucosa-associated lymphoid tissue lymphoma and immunoproliferative small intestinal disease have rarely been reported.
- The differential diagnosis includes primary small bowel carcinoma, metastasis, small bowel leiomyoma/gastrointestinal stromal tumor, and inflammatory bowel disease.

The gastrointestinal (GI) tract is the most common organ involved in extra-nodal lymphoma

H. J. Kim (✉)
Department of Internal Medicine, Gyeongsang National University College of Medicine, Jinju, South Korea

and almost all diagnosed lymphomas are non-Hodgkin's lymphoma, with approximately 5–20% lymphomas occurring in the GI tract [1]. Lymphomas of the Small intestinal lymphoma are not uncommon among the small intestinal neoplasms (incidence rate, 15–20%), followed by small bowel adenocarcinoma and small bowel neuroendocrine tumors. [1] The incidence of small bowel lymphoma is low, but it has gradually increased since the 1980s.

Previously, it was difficult to diagnose small bowel lymphoma, and most cases were diagnosed postoperatively using surgical samples obtained from patients with intestinal obstruction or GI bleeding. The development of imaging techniques, such as abdominal computed tomography (CT) and magnetic resonance imaging (MRI), and endoscopic techniques, such as capsule endoscopy (CE), small bowel enteroscopy, and ultrasound endoscopy, has led to relatively accurate diagnosis of small bowel lymphoma. However, the lesions that are difficult to diagnose with endoscopy are still diagnosed using surgical specimens. Treatments are also being diversified through the use of various chemotherapies, monoclonal antibodies, and bone marrow transplantation [2].

This chapter describes not only the systematic classification and characteristics of small bowel lymphoma but also useful diagnostic methods and treatments.

© Springer Nature Singapore Pte Ltd. 2022
H. J. Chun et al. (eds.), *Small Intestine Disease*, https://doi.org/10.1007/978-981-16-7239-2_46

Epidemiology

Small bowel lymphoma can occur at any age group (printed cases age range, 32–86 years); however, the incidence rate increases with age, and it is more prevalent in men than in women [2]. The clinical symptoms are unusual and non-specific. Although the clinical symptoms are vague and asymptomatic, the most common symptom is abdominal pain of varying intensity (approximately 70%), followed by ileal obstruction (38%), weight loss (29%), and hemorrhage (21%) [1]. In particular, an emergency operation is often necessary when small bowel lymphoma is associated with symptoms of intestinal obstruction.

Small intestinal lymphomas may be present in various locations, with the most common location being in the ileum (60–65%), particularly in the terminal ileum close to the ileocecal valve, followed by the jejunum (20–25%), the duodenum (6–8%), and other location sites (8–9%). Approximately half of the cases of small bowel lymphomas are single lesions and the other cases are multiple lesions. Simultaneous double lesions also can occur in the small bowel, and colonic lesions are more common than small bowel lesions in multiple simultaneous lesions involving small bowel lymphomas [1, 2].

A primary small bowel lymphoma is of a more heterogenous pathologic type than a gastric lymphoma. The most common pathologic type of small bowel lymphoma is the diffuse large B-cell lymphoma, followed by follicular lymphoma, Burkitt's lymphoma, and mantle cell lymphoma. Mucosa-associated lymphoid tissue (MALT) lymphoma and immunoproliferative small intestinal disease can also occur. B-cell origin small bowel lymphomas are the most common, whereas T-cell origin lymphomas and enteropathy-associated T-cell lymphomas (EATL) related to celiac disease rarely occur [3].

Morphologically, small bowel lymphomas are classified as polypoid/nodular, infiltrative, aneurysmal, exophytic mass, and stenosing mass. Pathological examination of tissue specimens is essential for accurate classification, and there is no correlation between morphological classification and histologic classification.

Diagnosis

The small bowel is a difficult organ to investigate. However, investigating the duodenum and terminal ileum has become relatively simpler using esophagogastroduodenoscopy and colonoscopy. Video CE and the double-balloon technique of push-and-pull enteroscopy have been established as new diagnostic, interventional, and therapeutic modalities. Advances in radiological techniques such as enteroclysis or CT enteroscopy have also contributed to improved diagnostic accuracy and reliability.

The small bowel series is a traditional small bowel evaluation method that is a relatively easy to use and is a less uncomfortable test; however, the sensitivity rate for determining a small tumor is as low as 30–44%.

Enteroclysis is highly sensitive to small bowel tumors and has a sensitivity of >90%, but it requires proficiency and has a relatively low sensitivity for small-sized tumors, subepithelial tumors, and smooth round tumors.

Abdominal CT is the most commonly performed procedure for small bowel tumors >1 cm in size, providing useful information concerning the small bowel mass, and is not only helpful in tumor staging at the time of diagnosis but is also useful in evaluating the treatment response during the follow-up period.

CT enterography shows detailed changes in the small bowel mucosa and small bowel wall thickness (94% sensitivity, 90% specificity, 91% positive prediction, and 95% negative prediction). However, for small bowel luminal dilatation, a timely intake of an additional hyperosmolar solution such as sorbitol solution is required.

Magnetic resonance enterography is possible without radiation exposure, providing more accurate tumor measurement and has high diagnostic accuracy (approximately 97%) for small bowel tumors; however, it is expensive and has a long procedural time with possible magnetic bias and motion artifacts.

CE non-invasively provides entire small bowel images and readily indicates a small bowel tumor. The only contraindication for using CE is small bowel obstruction, where there is a risk of capsule retention. In one multicentered CE analysis study, CE showed an exclusive diagnostic effect of 52% and led to exclusive therapeutic decisions in 12% of cases [4].

Small bowel endoscopy originated with both push enteroscopy and intraoperative enteroscopy. It has now developed into push-and-pull enteroscopy, also known as single- or double-balloon enteroscopy, and is useful for visualization of small bowel neoplasms and for performing biopsies. However, it has a long procedure time and requires costly endoscopic equipment.

The use of positron emission tomography-CT (PET-CT) is still under review concerning small bowel lymphoma, but some studies have reported its usefulness in diagnosing EATL.

At the time of confirmed diagnosis, taking a detailed history and careful physical examinations are important to provide information for determining the possible causes of specific lymphoma subtypes and to evaluate the overall physical condition of the patient. Laboratory tests including complete blood count, liver and renal function, lactate dehydrogenase, glucose, uric acid, calcium, phosphorus, and electrolyte tests are required in addition to bone marrow examination and serum electrophoresis.

Of the various staging systems available, the modified Ann Arbor classification or the Paris staging system is most commonly used. CT scans of the chest, abdomen, and pelvis are necessary for lymphoma staging. In some cases, PET-CT and/or Endoscopic Ultrasonography (EUS) may also be available for staging, and the international prognosis index (IPI) is useful for all non-Hodgkin's lymphoma subtypes.

Treatment

Previously, surgery has been the mainstay of treatment for small bowel lymphoma. However, this has changed with the recent development of combination chemotherapy and/or monoclonal antibodies. A high postoperative mortality rate has been reported previously, and chemotherapy provides greater survival benefits over surgery alone, but consideration should be given to the association with high postoperative mortality. Radiation therapy for small bowel lymphoma is less helpful as multiple lesions and metastatic lesions can be present at the time of diagnosis. Most studies have comprised small, retrospective, and epidemiologic studies rather than independent variable studies. The treatment outcome of primary small bowel lymphoma has been reported to be poorer than for other site lymphomas. Poor prognosis has been related to surgery undertaken for diagnosis and emergency operations for GI obstruction. In particular, primary duodenal lymphoma often requires performing difficult surgical operations such as a pancreaticoduodenectomy. In patients in whom initial therapy has failed, high-dose chemotherapy and stem cell transplantation can be used [5].

Low-grade B cell lymphoma of the small bowel (stage IE) is usually appropriate for surgical resection. For patients at an advanced stage, treatment that includes chemotherapeutic agents and targeted agents is important.

There are no treatment guidelines for small bowel MALT lymphoma, and some patients may benefit from eradication of *Helicobacter pylori*. Localized lymphoma can be treated using an endoscopic procedure or local resection; however, multiple advanced small bowel MALT lymphoma require chemotherapy.

For follicular lymphoma of the small bowel in the asymptomatic indolent stage, a policy of observation may be an option, and the symptomatic stage has various treatment options such as surgery, chemotherapy, and/or radiation therapy.

Mantle cell lymphoma has a poor prognosis except in cases with an excellent initial chemotherapeutic response. More recent clinical trials involving innovative medications and stem cell transplantations are being undertaken.

Prognosis

The prognosis of B-cell lymphoma is superior to that of T-cell lymphoma. [6] T-cell lymphoma is generally at a more advanced stage at the time of diagnosis and frequently requires emergency surgery [7]. Factors known to affect prognosis include age, gender, symptoms, lactic dehydrogenase level, and the IPI score; however, the precise influence of these factors remains unclear. One small study reported that the 5-year overall survival rate for surgery and chemotherapy is 79.5% (single chemotherapy, 13.9%) [8].

References

1. Schottenfeld D, Beebe-Dimmer JL, Vigneau FD. The epidemiology and pathogenesis of neoplasia in the small intestine. Ann Epidemiol. 2009;19:58–69.

2. Yin L, Chen CQ, Peng CH, et al. Primary small-bowel non-Hodgkin's lymphoma: a study of clinical features, pathology, management and prognosis. J Int Med Res. 2007;35:406–15.

3. Roggero E, Zucca E, Cavalli F. Gastric mucosa-associated lymphoid tissue lymphomas: more than a fascinating model. J Natl Cancer Inst. 1997;89:1328–30.

4. Cheung DY, Lee IS, Chang DK, et al. Capsule endoscopy in small bowel tumors: a multicenter Korean study. J Gastroenterol Hepatol. 2010;25:1079–86.

5. Beaton C, Davies M, Beynon J. The management of primary small bowel and colon lymphoma–a review. Int J Color Dis. 2012;27:555–63.

6. Chestovich PJ, Schiller G, Sasu S, Hiatt JR. Duodenal lymphoma: a rare and morbid tumor. Am Surg. 2007;73:1057–62.

7. Cheung MC, Housri N, Ogilvie MP, Sola JE, Koniaris LG. Surgery does not adversely affect survival in primary gastrointestinal lymphoma. J Surg Oncol. 2009;100:59–64.

8. Khosla D, Kumar R, Kapoor R, et al. A retrospective analysis of clinic pathological characteristics, treatment, and outcome of 27 patients of primary intestinal lymphomas. J Gastrointest Cancer. 2013;44(4):417–21.

Other Small Bowel Tumors

Duk Hwan Kim

Key Points

1. Malignant small bowel tumors, such as gastrointestinal stromal tumors and carcinoid tumors, should be treated even in the absence of clinical symptoms.
2. Tumor size and mitotic count were included in the risk classification system for gastrointestinal stromal tumors.
3. Carcinoid syndrome can occur in small intestinal carcinoid tumors, and surgical resection including lymph node dissection should be considered in case of multiple small bowel carcinoid tumors.

Introduction

Small bowel tumors, whether benign or malignant, are very rare in clinical practice and initially present with ambiguous symptoms, such as abdominal discomfort. With respect to malignant small bowel tumors, surgical emergencies such as intussusception or intestinal obstruction occur frequently, which are very challenging for physicians to manage. However, recent advances in techniques for diagnosing various small intestinal diseases, including capsule endoscopy or device-assisted enteroscopy, have increased the probability of detecting small bowel tumors. Therefore, this chapter aimed to discuss other small bowel tumors that are relatively uncommon.

Malignant Tumors

Gastrointestinal Stromal Tumor

Pathophysiology

Gastrointestinal stromal tumor (GIST) is a sarcoma derived from mesenchymal cells. Prior to the introduction of immunohistochemical diagnosis, all tumors comprising spindle cells were classified as either leiomyomas or leiomyosarcomas. Nonetheless, most of these tumors have been found to be lacking in smooth muscle differentiation, and interstitial cells of Cajal have been revealed as their precursor cells [1]. More than 80% of all GISTs have *c-KIT* (CD117) and *PDGFRα* gene mutations as an important pathogenesis [2].

Diagnosis

GISTs arise in the form of submucosal tumors because they originate from the muscle layer of the gastrointestinal tract (Fig. 1). GISTs are diagnosed incidentally in most cases, as they do not cause any distinctive symptoms until they become larger. However, an increase in their size may

D. H. Kim (✉)
Digestive Disease Center, CHA Bundang Hospital, CHA University School of Medicine, Seongnam, South Korea

© Springer Nature Singapore Pte Ltd. 2022
H. J. Chun et al. (eds.), *Small Intestine Disease*, https://doi.org/10.1007/978-981-16-7239-2_47

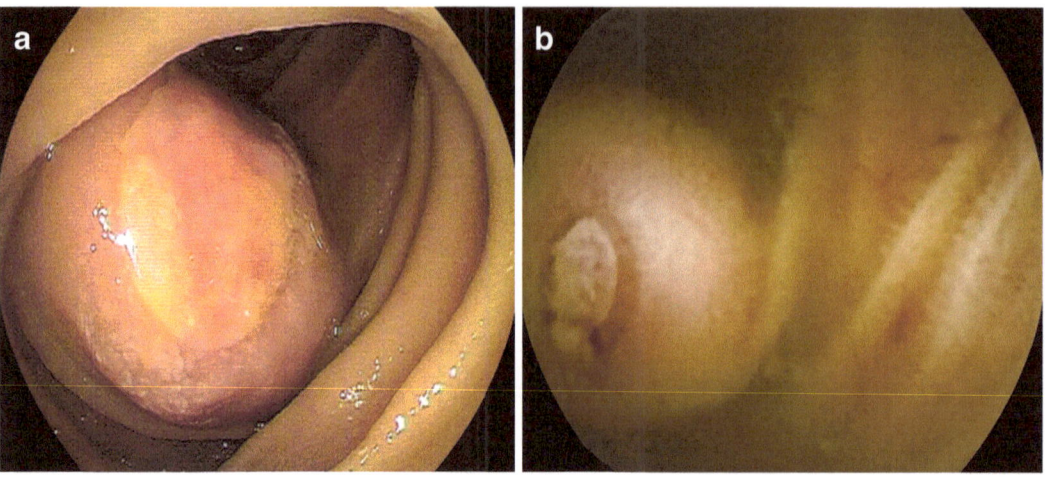

Fig. 1 Gastrointestinal stromal tumor in the small bowel. (a) Enteroscopy. (b) Capsule endoscopy

result in abdominal pain or obstruction, and gastrointestinal bleeding or anemia associated with surface ulceration may develop [3]. GISTs are known to be the most prevalent in the stomach, followed by the small intestine, colon, and esophagus. Although these tumors are generally considered benign, metastasis to other organs such as the liver and peritoneum may occur; hence, GIST staging should be established using abdominopelvic computed tomography (CT) at the time of diagnosis. If metastasis to organs other than the abdomen is suspected, other imaging tests can be performed. In this case, positron emission tomography (PET) can be used for diagnosis because GISTs show activity on PET scan. Pathologic diagnosis is established based on immunohistochemical staining results and cell morphology on histological examination. Spindle cell (70%), epithelioid (20%), and mixed-type (10%) GISTs are the most frequent cases [4]. Because more than 90% of GISTs immunohistochemically stain positive for CD117, this result serves as a powerful tool for exact diagnosis. Thus far, there is no recommendation on how to perform a biopsy for diagnosing small bowel GIST. Repeated endoscopic biopsy can be easily performed; nonetheless, it is more likely to be difficult in the limited small intestine environment and the diagnosis rate is not high owing to the characteristics of the tumor originating from the muscle layer. Partial tumor resection for diagnosis is not recommended because of the risk of tumor seeding that may occur during resection.

Treatment

Generally, GISTs in organs other than the stomach have a worse prognosis. Patients with resectable small bowel tumors with a high possibility of being GISTs are most preferable to undergo surgical resection because tracking the changes in the shape and size of the lesion in the small intestine is often difficult. While tumor size and mitotic index have traditionally been used as risk factors for recurrence according to National Institutes of Health classification system, an investigator has included nongastric tumor location such as small bowel and tumor rupture as factors predicting poor prognosis (Table 1) [5]. Imatinib, a tyrosine kinase inhibitor, can be used as medical treatment in patients with metastatic or unresectable small bowel GIST, whereas sunitinib may be administered as secondary treatment in patients whose GIST does not respond to imatinib.

Carcinoid Tumor

Pathophysiology

Carcinoid tumors are well-differentiated neuroendocrine tumors and represent the second most common malignant tumor in the small intestine

Table 1 Modified risk stratification of primary gastrointestinal stromal tumor

Risk category	Tumor size (cm)	Mitotic index (per 50 HPF)	Primary tumor site
Very low risk	≤2.0	≤5	Any
Low risk	2.1–5.0	≤5	Any
Intermediate risk	≤5.0	6–10	Gastric
	5.1–10.0	≤5	Gastric
High risk	Any	Any	Tumor rupture
	>10.0	Any	Any
	Any	>10	Any
	>5.0	>5	Any
	≤5.0	>5	Non-gastric
	5.1–10.0	≤5	Non-gastric

Adapted with permission from the author [5]

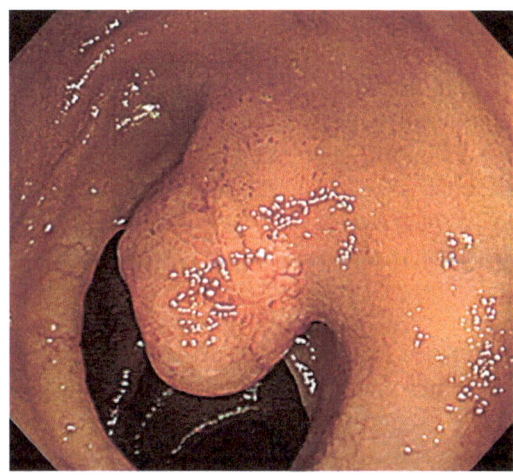

Fig. 2 Carcinoid tumor in the small bowel

after adenocarcinoma [6]. Carcinoid tumors can be classified as those occurring in the foregut, midgut, or hindgut depending on the embryological origin. Carcinoid tumor occurring in the midgut is most commonly found in the appendix but has low clinical significance. Most carcinoid tumors in the small intestine are found in the distal ileum.

Diagnosis

Carcinoid syndrome can occur as a result of the release of serotonin secreted by midgut carcinoid tumors into the systemic circulation, leading to symptoms such as flushing, abdominal pain, and diarrhea. Carcinoid tumors in the small bowel without carcinoid syndrome are usually asymptomatic owing to their very slow growth and are found in sizes of <1 cm. However, intestinal obstruction due to bowel adhesions can develop secondary to desmoplastic reactions. In rare cases, hemorrhage due to ulceration of the tumor surface may occur [7]. A carcinoid tumor can appear endoscopically as a light-yellowish submucosal tumor that is visible through the mucosa (Fig. 2). Multiple carcinoid tumors are detected in nearly one-third of all small bowel carcinoid tumors; in these cases, mesenteric involvement of the tumor through lymphatic dissemination should be confirmed. Patients usually present with severe carcinoid symptoms when the dis-

ease progresses, including multiple liver metastases. Evaluation of the entire gastrointestinal tract, including colonoscopy, should be performed for disease staging. Abdominopelvic CT scan can aid in assessing disease extent. However, contrast-enhanced CT is not diagnostic, as carcinoid tumors can be isodense with surrounding tissue [8]. As most neuroendocrine tumors contain somatostatin receptors, indium-111 octreotide scintigraphy can be useful for the localization of carcinoid tumors. PET scan may be performed for undifferentiated tumors. When carcinoid syndrome is suspected, measurement of 5-hydroxyindoleacetic acid by 24-hour urine test is diagnostic.

Treatment

In conformity with the 2018 recommendation by the National Comprehensive Cancer Network, surgical resection with lymph node dissection should be performed for resectable carcinoid tumors in the small intestine. If octreotide or lanreotide is to be administered, prophylactic cholecystectomy should be performed. In the case of locally advanced or metastatic carcinoid tumors, the 10-year survival rate has been reported to be 40–70% [9]. Even in the presence of hepatic metastasis, long-term survival remains possible through active surgical treatment. Therefore, tailored therapeutic planning is required in a multidisciplinary clinic.

Metastatic Small Bowel Tumors

Invasion of the small intestine typically occurs when malignant tumors originating from areas other than the gastrointestinal tract invade the gastrointestinal tract. Melanoma, lung cancer (Fig. 3), breast cancer, and kidney cancer are common primary cancers. Small intestinal involvement usually results from hematogenous spreading, although direct invasion from an adjacent organ is possible. Abdominal pain, hemorrhage, and intestinal obstruction may be present. Small bowel metastasis usually occurs at the terminal stage of the disease and shows poor prognosis.

Benign Tumors

Benign tumors in the small intestine include adenoma, lipoma (Fig. 4), hyperplastic polyp, leiomyoma, hemangioma (Fig. 5), and inflammatory fibroid polyp (Fig. 6). Benign small bowel tumors are usually reported to be less likely to become malignant because of the following reasons: (1) the transit time in the small intestine is relatively short, such that the effects of carcinogens exposed to the small intestinal mucosa are minimal; (2) large amounts of small intestinal secretions dilute the toxins and carcinogens; (3) relatively high intestinal pH inhibits the formation of bacterial colonies; and (4) benzyl peroxidase at high con-centration in the small intestine is involved in the degradation of carcinogens [10]. In the absence of symptoms, adenomas are considered to be pre-cancerous lesions of adenocarcinoma and should be removed endoscopically or surgically. When benign tumors are diagnosed, treatment is decided according to their size and symptoms. Opinions as to the treatment and follow-up for asymptomatic benign tumors are conflicting, and individual treatment is required for these tumors.

Conclusion

Small bowel endoscopic techniques have recently been advanced, and the frequency of small bowel tumors being diagnosed is increasing. Further studies on the diagnosis and treatment of various small bowel tumors as well as their prognostic factors are warranted because there is still lack of clinical data. Small bowel evaluation is relatively limited so far, and small bowel tumors often progress slowly in both benign and malignant. Moreover, most treatments are dependent on surgical removal. These features make it difficult to establish a therapeutic approach to small bowel tumors, particularly in the elderly population. Furthermore, considering the increasing number of cases treated by endoscopy to date, studies on the development and appropriateness of various endoscopic treatment modalities should be continued, and it is expected that a more precisely

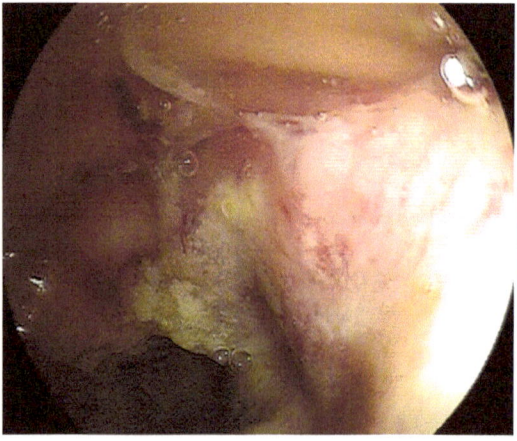 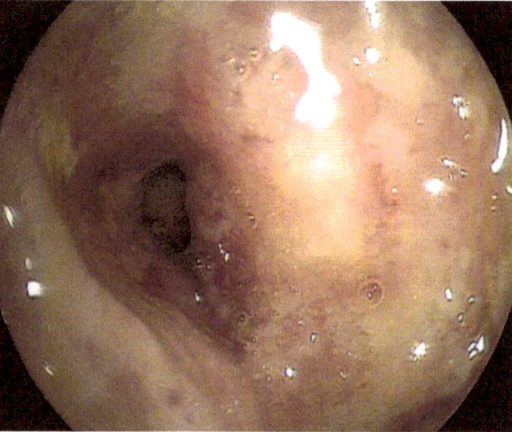

Fig. 3 Small bowel metastasis of the lung cancer

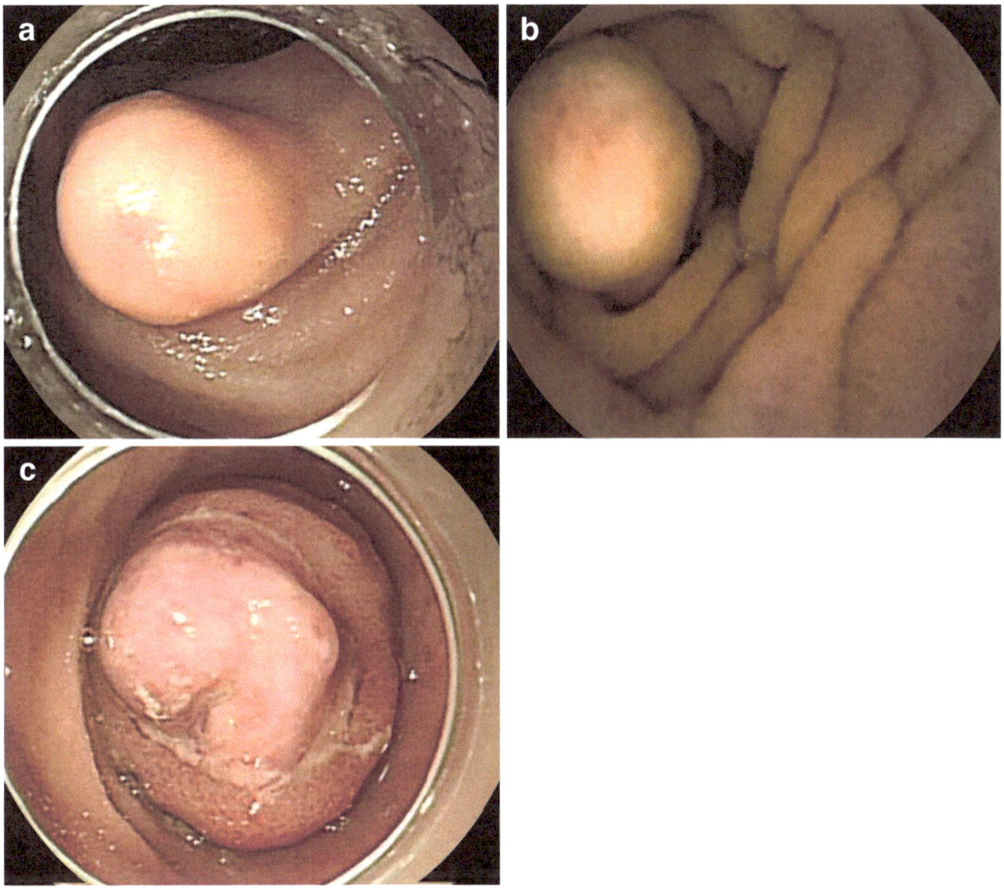

Fig. 4 Lipoma in the small bowel. (**a**) Enteroscopy. (**b**) Capsule endoscopy. (**c**) Lipoma with ulceration on the surface

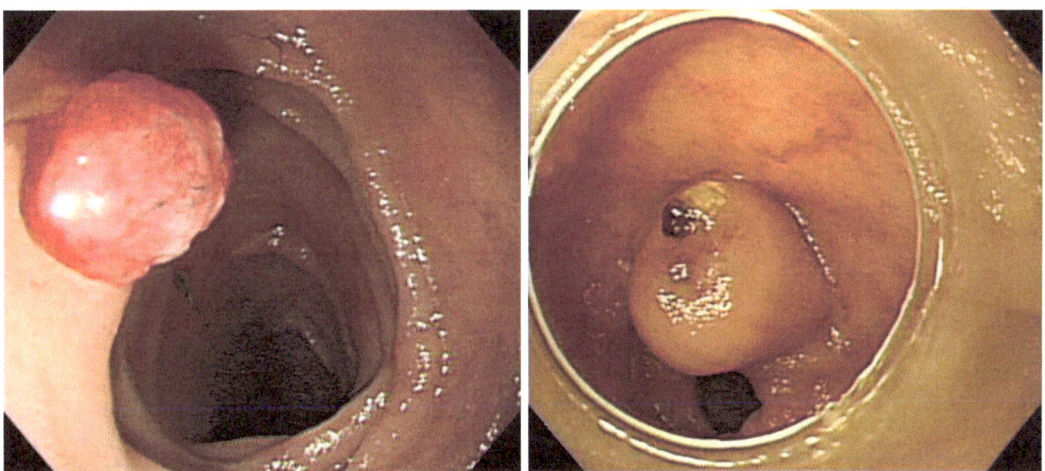

Fig. 5 Hemangioma in the small bowel

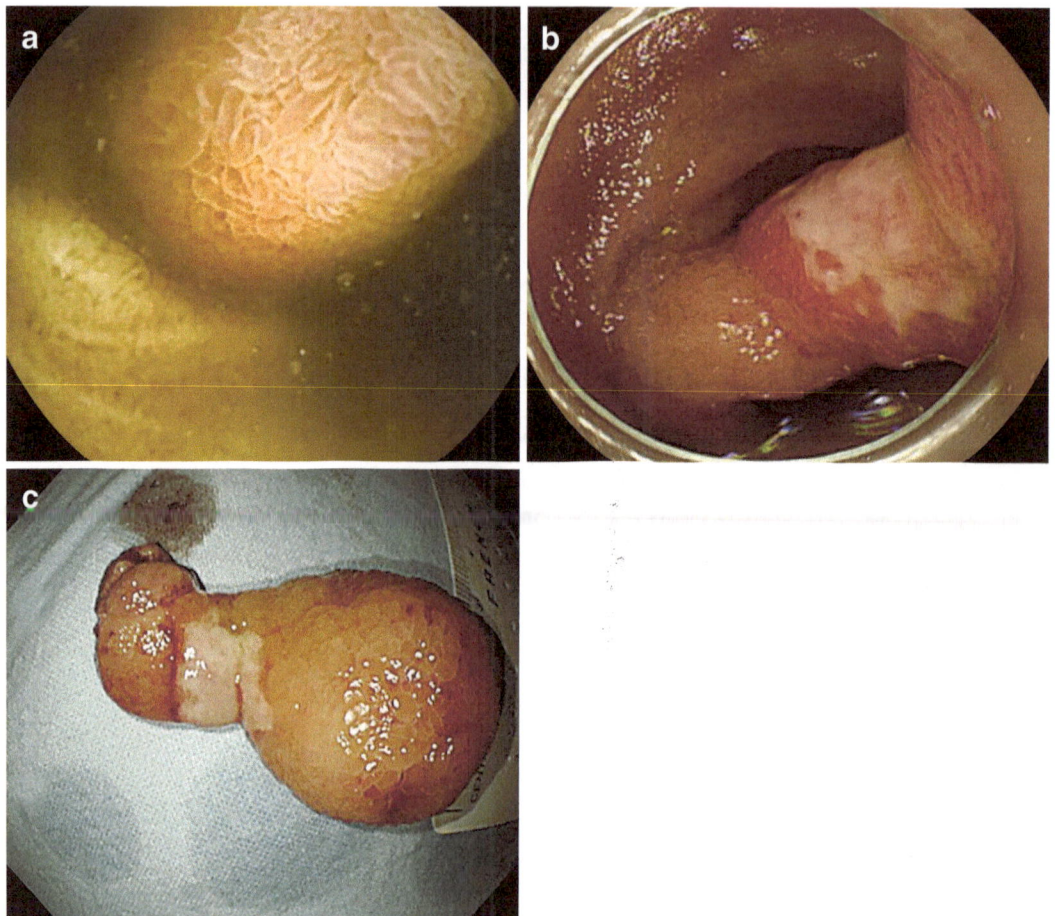

Fig. 6 Inflammatory fibroid polyps in the small bowel. (**a**) Capsule endoscopy. (**b**) Enteroscopy. (**c**) Gross pathology after endoscopic resection

tailored treatment for small bowel tumors will become possible.

References

1. Lasota J, Jasinski M, Sarlomo-Rikala M, Miettinen M. Mutations in exon 11 of c-Kit occur preferentially in malignant versus benign gastrointestinal stromal tumors and do not occur in leiomyomas or leiomyosarcomas. Am J Pathol. 1999;154:53–60.
2. Wong NA. Gastrointestinal stromal tumours–an update for histopathologists. Histopathology. 2011;59:807–21.
3. Miettinen M, Makhlouf H, Sobin LH, Lasota J. Gastrointestinal stromal tumors of the jejunum and ileum: a clinicopathologic, immunohistochemical, and molecular genetic study of 906 cases before imatinib with long-term follow-up. Am J Surg Pathol. 2006;30:477–89.
4. Miettinen M, Lasota J. Gastrointestinal stromal tumors: review on morphology, molecular pathology, prognosis, and differential diagnosis. Arch Pathol Lab Med. 2006;130:1466–78.
5. Joensuu H. Risk stratification of patients diagnosed with gastrointestinal stromal tumor. Hum Pathol. 2008;39:1411–9.
6. Donohue JH. Malignant tumours of the small bowel. Surg Oncol. 1994;3:61–8.
7. Makridis C, Rastad J, Oberg K, Akerstrom G. Progression of metastases and symptom improvement from laparotomy in midgut carcinoid tumors. World J Surg. 1996;20:900–6. Discussion 907
8. Sugimoto E, Lorelius LE, Eriksson B, Oberg K. Midgut carcinoid tumours. CT appearance Acta Radiol. 1995;36:367–71.
9. Kim MK, Warner RR, Roayaie S, et al. Revised staging classification improves outcome prediction for small intestinal neuroendocrine tumors. J Clin Oncol. 2013;31:3776–81.
10. Genta RM, Feagins LA. Advanced precancerous lesions in the small bowel mucosa. Best Pract Res Clin Gastroenterol. 2013;27:225–33.

Meckel's Diverticulum

Sehyun Jang and Bora Keum

Key Points

- The prevalence rate of Meckel's diverticulum is approximately 2%, and most patients are asymptomatic. The incidence of complications decreases with age. The most common complication in adults is intestinal obstruction.
- A high degree of suspicion is important in diagnosing Meckel's diverticulum. 99 m-Tc-pertechnetate scintigraphy is the most sensitive diagnostic tool.
- Laparoscopic surgical resection is the primary treatment when complications are present.

Introduction

Meckel's diverticulum is the most prevalent congenital anomaly of the gastrointestinal tract [1]. This condition was named after Johan Friedrich Meckel, who first described the developmental characteristics of the anomaly in 1809. Meckel's diverticulum is a true diverticulum outpouching of the ileum in the anti-mesenteric side due to incomplete obliteration of the omphalomesenteric duct at the seventh week of gestation. This anomaly is said to follow the "rule of twos": it is

S. Jang · B. Keum (✉)
Korea University Anam Hospital, Seoul, South Korea

found in 2% of the population, is twice as common in men than in women, is located in the proximal 2 ft. (60 cm) of the ileocecal valve, is about 2 in (5 cm) long, and its symptoms occur before the age of 2 years.

Clinical Features

Most affected individuals are asymptomatic. The overall symptom manifestation rate is 4–6%. In most patients, the manifestation of symptoms occurs in childhood. Generally, 45% of patients show symptoms before the age of 2 years. It is well known that the incidence rate decreases with age. The clinical presentation also varies with age. The most common presentation of Meckel's diverticulum in children is painless gastrointestinal bleeding, whereas symptoms associated with intestinal obstruction are more common in adults [2].

Gastrointestinal Bleeding

It is reported that approximately 55.5% of children with symptoms experience gastrointestinal bleeding, which mainly involves acute or chronic painless rectal hemorrhage. The bleeding is commonly characterized as dark red or reddish-brown or melena. Gastrointestinal bleeding has been primarily associated with ectopic tissues, such as ectopic gastric mucosa or ectopic pancreatic mucosa. An acidic or alkaline substance secreted by the ectopic mucosa forms ulceration in the adjacent mucosa, resulting in bleeding. The ectopic gastric mucosa is common (incidence, 60–65%), whereas ectopic pancreatic mucosa is observed in 5% [3]. Ulcers are located adjacent to or slightly distal to the diverticulum.

Intestinal Obstruction

The most common symptom manifesting in adults is intestinal obstruction caused by Meckel's diverticulum. Intestinal obstruction is the second most common complication in children. There are many causes of obstruction, and some of them are described below.

Meckel's diverticulum is the most common anatomical leading point of ileocecal intussusception and can cause repetitive intestinal obstruction. Volvulus resulting from a Meckel's diverticulum can also cause intestinal obstruction. Volvulus is caused by twisting of the bowel around the persistent vitelline duct. The mesodiverticular band, which is the remnant of the vitelline artery, forms a fibrous band between the diverticular end and the mesentery. Obstruction can also occur when the ileum is trapped in the space between the diverticulum and the lower part of the mesodiverticular band. Littre's hernia includes any type of hernia in which Meckel's diverticulum is involved. The major types of Littre's hernia are inguinal and femoral hernias. Strangulated Littre's hernia causes intestinal obstruction. If not treated immediately, this complication will result in strangulation and eventually lead to small-intestinal necrosis. Therefore, prompt surgical resection including the diverticulum and part of the small intestine is needed.

Meckel's Diverticulitis

Diverticulitis accounts for 10–20% of complications and is mainly seen in elderly patients. Diverticulitis has similar clinical characteristics to acute appendicitis and may lead to perforation, resulting in peritonitis. Therefore, it has been called a "second appendix." Enterolith in the diverticulum, food, or foreign body promotes inflammation. Edward's syndrome (trisomy 18) is known to increase the risk of Meckel's diverticulitis.

Tumor

It is rare for a tumor to occur in Meckel's diverticulum. Most tumors are benign, such as lipoma, neurofibromatoma, and angioma. Malignant tumors are also reported, with carcinoid tumor being the most common, followed by adenocarcinoma and gastrointestinal stromal tumors.

Diagnosis

The majority of patients with Meckel's diverticulum are asymptomatic. Meckel's diverticulum without symptoms is not well detected. The diagnosis begins with a suspicion of Meckel's diverticulum when complications such as bleeding and intestinal obstruction occur. The diagnostic approach varies depending on the symptoms. In patients with gastrointestinal bleeding, Meckel's scan (technetium-99 m pertechnetate scintigraphy) is the most sensitive diagnostic tool. Meckel's scan is the most effective diagnostic method in children with gastrointestinal bleeding, with 80–90% sensitivity, 95% specificity, and 90% accuracy. However, in adult patients, the sensitivity decreases to 62%, specificity to 9%, and accuracy to 46%. Pentagastrin, H2 blockers, and glucagon can be injected to increase the sensitivity. Technetium-99 m pertechnetate is absorbed from the parietal cells of the gastric mucosa. Nuclear imaging reveals ectopic mucosa in Meckel's diverticulum after the intravenous infusion of 99 m-Tc pertechnetate (Fig. 1). If there is very little or no ectopic mucosa in the diverticulum, scintigraphic activity is diminished when gastrointestinal bleeding or bowel hypersecretion is present, therefore false-negative results may occur. False-positive results may occur when ectopic mucosa is present elsewhere besides the Meckel's diverticulum, as well as when angiodysplasia, small-intestinal ulcers,

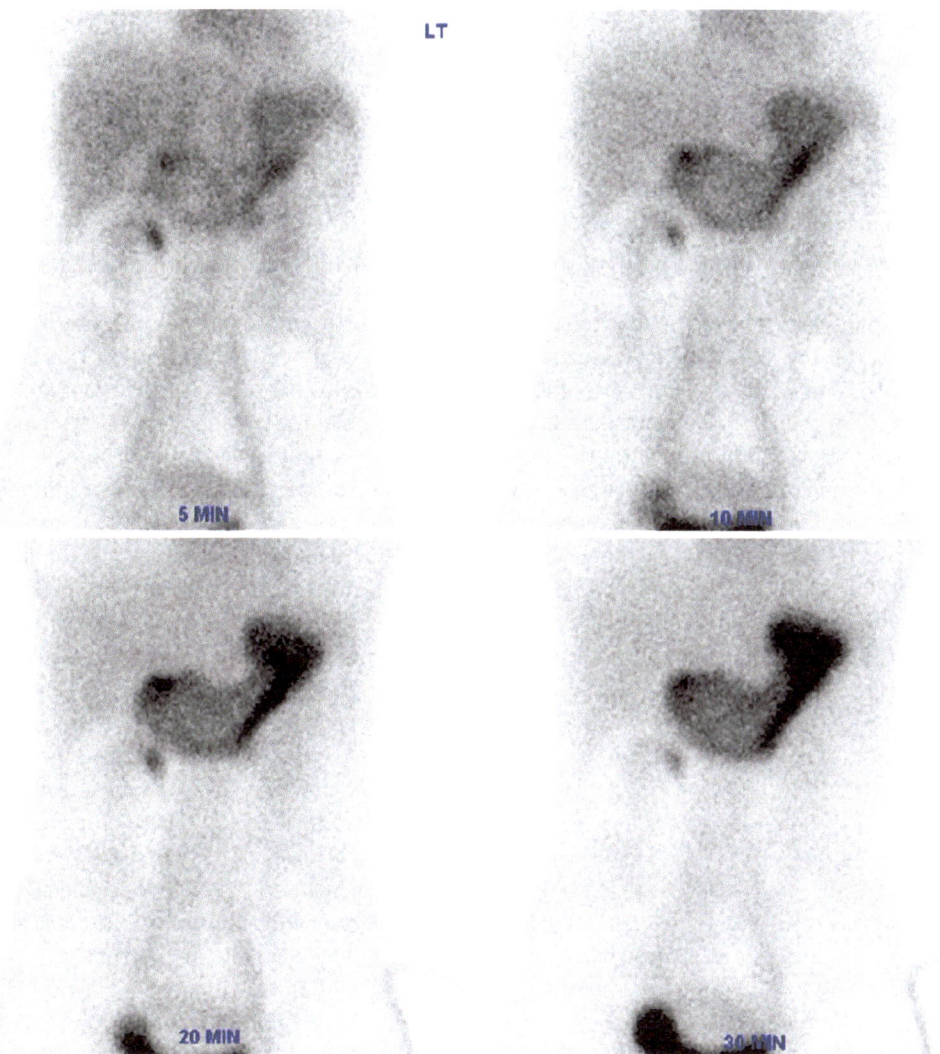

Fig. 1 Meckel's diverticulum detected in the right upper quadrant on technetium-99 m pertechnetate scanning

intussusception, inflammatory bowel disease, adhesion, and hydronephrosis are present. 99 m-Tc-pertechnetate is excreted in the kidney; thus, the kidney, ureter, and bladder can be visualized during the evaluation [4].

Another diagnostic method, such as capsule endoscopy or double-balloon enteroscopy, can be helpful in patients with unexplained gastrointestinal bleeding. The positive prediction rate of capsule endoscopy is about 80–85%. Capsule retention is very rarely reported in patients with Meckel's diverticulum. Double-balloon enteroscopy performed by experienced endoscopists is

considered a safe diagnostic tool and can be applied if Meckel's diverticulum is suspected but could not be diagnosed. Considering the anatomical characteristics, it is recommended to consider retrograde double-balloon enteroscopy first. The advantage of double-balloon enteroscopy is that it is able to directly inspect lesions and to accurately localize the lesion so that biopsy and therapeutic procedures, such as cauterization, can be performed if needed. Although controversial, it has been suggested that even if the results of Meckel scans or capsule endoscopy are negative, double-balloon endoscopy is still essential to completely rule out Meckel's diverticulum. Angiography may also be an option in the diagnosis of gastrointestinal bleeding with a suspicion of Meckel's diverticulum. The remnant omphalomesenteric artery, which receives blood flow from the superior mesenteric artery, is shown on angiography. Angiography has a 59% accuracy and is useful if the bleeding rate is >2–3 mL/min [5].

Ultrasonography and computed tomography (CT) are non-invasive diagnostic methods in patients without bleeding. Ultrasonography is mainly used in pediatric patients with right lower abdominal pain because of its non-invasiveness. It is effective in detecting a thickened bowel wall due to inflammation or intra-abdominal abscess. CT is less accurate in distinguishing Meckel's diverticulum from the normal small intestine in cases without accompanying complications. However, when complications are present, CT is more specific than ultrasonography and is particularly helpful in detecting fluid- or gas-filled structures (Fig. 2).

Treatment

The treatment of choice for Meckel's diverticulum with complications is laparoscopic resection. (Fig. 3). In case of gastrointestinal bleeding, surgical resection of Meckel's diverticulum can prevent further bleeding. It is mandatory to completely resect the ectopic mucosa. Otherwise, ulcers or bleeding may recur. There is yet no consensus about the treatment of asymptomatic Meckel's diverticulum that is incidentally discovered. Some argue that persons with Meckel's diverticulum have a 5–6% chance of developing complications throughout their lives, whereas some argue that surgical resection is necessary because preventive surgical resection has a low complication rate of about 1% [5]. However, currently, the majority opinion is that close follow-up is necessary for patients with no symptoms. As mentioned above, Meckel's diverticulum has a decreasing chance of symptomatic presentation with age. Some authors argue that surgical resection is needed depending on the type of diverticulum and the age of the patient even when there are no symptoms. Some surgeons suggest that surgical resection should be considered based on a cut-off point of 2 cm. Other surgeons recommend that the width of Meckel's diverticulum should be the main factor to consider in deciding the need for resection. However, no clear standards have been established thus far. If Meckel's diverticulum is incidentally detected during surgery for another condition, some have suggested preventive resection because of the risk of complications and others recommend no further intervention.

Summary

Meckel's diverticulum is the most common congenital anomaly of the gastrointestinal tract. Most affected individuals are asymptomatic. Meckel's diverticulum has a decreasing chance of symptomatic presentation with age. However, in patients with small-bowel symptoms such as small-intestinal bleeding or intestinal obstruction that are challenging to be diagnosed, Meckel's diverticulum should be suspected as one of the causes. Particularly, in young patients with gastrointestinal bleeding or intestinal obstruction which are unexplained and recurrent, it is important to consider the possibility of Meckel's diverticulum and the appropriate diagnostic method should be carried out.

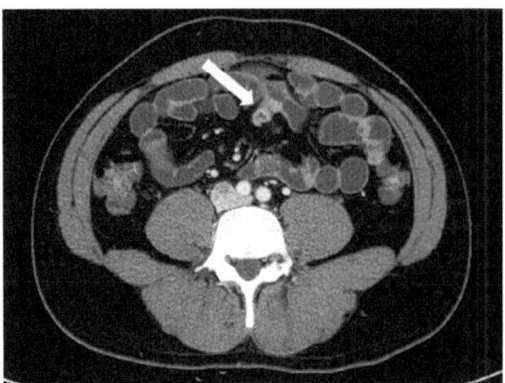

Fig. 2 Meckel's diverticulum in abdominal computed tomography scan of a 34-year-old man with hematochezia. A protruding structure of the small-bowel loop is observed, and the contrast-enhanced bowel wall is visible inside (arrowed)

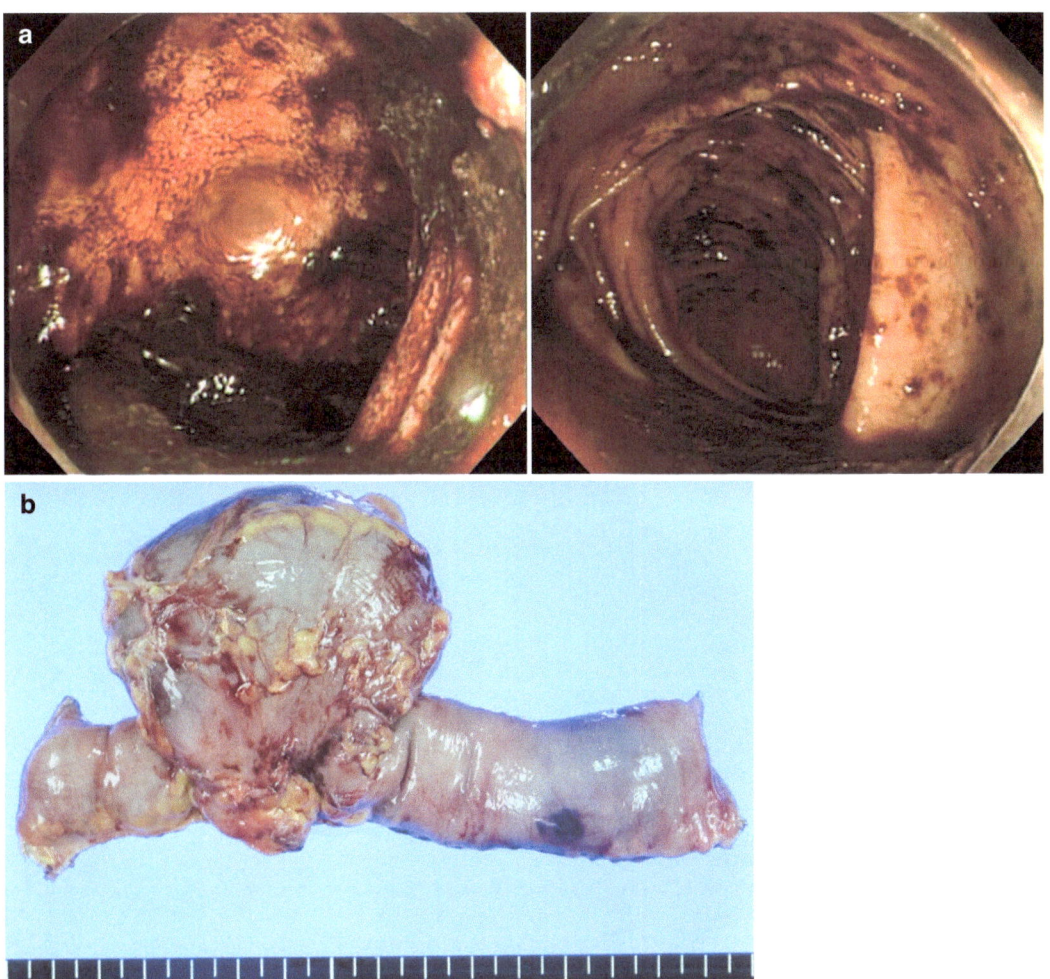

Fig. 3 A 30-year-old female patient with hematochezia. (**a**) a colonoscopy shows that no bleeding focus was found in the terminal ileum and colon, (**b**) laparoscopic surgery was performed to resect the large Meckel's diverticulum

References

1. Sagar J, Kumar V, Shah DK. Meckel's diverticulum: a systematic review. J R Soc Med. 2006;99(10):501–5.
2. Uppal K, Tubbs RS, Matusz P, Shaffer K, Loukas M. Meckel's diverticulum: a review. Clin Anat. 2011;24(4):416–22.
3. St-Vil D, Brandt ML, Panic S, Bensoussan AL, Blanchard H. Meckel's diverticulum in children: a 20-year review. J Pediatr Surg. 1991;26(11):1289–92.
4. Lin S, Suhocki PV, Ludwig KA, Shetzline MA. Gastrointestinal bleeding in adult patients with Meckel's diverticulum: the role of technetium 99m pertechnetate scan. South Med J. 2002;95(11):1338–41.
5. Malik AA, Shamsul B, Wani KA, Khaja AR. Meckel's diverticulum-Revisited. Saudi J Gastroenterol. 2010;16(1):3–7.

Amyloidosis of the Small Bowel

Sun Hyung Kang

Key Points
- Gastrointestinal (GI) amyloidosis can induce various symptoms depending on the type of proteins and invasion site and is very difficult to diagnose in the absence of a physician's clinical suspicion.
- The most common invasion site of GI amyloidosis is the small bowel and various symptoms may appear depending on invasion depth.
- Systemic chemotherapy, symptomatic therapy, and surgical treatment can be applied depending on the type of deposited protein.

Introduction

Amyloidosis represents a rare disease that induces systemic amyloid deposition in multiple organs, particularly the heart and kidneys, as well as the nerves, soft tissues, and digestive tract, which are among the most frequently affected sites. Amyloid proteins are abnormally deposited in the extracellular matrix, leading to organ dysfunction. Gastrointestinal (GI) amyloidosis can induce various symptoms depending on the type of proteins and invasion site and is very difficult to diagnose in the absence of a physician's clinical suspicion. More than 31 types of proteins are recognized as the precursors of amyloid protein; nonetheless, only some types of proteins are considered to be of clinical significance. This article aimed to review the pathologic, clinical, and endoscopic features of GI amyloidosis.

Types of Amyloidosis

Amyloidosis is classified into two types according to the cause of amyloid deposition—namely, primary and secondary amyloidosis. Primary amyloidosis is the most common type of monoclonal immunoglobulin light chain (AL) deposition and is associated with plasma cell abnormalities, including multiple sclerosis [1]. Secondary amyloidosis mainly results from the deposition of serum amyloid A proteins (SAAs), which are circulating acute-phase reactants, and is often due to chronic inflammatory diseases such as rheumatoid arthritis, Crohn's disease, leprosy, and tuberculosis [2]. Furthermore, transthyretin amyloidosis, which is associated with $\beta2$ microglobulin amyloidosis or familial amyloidotic polyneuropathy (FAP), is commonly encountered in clinical practice. Amyloidosis is often difficult to diagnose because of its diverse clinical manifestations, which can depend on the deposition patterns of each protein.

S. H. Kang (✉)
Division of Gastroenterology, Department of Internal Medicine, Chungnam National University School of Medicine, Daejeon, South Korea

Clinical Features and Histopathology

Determination of clinical features may vary according to the amount and distribution of amyloid deposits. If protein distribution is chiefly confined to the mucosal layer, diarrhea or absorptive disorder may be a major symptom. If proteins are deposited in the muscle layer, this may lead to intestinal obstruction. GI bleeding can mainly occur when protein deposition invades the mucosal and submucosal layers. The primary mechanism of GI bleeding is vascular occlusion and weakening of the blood vessel. Vascular occlusion results from protein deposition in the vessel, and amyloid deposition may lead to ischemia, ulceration, wall infarction, and finally weakening of the blood vessel.

In primary amyloidosis, the AL protein mainly invades the mucosal layer and proper muscle layer. Therefore, it may appear as a protrusion of the mucous membrane or thickened wrinkles on endoscopic examination. The AL protein is predominantly involved in the proximal small bowel in older male patients and is thus more likely to appear as a duodenal lesion on duodenoscopy (Fig. 1).

In secondary amyloidosis, the SAA protein is mainly confined to the mucosal and submucosal layers and may cause diarrhea, absorption disorder, GI bleeding, and intestinal obstruction. Secondary amyloidosis can occur mainly in the form of fine granular mucosal pattern and mucosal friability on endoscopy (Fig. 2). Secondary amyloidosis accompanying FAP may lead to diarrhea, constipation, or early satiety owing to protein deposition in the submucosal layer and intestinal nerve plexus. Normal or nonspecific mucosal change can be observed, but fine granular mucosal change or mucosal friability, as seen with the SAA protein, may also occur.

There exist few reports on amyloidosis in Korea. In one Korean single-center study, 24 (15.5%) out of 155 patients showed GI involvement, whereas only 1 patient had small bowel involvement. Diagnosing amyloidosis based solely on patients' symptoms is difficult because various nonspecific GI symptoms (e.g., GI bleeding, weight loss, dyspepsia, abdominal pain, constipation, diarrhea) may appear [3].

Diagnosis and Treatment

As mentioned above, diagnosing amyloidosis is very difficult if there exists no positive suspicion of amyloidosis because most patients present with nonspecific symptoms. Active diagnostic evaluation is needed for patients with unex-

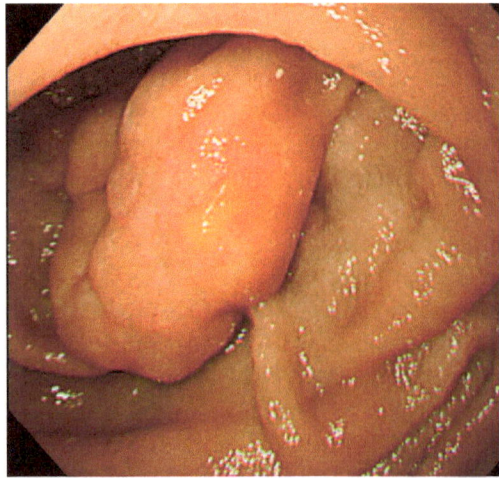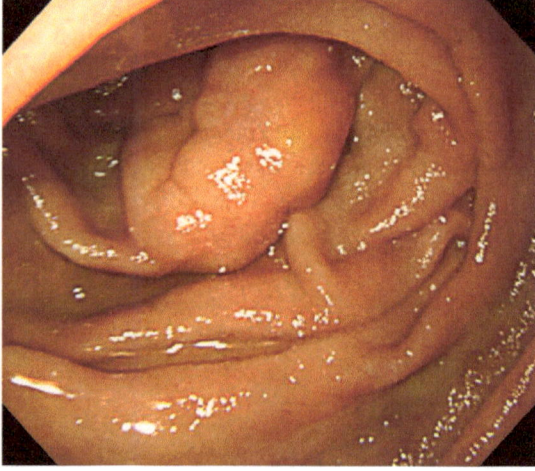

Fig. 1 A 59-year-old male patient with small bowel amyloidosis. Elevated mucosal change was detected on duodenoscopy

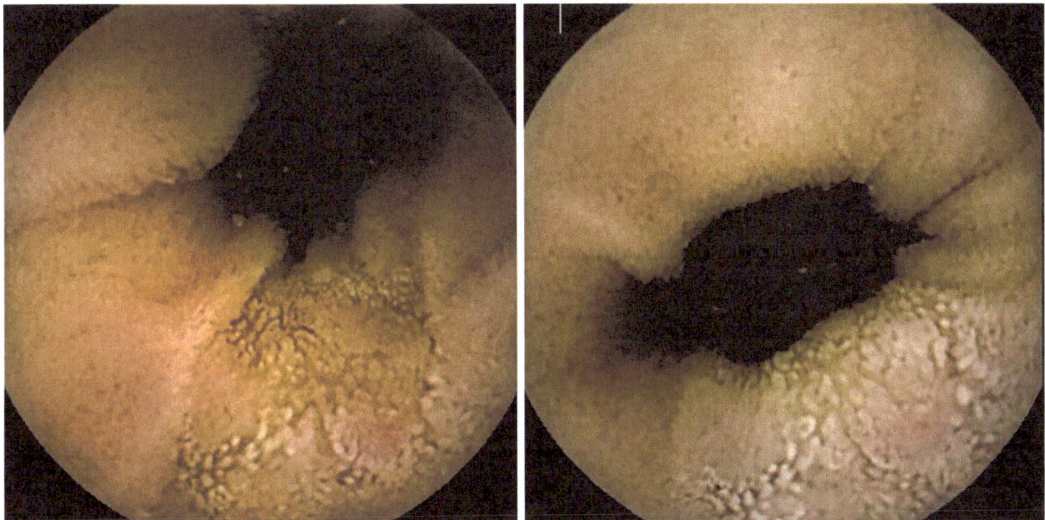

Fig. 2 Fine granular mucosal change, as detected on capsule endoscopy

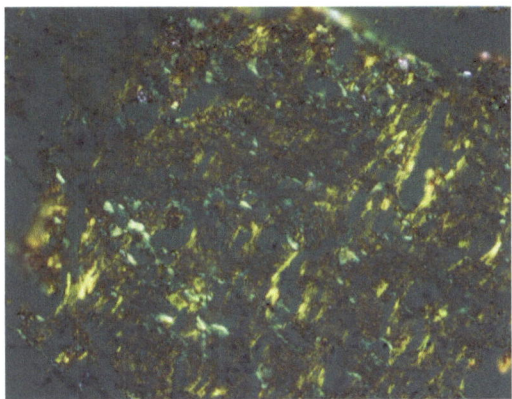

Fig. 3 Amyloid deposition, which was confirmed by Congo red staining

plained GI symptoms and underlying amyloidosis-associated disease. Amyloidosis can be diagnosed when the amyloid deposition is proved by histologic examination of the involved organs. Amyloid deposition can be clearly observed using Congo red stain (Fig. 3). Abdominal fat or gingival biopsy may be helpful in patients with inaccessible target organs. On endoscopy, multiple elevated mucosae and fine granular patterns may be present in various forms depending on the type and distribution of the deposited proteins (Figs. 1 and 2). Computed tomography (CT) may be helpful in some cases.

On CT, the blood supply is reduced; hence, the mucosa is thickened and the center of the lesion may appear as a low-density area (Fig. 4) [4].

Treatment depends on the underlying cause and type of protein. Chemotherapy and stem cell transplantation are useful for AL amyloidosis. As for SAA amyloidosis, it is important to correct the underlying disease. Prokinetic agents can be useful in patients with nausea and dysmotility symptoms. In case of severe diarrhea and protein-losing enteropathy, octreotide, corticosteroid, loperamide, and opiate may be helpful. Furthermore, antibiotics for small intestinal bacterial overgrowth may be a therapeutic option for severe diarrhea, and surgical resection for a localized disease may be considered.

Conclusion

Because small bowel amyloidosis is a rare disease and may have nonspecific symptoms, there is no way to make a quick diagnosis, except when the treating doctor suspects the disease. As nonspecific mucosal changes alone can be observed on endoscopy, an aggressive biopsy may aid in diagnosing amyloidosis in case of suspicious endoscopic findings.

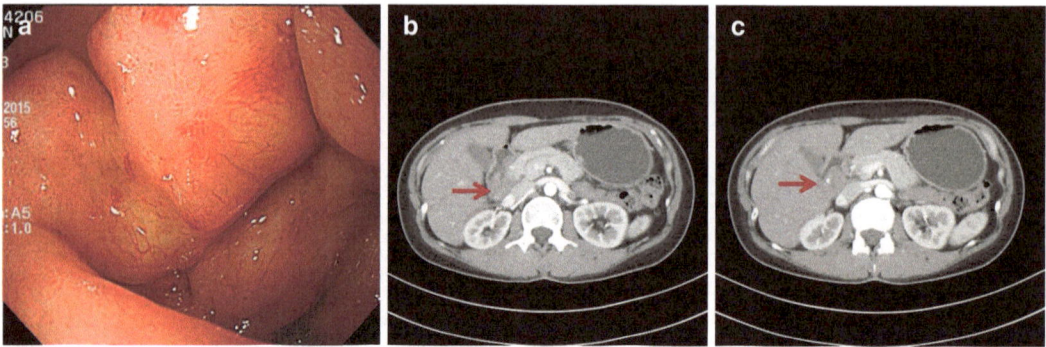

Fig. 4 A 46-year-old female patient. (**a**) Luminal narrowing due to elevated mucosal change was observed. (**b, c**) Low-attenuation polypoid lesion with calcification was detected on CT scan

References

1. Bansal R, Syed U, Walfish J, Aron J, Walfish A. Small bowel amyloidosis. Curr Gastroenterol Rep. 2018;20:11.
2. Hokama A, Kishimoto K, Nakamoto M, et al. Endoscopic and histopathological features of gastrointestinal amyloidosis. World J Gastrointest Endosc. 2011;3:157–61.
3. Lim AY, Lee JH, Jung KS, et al. Clinical features and outcomes of systemic amyloidosis with gastrointestinal involvement: a single-center experience. Korean J Intern Med. 2015;30:496–505.
4. Kala Z, Valek V, Kysela P. Amyloidosis of the small intestine. Eur J Radiol. 2007;63:105–9.

Small-bowel Involvement of Connective Tissue Diseases

Byoung Wook Bang

Key Points
- Small-bowel involvement of connective tissue diseases is rarely seen in systemic sclerosis, systemic lupus erythematosus, Henoch–Schönlein purpura, inflammatory myopathy, mixed connective tissue disease, and rheumatoid arthritis, and is known to involve a variety of etiologies.
- The major causes include (i) excessive accumulation of collagen; (ii) gastrointestinal motility disorder caused by muscle atrophy; and (iii) mucosal erosion, ulcer, and small-bowel ischemia caused by vasculitis.

Involvements of connective tissue diseases (CTDs) are not common in clinical practice, and most of the symptoms are non-specific and often overlooked. In the case of gastrointestinal (GI) anomalies associated with CTD, three etiologies can be considered. First, excessive accumulation of collagen in the submucosal tissue of the intestine, bowel wall fibrosis, and muscle atrophy can lead to GI motility disorders. Second, arteritis or vasculitis may involve the small intestine. In this case, mucosal erosion and ulceration may occur, and, although rare, small-intestinal ischemia or necrosis occurs depending on the size of the affected blood vessels (Table 1). Finally, even if CTD does not directly involve the GI tract, GI symptoms caused by non-steroidal anti-inflammatory drugs (NSAIDs) or steroids used for the treatment of CTD may develop. GI involvement due to collagen accumulation occurs mainly in scleroderma and dermatomyositis, whereas vasculitis-induced GI disturbances may occur in systemic lupus erythematosus (SLE), rheumatoid arthritis, and polyarteritis nodosa. It is not uncommon for those two causes to overlap (Table 2).

Systemic Sclerosis (SSc)

SSc is an autoimmune disease characterized by systemic inflammation, microangiopathy, and fibrosis. The main symptom is progressive dermatofibrosis; however, it also involves the internal organs, and the GI tract is the most frequently affected organ after the skin. SSc can be divided into two types: limited cutaneous SSc, in which vascular involvement is predominant, and diffuse cutaneous SSc, in which collagen accumulation is predominant. Both types can involve the GI tract, and the extent of skin lesions and GI involvement may not match. The small intestine is the second most commonly affected digestive organ after the esophagus, and 40% of patients

B. W. Bang (✉)
Inha University College of Medicine,
Incheon, South Korea

Table 1 Small-intestinal involvement associated with vasculitis

Vasculitis	Characteristics	Symptoms
Large-vessel vasculitis		
Takayasu arteritis	Small-bowel ischemia (rare)	
Giant-cell arteritis	Mesenteric arteritis (rare)	Abdominal pain
Middle-vessel vasculitis		
Polyarteritis nodosa	Mesenteric vasculitis or necrosis associated with hepatitis B	Nausea, vomiting, hematochezia, melena
Small-vessel vasculitis		
ANCA-associated vasculitis 1) Microscopic polyangiitis. 2) Granulomatosis polyangiitis 3) Eosinophilic granulomatosis with polyangiitis	Mucosal ulcer, bowel ischemia, infarction, perforation, bowel obstruction	
IgA vasculitis (Henoch–Schönlein purpura)	Mucosal purpura with gastrointestinal bleeding	Abdominal pain, vomiting, GI bleeding
Cryoglobulinemic vasculitis	Bowel ischemia associated with hepatitis C	
Behcet's disease	Ileal and cecal ulcer	Abdominal pain, GI bleeding
Vasculitis associated with systemic disease		
Rheumatoid vasculitis	Mesenteric vasculitis/ischemia	
Lupus vasculitis		

ANCA anti-neutrophil cytoplasmic antibody; *IgA* immunoglobulin A; *GI* gastrointestinal

Table 2 Representative small-bowel diseases according to connective tissue disease

Connective tissue disease	Small-bowel disease
Systemic sclerosis	Bowel movement disorder, chronic pseudo-obstruction, small-bowel bacterial overgrowth
Systemic lupus erythematosus	Mesenteric vasculitis, chronic pseudo-obstruction, protein-losing enteropathy
Henoch–Schönlein purpura	Hemorrhagic enteritis
Inflammatory myopathy	Pneumatosis cystoides, bowel movement disorder, chronic pseudo-obstruction, celiac disease
Mixed connective tissue disease	Vasculitis, vascular ischemia
Rheumatoid arthritis	Rheumatoid vasculitis, celiac disease, amyloidosis associated with inflammatory bowel disease

have been reported to show decreased GI motility [1, 2]. The mechanism of small-intestinal involvement is not clear; however, it is known that vascular damage, excessive accumulation of collagen, and abnormal immune response are involved [2]. In the early stages, there are no symptoms. As the disease progresses, GI motility deteriorates, causing abdominal distension, vomiting, abdominal pain, and diarrhea. Further progression of the disease may result in pseudo-obstruction or small-bowel bacterial overgrowth, which is a major cause of malabsorption. The findings of small-bowel follow-through include reduced peristalsis, dilated bowel, and prominent small-bowel folds (hidebound bowel sign). Abdominal computed tomography (CT) also shows a dilated small bowel and pseudo-obstruction, similar to that in small-bowel follow-through (Fig. 1). Treatment with metronidazole (500 mg twice a day) or ciprofloxacin (500 mg twice a day) can be applied for 2–4 weeks if small-bowel bacterial overgrowth occurs. Involvement of the GI tract in SSc is not as fatal as other organ involvements but has a large influence on the quality of life.

SLE

SLE is an autoimmune disease that affects the systemic organs in relation to the production of autoantibodies. Digestive symptoms are com-

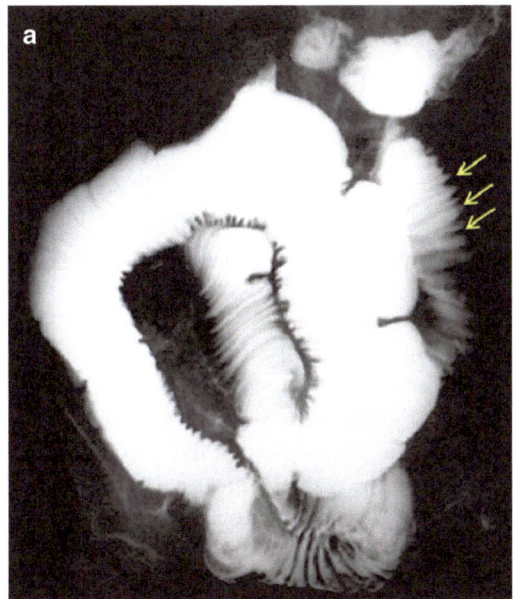
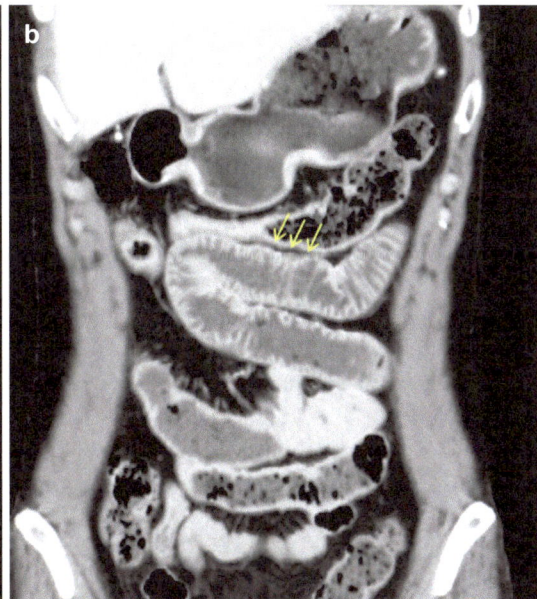

Fig. 1 (**a**) Small-bowel follow-through image showing a dilated, atonic small bowel and closely spaced, thin transverse folds (**b**) Abdominal computed tomography scan showing diffuse wall thickening and dilated proximal jejunum, which are classic features of scleroderma with pseudo-obstruction.

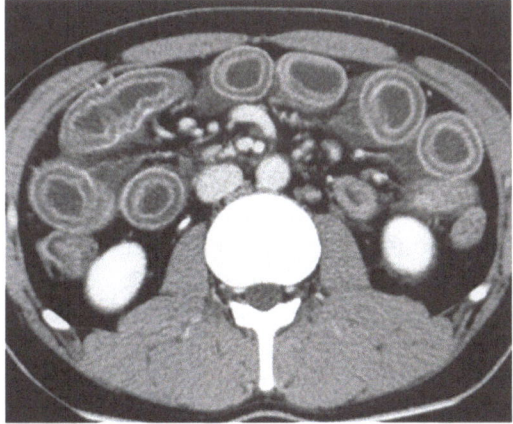

Fig. 2 Abdominal computed tomography scan with intravenous contrast demonstrating diffuse bowel thickening with wall enhancement, appearing as a "target" sign

monly observed in 25–40% of patients with SLE. Most of the digestive symptoms can be due to vasculitis or complications caused by therapeutic drugs. The small-bowel diseases associated with SLE are enumerated below.

1. *Mesenteric vasculitis*

   Mesenteric vasculitis is a life-threatening SLE complication that causes ischemic changes in the mesenteric artery due to vasculitis, leading to GI symptoms such as postprandial abdominal pain, food aversion, weight loss, vomiting, and diarrhea. It usually affects the small and large intestines, especially in the distal ileum and cecum. In the case of mesenteric thrombosis or infarct, it can lead to acute abdominal pain due to intestinal perforation and peritonitis. The diagnosis is based on abdominal CT findings, including (i) thickening of the wall, (ii) appearance of a "target" sign, (iii) dilatation of the bowel segment, and (iv) mesenteric fat infiltration (Fig. 2). Patients with mesenteric vasculitis without perforation can be administered high-dose steroids and may be considered for immunosuppressant therapy.

2. *Protein-losing enteropathy*

   SLE rarely causes protein-losing enteropathy, characterized by severe diarrhea and hypoalbuminemia without proteinuria. In these patients, villous atrophy and submucosal edema accompanied by inflammatory cell infiltration are observed in histologic findings. Protein-losing enteropathy occurs especially in patients with severe SLE with multiple-organ involvement.

3. *Pseudo-obstruction*

Pseudo-obstruction may be suspected when patients with SLE complain of abdominal pain or abdominal distension. Pseudo-obstruction is a rare complication of SLE, which manifests as signs and symptoms of mechanical obstruction in the small and large intestines, without anatomical obstruction. Most cases occur in patients with active SLE, although it may occur at the onset of the disease and may appear as acute, recurrent, or chronic. The etiology of SLE-related pseudo-obstruction is unknown; however, it may be due to immune complex deposition in smooth muscle cells, chronic ischemia due to vasculitis, and decreased GI motility. Radiologic examination shows dilated bowel and decreased intestinal motility. Treatment with high-dose steroids or immunosuppressive agents to control SLE itself, in addition to nutritional support and prokinetics, can be used.

Henoch–Schönlein Purpura (HSP)

HSP is a systemic leukocytoclastic vasculitis syndrome associated with abdominal pain, hematuria, arthritis, and purpura in the hips and legs [3]. The mechanism by which HSP involves the digestive system is related to the deposition of immunoglobulin A complex on the small blood vessel wall and the infiltration of leukocytes into the blood vessel periphery. This causes submucosal bleeding and edema, resulting in abdominal pain. GI symptoms are typically reported to occur from the eighth day after the onset of purpura, although they occasionally occur weeks to months after the onset of purpura. It has been reported that 15–35% of cases may have GI symptoms before the onset of purpura and that cases with GI symptoms without purpura may be difficult to diagnose. Therefore, endoscopy is necessary if there is abdominal pain, hematemesis, or melena, regardless of the skin lesion. Mucosal lesions may occur anywhere in the GI tract; however, the small intestine is the most frequent site. In the small intestine, mucosal hyperemia, hemorrhagic erosion, and small ring-shaped lesions are observed. The most characteristic findings are severe hemorrhagic and erosive duodenitis (Fig. 3) [4]. Although most cases can be diagnosed with upper endoscopy and colonoscopy, capsule endoscopy is the best diagnostic method that allows a good view of the small-intestinal lesions of HSP. The CT findings are non-specific but can reveal intestinal wall thickening, lymphadenopathy, and mesenteric edema. Although most HSPs spontaneously resolve, steroid therapy has been reported to help improve HSP-related digestive symptoms [5]. Other complications of HSP include small-intestinal perforation, intussusception, ischemic vasculitis, or protein-losing enteropathy.

Inflammatory Myopathies

Inflammatory myopathy is an autoimmune disease that causes muscle weakness. It is divided into polymyositis and dermatomyositis. Polymyositis is a disease that affects the proximal muscles and causes muscle weakness. Dermatomyositis is a condition accompanied by characteristic skin lesions in the face, hand, and trunk, with symptoms of myositis. With respect to small-intestinal involvement, vasculitis or ischemia due to thrombosis (resulting in abdominal pain, vomiting, and melena) and, in severe cases, perforation may occur. Very rarely, inflammatory myopathy causes pseudo-obstruction. In small-bowel follow-through, inflammatory myopathy mainly affects the duodenum and jejunum. Moreover, the intestine is dilated and shows segmental intestinal obstruction, which is distinguishable from the intestinal involvement of SSc. In addition, inflammatory myopathy is reported to be associated with pneumatosis cystoides and celiac disease [6].

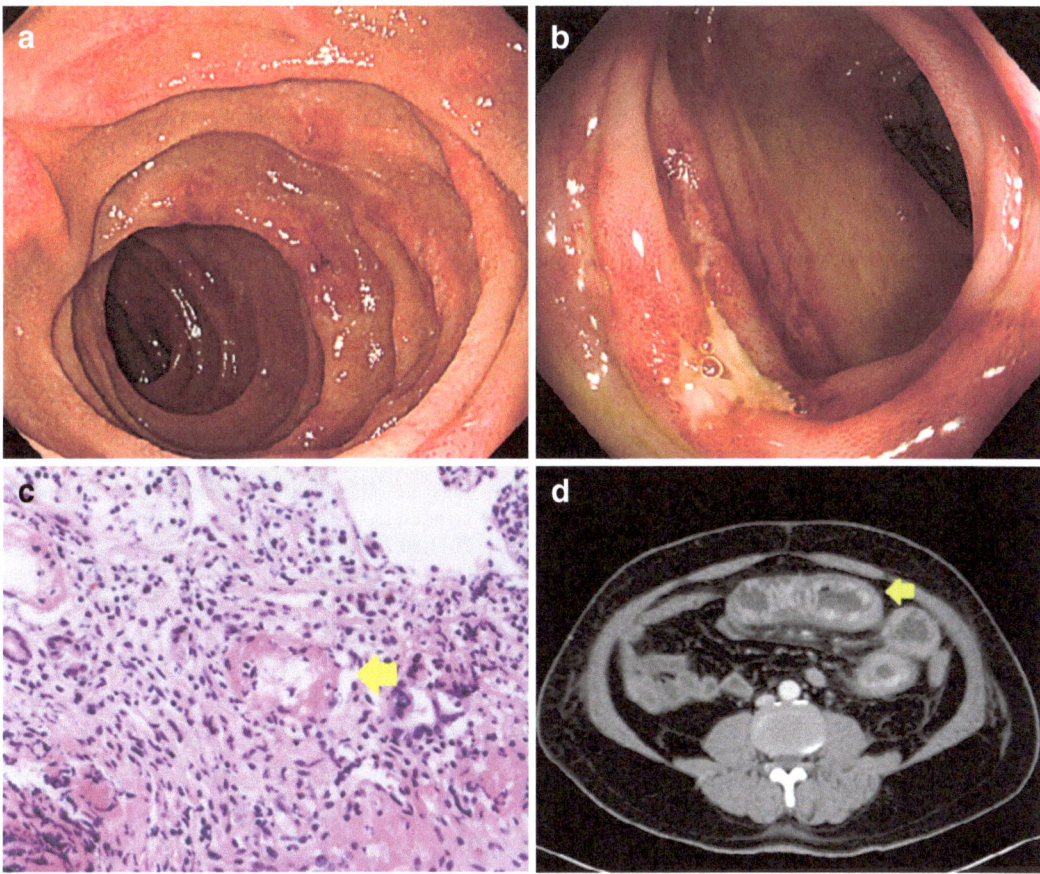

Fig. 3 (**a**, **b**) Endoscopic images showing multiple hemorrhagic erosions and patches in the duodenum (**a**) and terminal ileum (**b**). (**c**) Histologic image showing mucosal erosion and hemorrhage due to leukocytoclastic vasculi-tis, consistent with the involvement of Henoch–Schönlein purpura. (**d**) Abdominal computed tomography scan showing non-specific small-bowel edema and dilatation

Mixed CTD (MCTD)

MCTD is diagnosed when the clinical manifestations of various CTDs, such as SLE, multiple myositis, SSc, and rheumatoid arthritis, overlap and anti-U1-RNP antibody shows a high titer in the serum. The main mechanism of GI involvement of MCTD is vasculitis, which may result in various clinical symptoms depending on the size of the involved blood vessels. When a large vessel is involved, ischemia, infarction, or bleeding occurs, whereas small-vessel involvement causes inflammation or capillary hemorrhage. As the disease progresses, it may lead to intestinal obstruction or thrombosis [7].

Rheumatoid Arthritis

Rheumatoid arthritis is an autoimmune chronic inflammatory disease characterized by multiple arthritis. Initially, the synovial membrane surrounding the joint is inflamed. When it progresses, it causes joint destruction and deformation. Approximately 1–5% of patients with rheumatoid arthritis develop rheumatic vasculitis, which shows GI involvement in 10–38% of the cases [8]. Abdominal pain is the most common symptom of rheumatic vasculitis due to GI involvement, and other symptoms such as vomiting, nausea, and melena are present. Although very rare, severe cases can also lead to bowel ischemia, infarction, and perforation. Although there is no established treatment, the combination therapy of cyclophosphamide and steroid is the most commonly used [9]. However, symptoms due to rheumatoid arthritis or related GI tract involvement are very rare, and most GI symptoms of patients with rheumatoid arthritis are caused by adverse effects of most therapeutic agents, including NSAIDs, steroids, immunosuppressants, and various biological agents [9].

References

1. Savarino E, Furnari M, de Bortoli N, et al. Gastrointestinal involvement in systemic sclerosis. Presse Med. 2014;43:e279–91.
2. Tian XP, Zhang X. Gastrointestinal complications of systemic sclerosis. World J Gastroenterol. 2013;19:7062–8.
3. Park SH, Lee MH, Kim HS, et al. A case of henoch-schoenlein purpura involving GI tract. Korean Journal of Gastrointestinal Endoscopy. 1996;16:94–101.
4. Esaki M, Matsumoto T, Nakamura S, et al. GI involvement in henoch-schönlein purpura. Gastrointest Endosc. 2002;56:920–3.
5. Ronkainen J, Koskimies O, Ala-Houhala M, et al. Early prednisone therapy in henoch-schonlein purpura: A randomized, double-blind, placebo-controlled trial. J Pediatr. 2006;149:241–7.
6. Gadiparthi C, Hans A, Potts K, Ismail MK. Gastrointestinal and hepatic disease in the inflammatory myopathies. Rheum Dis Clin N Am. 2018;44:113–29.
7. Li M, Luo W, Li P, Luo J, Huo J, Li Y. Connective tissue disease-induced gastrointestinal vasculitis: A clinical analysis of 14 cases. Int J Clin Exp Pathol. 2016;9:2091–8.
8. Ebert EC, Hagspiel KD. Gastrointestinal and hepatic manifestations of rheumatoid arthritis. Dig Dis Sci 2011;56:295–302.
9. Craig E, Cappelli LC. Gastrointestinal and hepatic disease in rheumatoid arthritis. Rheum Dis Clin. 2018;44:89–111.

Celiac Disease

Soon Man Yoon

Key Points
- Celiac disease is a gluten-induced immune-mediated enteropathy.
- Celiac disease has a worldwide distribution and an increasing incidence.
- Celiac disease is characterized by abnormal small-intestine histopathology and clinical improvement after a gluten-free diet.

Introduction

Celiac disease is a chronic immune-mediated enteropathy of the small intestine that is triggered by the ingestion of gluten in genetically susceptible individuals [1]. Although celiac disease was originally considered largely a disease of Caucasians, recent observations have established that it has a worldwide distribution and that its incidence has increased [2]. Celiac disease has had several other names, including celiac sprue, gluten-sensitive enteropathy, nontropical sprue, celiac syndrome, and adult celiac disease [1]. The etiology of celiac disease is not known; however, environmental, genetic, and immunologic factors seem to contribute to the disease [1–3]. Celiac disease is characterized by villus atrophy of the small-intestinal mucosa associated with malabsorption of nutrients, which shows prompt clinical and subsequent histologic improvement after the elimination of gluten from the diet [2].

Epidemiology

Epidemiologic studies using specific celiac serology testing have indicated that celiac disease has a wide geographic distribution and affects individuals from multiple and diverse ethnic and racial backgrounds [1–3]. The overall prevalence of celiac disease in Europe has been estimated to be 1%, and a female predominance has been noted [1, 3]. Globally, the prevalence of celiac disease is increasing. Recently, there have been several reports of celiac disease cases in Asia including Korea [4].

Pathogenesis

1. *Environmental factors*

    With respect to environmental factors, there is a clear association of celiac disease with gliadin, a component of gluten that is present in wheat, barley, and rye. Gliadin peptides interact with gliadin-specific T cells that mediate tissue injury and induce the release of

S. M. Yoon (✉)
Department of Gastroenterology, Chungbuk National University College of Medicine,
Cheongju-si, South Korea
e-mail: smyoon@chungbuk.ac.kr

© Springer Nature Singapore Pte Ltd. 2022
H. J. Chun et al. (eds.), *Small Intestine Disease*, https://doi.org/10.1007/978-981-16-7239-2_51

one or more cytokines (e.g., interferon γ) that cause tissue injury [1–3].

2. *Genetic factors*

Family studies have demonstrated the frequent intrafamilial occurrence of celiac disease and a high concordance in first-degree relatives of patients with celiac disease (range 8–18%). More than 90% of patients with celiac disease express the HLA-DQ2 allele; most of the others express the HLA-DQ8 allele, and a minority of the patients are DQ2/DQ8 positive [1–3].

3. *Immunologic factors*

Serum anti-tissue transglutaminase (tTG) antibody, anti-endomysium antibody, and anti-gliadin antibody are specifically present in untreated celiac disease patients. The sensitivity and specificity of anti-endomysial antibody are 90–95% in patients with celiac disease [1–3].

Symptoms

Celiac disease exhibits a wide spectrum of clinical presentations, from signs and symptoms of malabsorption such as diarrhea, steatorrhea, abdominal discomfort, weight loss, and the consequences of nutrient depletion (i.e., anemia and metabolic bone disease) to the total absence of gastrointestinal symptoms despite evidence of depletion of a single nutrient (e.g., iron or folate deficiency, osteomalacia, edema from protein loss) [1, 2, 5]. The onset of symptoms can occur at any time from the first year of life through adulthood. A large number of patients are essentially asymptomatic despite abnormal small-intestinal histopathology and serologies [1, 2]. The symptoms of celiac disease may appear with the introduction of cereals into an infant's diet, although spontaneous remissions often occur during the second decade of life, which may be either permanent or followed by the reappearance of symptoms over several years [2]. Alternatively, the symptoms of celiac disease may first become evident at almost any age throughout adulthood. In many patients, frequent spontaneous remissions and exacerbations occur [2].

Diagnosis

The diagnosis of celiac disease requires the detection of characteristic histologic changes on small-intestinal biopsy together with a prompt clinical and histologic response after the institution of a gluten-free diet [1, 2]. A biopsy should be performed when patients have symptoms and laboratory findings suggestive of nutrient malabsorption and/or deficiency as well as a positive tTG antibody test. As the presentation of celiac disease is often subtle, without overt evidence of malabsorption or nutrient deficiency, a relatively low threshold for biopsy performance is important [1, 2, 3]. Multiple biopsies should be accomplished (e.g., a total of six to eight biopsies from the second and third portions of the duodenum). Although the endoscopic features of celiac disease often appear normal, scalloping or absence and flattening of duodenal folds, multiple fissures, or a mosaic-like appearance have been noted in some patients with celiac disease. However, these findings are not specific to celiac disease [1]. The classic changes seen on duodenal/jejunal biopsy are restricted to the mucosa and include (i) an increase in the number of intraepithelial lymphocytes; (ii) absence or a reduced height of villi, which causes a flat appearance with increased crypt cell proliferation resulting in crypt hyperplasia and loss of villous structure, with consequent villous, but not mucosal, atrophy; (iii) a cuboidal appearance and nuclei that are no longer oriented basally in surface epithelial cells; and (iv) increased numbers of lymphocytes and plasma cells in the lamina propria [1, 2]. Although these features are characteristic of celiac disease, they are not diagnostic because a similar appearance can be observed in tropical sprue, eosinophilic enteritis, milk-protein intolerance, lymphoma, bacterial overgrowth, Crohn's disease, and gastrinoma with acid hypersecretion. However, the characteristic histologic appearance that reverts to normal after the initiation of a gluten-free diet establishes the diagnosis of celiac disease [2].

Treatment

Removal of gluten from the diet is essential for treating patients with celiac disease [1–3]. More than 90% of patients who have the characteristic findings of celiac disease respond to complete dietary gluten restriction. The most common cause of persistent symptoms in a patient is a continued intake of gluten [2]. As gluten is ubiquitous, significant effort must be made to exclude all gluten from the diet [1–3]. Other therapeutic approaches include the use of systemic glucocorticoids. Moreover, peptidases that can inactivate toxic gliadin peptides and small molecules that can block toxic peptide uptake across intestinal tight junctions are being developed [1–3].

Prognosis

Celiac disease has an excellent prognosis if diagnosed early and if the patient will adhere to a lifelong gluten-free diet. Conversely, if it is not recognized and properly treated, patients can develop marked malnutrition and complications including infection and malignancy such as lymphoma [1].

References

1. Feldman M, Friedman LS, Brandt LJ. Sleisenger and Fordtran's gastrointestinal and liver disease: pathophysiology, diagnosis, management. 10th ed. Saunders-Elsevier; 2016.
2. Jameson JL, Fauci AS, Kasper DL, Hauser SL, Longo DL, Loscalzo J. Harrison's principles of internal medicine. 20th ed. McGraw-Hill; 2018.
3. Lebwohl B, Sanders DS, Green PHR. Coeliac disease. Lancet. 2018;391:70–81.
4. Ham H, Lee BI, Oh HJ, et al. A case of celiac disease with neurologic manifestations misdiagnosed as amyotrophic lateral sclerosis. Intest Res. 2017;15:540–2.
5. Leonard MM, Sapone A, Catassi C, Fasano A. Celiac disease and nonceliac gluten sensitivity: a review. JAMA. 2017;318:647–56.

Small-Bowel Behcet's Disease

Yehyun Park and Jae Hee Cheon

Key Points

- When to suspect intestinal Behcet's disease (BD): Intestinal BD is suspected if ulcerative lesions in the gastrointestinal tract are present in patients with systemic BD, characterized by recurrent oral ulcers, genital ulcers, uveitis, and skin lesions, or a single or a few deep round to oval ulcers with discrete margins in the ileocecal area.
- Involved sites: Involvement of the ileocecal region is common, but all digestive organs from the mouth to the anus can be affected. Erythema, erosions, and ulcers can be observed in the small intestine.
- Symptoms: Abdominal pain, diarrhea, hematochezia, vomiting, changes in bowel habits, weight loss, fever, and abdominal mass may be present.
- Diagnostic tests: Colonoscopy, upper gastrointestinal endoscopy, capsule endoscopy, computed tomography enterography, blood test, and stool test can be performed.
- Differential diagnosis: The differential diagnoses include Crohn's disease, intestinal tuberculosis, drug-induced enteritis, cytomegaloviral enteritis, amoebiasis, and *Salmonella* enteritis.
- Disease course: It has a chronic recurrent disease course. Complications may include massive bleeding, fistula, perforation, and intestinal obstruction, which may need surgery.
- Treatment: The treatment, which may include 5-aminosalicylic acid, steroids, immunomodulators, biological agents, colchicine, thalidomide, and surgery, is determined by the clinical severity of the disease.

Introduction

Behcet's disease (BD) is a chronic recurrent inflammatory disease involving multiple organs, characterized by oral ulcers, genital ulcers, uveitis, and skin lesions.

If there is a typical ulcerative lesion in the gastrointestinal tract in patients with BD, it is defined as intestinal BD. The incidence of intestinal involvement in patients with BD is reported to vary from 0% to 35%, and it is known that the prevalence is high in East Asia including Korea

Y. Park · J. H. Cheon (✉)
Department of Internal Medicine, Institute of Gastroenterology, Yonsei University College of Medicine, Seoul, South Korea
e-mail: geniushee@yuhs.ac

and Japan. In general, the presence of bowel involvement in patients with BD is associated with a poor prognosis.

The genetic factors of BD are known to be related to the *human leukocyte antigen (HLA)-B*51* allele and *major histocompatibility complex (MHC) class I related gene A. Interleukin (IL)-10, IL-23R,* and *IL-12RB2* gene mutations have also been associated with BD. However, genetic factors associated with the development of intestinal BD are still being studied.

Clinical Presentation

The clinical manifestations of intestinal BD are diverse, ranging from mild abdominal discomfort to severe abdominal pain, hematochezia or melena, fistulas, and perforations. The most common symptom is abdominal pain in about 90%. Especially, right lower quadrant pain and rebound pain can be present, and diarrhea, bloody stool, vomiting, change in bowel habit, weight loss, fever, or abdominal mass can occur as accompanying symptoms. Generally, gastrointestinal symptoms occur 4.5–6 years after the appearance of oral ulcers; however, in some patients, intestinal lesions precede extraintestinal symptoms [1].

Intestinal BD most commonly involves the ileocecal area; however, it can involve all digestive organs, from the mouth to the anus, similar to Crohn's disease. However, anorectal involvement in intestinal BD is rare unlike in Crohn's disease. Although small-intestinal involvement in intestinal BD is known to be less common than in Crohn's disease, recent studies on small-intestinal involvement evaluated using capsule endoscopy have shown that various lesions, such as erythema, erosions, and ulcers, can occur in the small intestine, and erythema can be seen in >90% of patients [2].

When patients with intestinal BD were followed up for 5 years, most (71.6%) had mildly active disease, whereas the rest (28.4%) had multiple recurrences or chronic symptoms. Intestinal BD may require surgery because of massive hemorrhage, fistula, perforation, and intestinal obstruction, and the cumulative operation rate is reported to be approximately 30% at 5 years and 40% at 10 years. The recurrence rate after surgery was reported to be 50–70% at 5 years [3].

Diagnostic Evaluation

Blood Tests

Blood tests may show leukocytosis, elevated erythrocyte sedimentation rate or C-reactive protein levels, anemia (iron deficiency), thrombocytosis, and hypoalbuminemia. Although the specific serologic markers, like in Crohn's disease and ulcerative colitis, have not yet been identified, the presence of the *HLA-B*51* allele in the blood can be detected.

In a recent genome-wide association study, *HLA-B*51* was identified in 59.1% of the BD group and in 29.3% of the control group (odds ratio, 3.49) [4].

Endoscopy

The characteristic endoscopic findings of intestinal BD are mainly a single or a few large round or ovoid deep ulcers that are confined to the ileocecal region. The margin of the ulcer is elevated; the boundary with the surrounding normal mucosa is clear, and the base of the ulcer is covered with whitish exudate. However, various lesions can be found, from small aphthous ulcers to multiple irregularly shaped ulcers. The characteristics of ulcers observed in intestinal BD can be divided into the typical and atypical types (Table 1, Fig. 1).

Table 1 Characteristics of ulcers in intestinal Behcet's disease

Typical ulcers
1. Single or a few large ulcers in the ileocecal area.
2. Round or ovoid deep ulcers.
3. Ulcers with discrete and elevated margins.
4. Ulcer base covered with exudate.
Atypical ulcers
1. Aphthous or geographic ulcers.
2. Multiple segmental or diffuse ulcers.

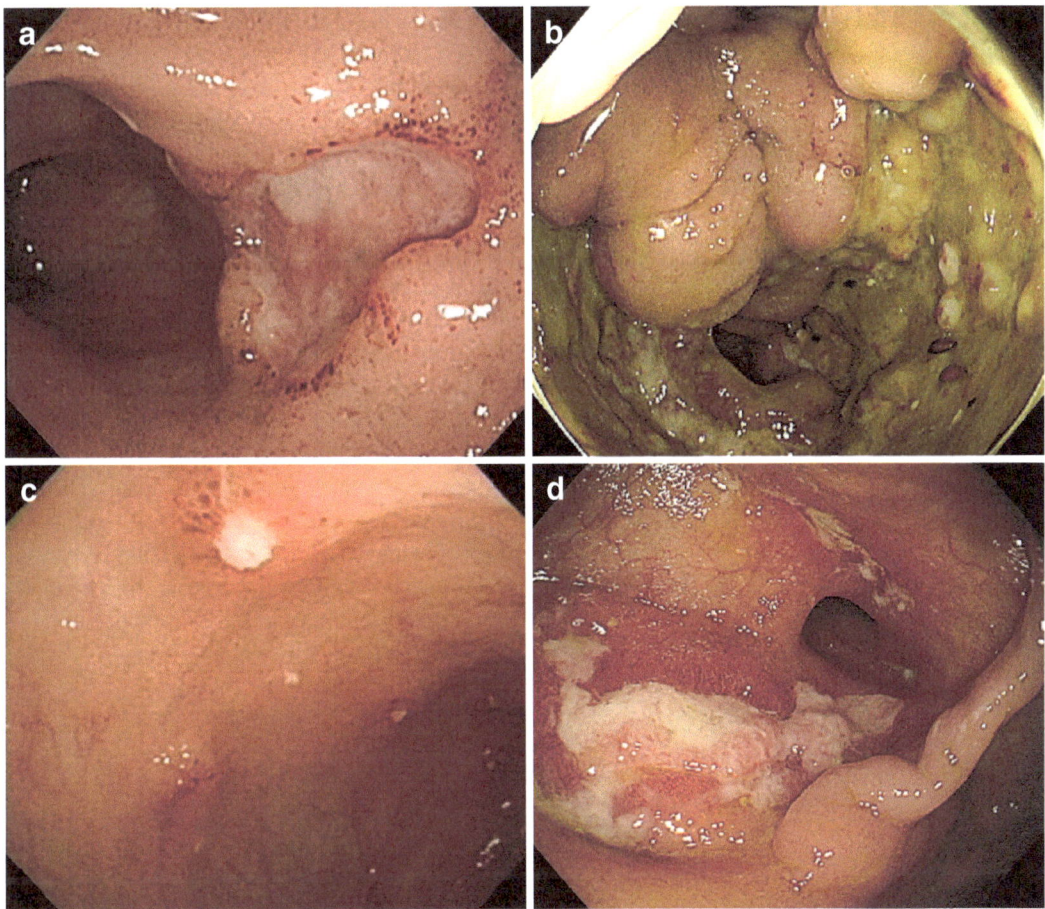

Fig. 1 Ileocecal ulcer in intestinal Behcet's disease. (**a, b**) Typical ulcer. (**c, d**) Atypical ulcer

Imaging

The small-bowel series of intestinal BD shows single or multiple discrete ulcers in the terminal ileum, with enlarged mucosal folds, deformity, and stenosis. The capsule endoscopic findings vary from non-specific erythema to erosions and ulcers. The findings of computed tomography (CT) enterography include large and deep penetrating ulcers with bowel wall thickening, mural hyperenhancement, and surrounding mesenteric infiltration. Occasionally, intestinal BD mani-

fests as a cecal mass or an aneurysmal dilatation of the terminal ileum [5].

Histopathology

Histologically, leukocyte or lymphocyte infiltration is accompanied by perivascular inflammation, but typical findings are observed in <50% of cases. Further, biopsy specimens often show nonspecific inflammatory findings.

Diagnosis and Differential Diagnosis

Diagnosis

The diagnosis of intestinal BD is based on the combination of clinical features, endoscopic findings, biopsy, and imaging. If a diagnosis is made or intestinal BD is suspected on the basis of colonoscopy and biopsy findings, the tests shown in Table 2 are performed. Upper gastrointestinal endoscopy can be performed to detect the presence of esophageal or gastric invasion, and small-bowel series, capsule endoscopy, or CT enterography is performed to determine the presence of small-intestinal involvement [6].

The diagnostic algorithm for intestinal BD based on endoscopic findings and systemic symptoms using the modified Delphi approach is shown in Figure 2 [7].

According to the diagnostic criteria, in the presence of a diagnosis of systemic BD and a typical ulcer on endoscopy, a definite diagnosis of intestinal BD (confirmed type) can be made. If there is an atypical ulcer in patients with systemic BD, or there is a typical ulcer in patients with oral ulcers or other symptoms of systemic BD but do not satisfy the diagnostic criteria for systemic BD, it is classified as the probable type. If a typical ulcer is present but there are no systemic symptoms, it is classified as the suspicious type. In this algorithm, the diagnostic criteria for systemic BD established by the Japanese Society for Behcet's Disease Study in 1987 were used. Probable and suspicious cases should be periodically checked against the criteria for a definitive diagnosis through a careful follow-up.

Table 2 Diagnostic workup for intestinal Behcet's disease

Colonoscopy
Upper gastrointestinal endoscopy
Small-bowel series, capsule endoscopy, CT enterography
Blood test (whole blood, routine chemistry, ESR, CRP)
Stool study (parasites, stool WBCs, bacteria, calprotectin, etc.)
Dermatologic (including pathergy test), ophthalmologic, neurologic, and rheumatologic evaluation

CT computed tomography; *ESR* erythrocyte sedimentation rate; *CRP* C-reactive protein; *WBCs* white blood cells

Differential Diagnosis

The differential diagnoses of intestinal BD include Crohn's disease, intestinal tuberculosis, drug-induced enteritis, cytomegaloviral enteritis, amoebiasis, and *Salmonella* enteritis, among which the differential diagnosis of Crohn's disease is especially important in clinical practice (Table 3). Crohn's disease has a segmental or diffuse distribution, but intestinal BD is mostly localized in the ileocecal area. The appearance of ulcers in Crohn's disease is predominantly irregular or longitudinal;

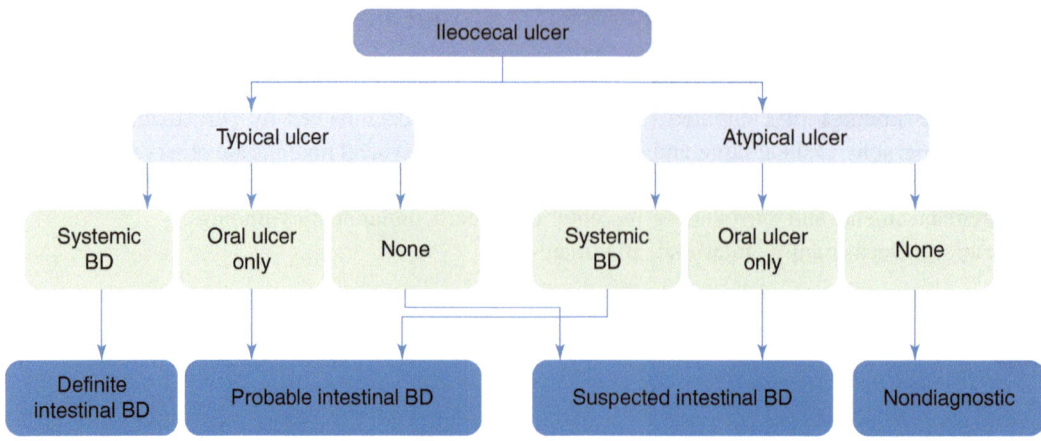

Fig. 2 Diagnostic algorithm for intestinal Behcet's disease

Table 3 Differential diagnosis between Crohn's disease and intestinal Behcet's disease

	Crohn's disease	Intestinal BD
Extraintestinal manifestation	Iritis, episcleritis	Oral and genital ulcer, papule and pustule, nerve and arterial involvement
Anal lesion (fissure, fistula)	Common	Rare
Stenosis, fistula, abscess	More common	Less common
ASCA positivity	41–76%	0–44.3%
Endoscopic finding	Irregular longitudinal ulcer, cobblestone appearance, aphthous ulcer	Round to oval shape, > 1 cm, localized, < 5 ulcers
Histopathology	Non-caseating granuloma (15–36%)	Perivasculitis with neutrophil and lymphocyte infiltration

BD Behcet's disease; *ASCA* anti-*Saccharomyces cerevisiae* antibody

however, in intestinal BD, ulcers are often round or oval, deep, and well defined. In a study comparing the colonoscopy findings of intestinal BD with those of Crohn's disease, it was found that a circular ulcer, fewer than five lesions, local distribution, and absence of aphthous ulcer or a cobblestone appearance suggest intestinal BD more than Crohn's disease. Thereby, differentiation between intestinal BD and Crohn's disease was possible in 92% of the cases [8].

Assessment of Disease Activity

Because intestinal BD has a variable clinical course with repeated relapse and remission, the clinical disease activity should be periodically assessed. The disease activity index for intestinal BD (DAIBD) can be used (Table 4) [9]. It has eight items in total, scored from 0 to 325, in which DAIBD ≤19 is classified as remission, 20 to <40 as mild, 40 to <75 as moderate, and ≥75 as severe.

Table 4 Disease activity index for intestinal Behcet's disease

Contents		Score
General Well-being	Well	0
	Fair	10
	Poor	20
	Very poor	30
	Terrible	40
Fever	< 38 °C	0
	≥ 38 °C	10
Extraintestinal manifestations	Oral ulcer, genital ulcer, eye lesion, skin lesion, or arthralgia	5 per item
	Vascular involvement or central nervous system involvement	15 per item
Abdominal pain in 1 week	None	0
	Mild	20
	Moderate	40
	Severe	80
Abdominal mass	None	0
	Palpable mass	10
Abdominal tenderness	None	0
	Mildly tender	10
	Moderately or severely tender	20
Intestinal complications	Fistula, perforation, abscess, or intestinal obstruction	10 per item
No. of liquid stools in 1 week	0	0
	1–7	10
	8–21	20
	22–35	30
	≥ 36	40

Treatment

There is no standard treatment based on a well-designed randomized controlled study of intestinal BD. The use of 5-aminosalicylic acid (5-ASA), steroids, immunomodulators, biological agents, colchicine, thalidomide, and surgery is determined according to the clinical severity of the disease. The treatment algorithm for intestinal BD is shown in Figure 3 [10].

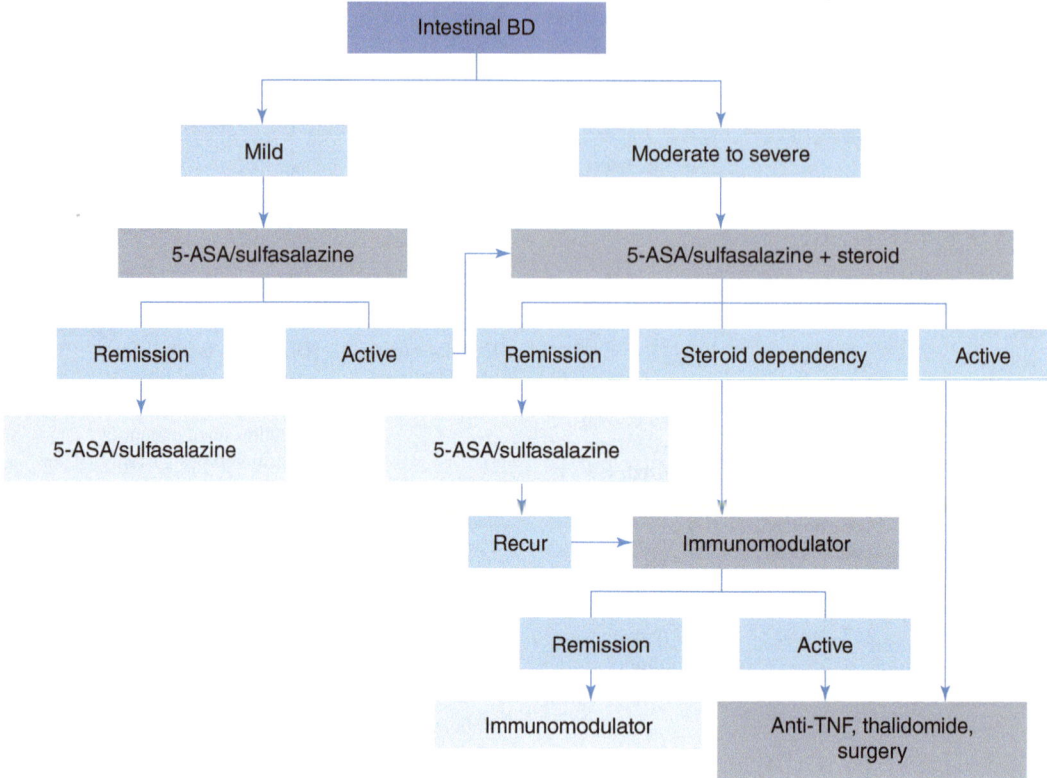

Fig. 3 Treatment algorithm for intestinal Behcet's disease

Conclusion

BD is a chronic recurrent inflammatory disease of the whole body. The characteristic endoscopic findings of intestinal BD are mainly a single or a few large round or ovoid deep ulcers limited to the ileocecal region. The edge of the ulcer is elevated compared with the surrounding area; the boundary with the surrounding normal mucosa is clear, and the ulcer base is covered by thick exudate. In the small intestine, erythema, erosion, and ulcers can be observed. Differentiation of intestinal BD with inflammatory bowel disease, especially Crohn's disease, is occasionally challenging because these diseases are similar in many aspects including genetic factors, clinical features, and treatment. In diagnosing intestinal BD, the presence of symptoms of systemic BD and typical endoscopic lesions is important. The goal of treatment is to induce and maintain clinical remissions to reduce complications, the need for surgery, and hospitalization, as well as to improve the quality of life. 5-ASA, steroids, immunomodulators, and biological agents are used as treatments. In cases of medically refractory disease, surgery may be considered.

References

1. Kim DH, Cheon JH. Intestinal Behcet's disease: a true inflammatory bowel disease or merely an intestinal complication of systemic Vasculitis? Yonsei Med J. 2016;57:22–32.
2. Arimoto J, Endo H, Kato T, et al. Clinical value of capsule endoscopy for detecting small bowel lesions in patients with intestinal Behcet's disease. Dig Endosc. 2016;28:179–85.
3. Jung YS, Cheon JH, Park SJ, Hong SP, Kim TI, Kim WH. Long-term clinical outcomes of Crohn's disease and intestinal Behcet's disease. Inflamm Bowel Dis. 2013;19:99–105.

4. Remmers EF, Cosan F, Kirino Y, et al. Genome-wide association study identifies variants in the MHC class I, IL10, and IL23R-IL12RB2 regions associated with Behcet's disease. Nat Genet. 2010;42:698–702.

5. Park MJ, Lim JS. Computed tomography enterography for evaluation of inflammatory bowel disease. Clin Endosc. 2013;46:327–66.

6. Cheon JH, Shin SJ, Kim SW, Lee KM, Kim JS, Kim WH. Diagnosis of intestinal Behcet's disease. Korean J Gastroenterol. 2009;53:187–93.

7. Cheon JH, Kim ES, Shin SJ, et al. Development and validation of novel diagnostic criteria for intestinal Behcet's disease in Korean patients with ileocolonic ulcers. Am J Gastroenterol. 2009;104:2492–9.

8. Lee SK, Kim BK, Kim TI, Kim WH. Differential diagnosis of intestinal Behcet's disease and Crohn's disease by colonoscopic findings. Endoscopy. 2009;41:9–16.

9. Cheon JH, Han DS, Park JY, et al. Development, validation, and responsiveness of a novel disease activity index for intestinal Behcet's disease. Inflamm Bowel Dis. 2011;17:605–13.

10. Cheon JH, Kim WH. An update on the diagnosis, treatment, and prognosis of intestinal Behcet's disease. Curr Opin Rheumatol. 2015;27:24–31.

Primary Intestinal Lymphangiectasia

Young Kwan Cho

Introduction

Primary intestinal lymphangiectasia was first reported by Waldmann et al. in 1961 as "idiopathy hyperplasia." [1] Waldmann et al. reported 18 cases and proposed the term "intestinal lymph-adenopathy" for diseases with loss of gastrointestinal protein and expansion of the lymphatic vessels in the mucosa of the small intestine. Intestinal lymphangiectasia is a rare disease that causes obstruction of lymph drainage owing to pressure increase in the lymphatic drainage of congenital anomalies or barriers. Elevated pressure in lymphatic drainage causes dilatation and rupture of lymphatic vessels, as well as leakage of lymph [2]. As lymph fluid consists of protein, fat, and lymphocytes, its leakage leads to hypoproteinemia, hypoalbuminemia, hypogammaglobulinemia, and lymphocytopenia. Therefore, intestinal lymphangiectasia is often referred to as protein-losing enteropathy [3].

Definition

Primary intestinal lymphangiectasia is characterized by abnormal dilatation of the gastric mucosa, submucosa, or draining lymphatic vessels. Lymphatic fluid, which is rich in plasma protein, hemoglobin, and lymphocytes, flows into the intestinal tract and causes edema, diarrhea, ascites, peripheral edema, and lymphocytopenia.

Pathophysiology

The pathophysiology of primary intestinal lymphangiectasia is hypothesized as follows: plasma protein is excreted through the mucosal epithelial

Y. K. Cho (✉)
Division of Gastroenterology and Hepatology, Department of Internal Medicine, Gangnam CHA Medical Center, Seoul, South Korea

© Springer Nature Singapore Pte Ltd. 2022
H. J. Chun et al. (eds.), *Small Intestine Disease*, https://doi.org/10.1007/978-981-16-7239-2_53

cell gap because of increased lymphatic pressure, and lymphatic fluid leaks into the intestinal tract with rupture of the enlarged lymphatic mucosa; however, the exact pathophysiology is unknown [1]. It was hypothesized that vascular endothelial growth factors such as vascular endothelial growth factor receptor-3, LYVE-1, vascular endothelial growth factor-C, and vascular endothelial growth factor-D are associated with lymphangiogenesis [4]. Several studies have suggested genetic susceptibility as a cause of intestinal lymphangiectasia and postulated that FOXC2 gene mutation, pik3ri gene deletion, and chromosome 4 deletion are involved [4].

Classification

Intestinal lymphangiectasia is classified into primary intestinal lymphangiectasia and secondary intestinal lymphangiectasia (Table 1). Primary intestinal lymphangiectasia is caused by congenital anomalies of the lymphatic vessels and can be diagnosed by excluding the underlying disease-causing secondary intestinal lymphangiectasia. Primary intestinal lymphangiectasia tends to occur in pediatric and young adults. The Von Recklinghausen, Turner, Noonan, Klippel-Trenaunay, and Hennekam syndromes are associated with primary intestinal lymphangiectasia [2]. Secondary intestinal lymphangiectasia is caused by an underlying disease that increases lymphatic occlusion or pressure in the lymphatic vessels. Secondary intestinal lymphadenopathy is especially caused by heart failure due to right-heart dysfunction, chemotherapy, and retroperitoneal lymph node enlargement due to infection in adults. Secondary lymphangiectasia is caused by liver cirrhosis, portal hypertension, or hepatic venous drainage disorders due to high pressure in lymph drainages. Further, secondary lymphangiectasia is caused by infections such as mesenteric tuberculosis, neoplasms involving the mesenteric lymphatic vessels, or malignant tumors associated with mesenteric sarcoma. In addition, secondary lymphangiectasia is caused by chronic pancreatitis with pseudocysts, Crohn's disease, and Whipple's disease [4].

Symptoms

Primary intestinal lymphangiectasia has variable clinical manifestations; however, it may also be asymptomatic. The most common symptoms are diarrhea, nausea, and vomiting. Hypoalbuminemia or abnormal lymphatic drainage results in varying degrees of peripheral edema of the lower extremities, face, and external genitalia [2]. Chylothorax or chylous ascites can also occur [5]. Gastrointestinal bleeding and abdominal mass are reported as manifestations of intestinal lymphangiectasia [6, 7]. Tetany due to steatorrhea, hypocalcemia, and hypomagnesemia may also occur. Hypoproteinemia, hypoalbuminemia, hypogammaglobulinemia, lymphocytopenia, hypocalcemia, hypomagnesemia, and reduction of fat-soluble vitamin concentration are observed in blood examination.

Diagnosis

In the presence of excessive protein loss through the gastrointestinal tract due to abnormally enlarged lymphatic vessels, primary intestinal lymphangiectasia can be diagnosed without other underlying diseases [4]. In the past, the amount of radioactive isotopes excreted in feces was measured by collecting stools for several days after the intravenous injection of radioactive isotope-conjugated polymer material; however, this method is no longer used recently owing to the

Table 1 Examination methods for primary intestinal lymphangiectasia

Examination methods for primary intestinal lymphangiectasia
Enteroscopy
Capsule endoscopy
Small-bowel series
Albumin scintigraphy
Ultrasonography
Computed tomography
Lymphangiography
Lymphatic scintigraphy

shortage of stools and the high cost of the procedure. Primary intestinal lymphangiectasia is diagnosed with endoscopic biopsy or on the basis of the pathologic findings of specimens obtained from surgical resection. A typical pathologic finding of primary intestinal lymphangiectasia is an enlarged lymphatic duct containing proteinaceous fluid (Fig. 1) [5]. There are three main endoscopic findings of primary intestinal lymphangiomatosis: scattered white spots, white villi, and mucinous covering [8]. Recently, a case of primary intestinal lymphangiectasia was diagnosed by biopsy during a double-balloon enteroscopy (Fig. 2) [5]. Dual

balloon enteroscopy has the advantage of easy tissue acquisition; however, the procedure takes a long time. Capsule endoscopy has been reported as a diagnostic tool in some studies [4]. Although capsule endoscopy cannot make a pathologic confirmation, it is useful for patients in whom endoscopy is difficult to perform (e.g., pediatric patients) and can help locate lesions to exclude other diseases. Other diagnostic tests include small bowel series, albumin scintigraphy, ultrasonography, computed tomography, lymphangiography, and lymphatic scintigraphy (Table 2, Fig. 3) [5].

Treatment

The primary treatment modality for primary intestinal lymphangiectasia is dietary therapy (low-fat, high-protein, and medium-chain triglyceride diet). Because medium-chain triglyceride is not absorbed through the small intestine but is absorbed into the portal by bypassing the lymphatic vessels, fat intake requires medium-chain triglycerides. Some patients require additional supplementation of calcium, magnesium, and fat-soluble vitamins. If there is no response to dietary therapy, parenteral nutritional support may be helpful. Because dietary therapy is more effective in children than in adults, early diagnosis of primary intestinal lymphangiectasia

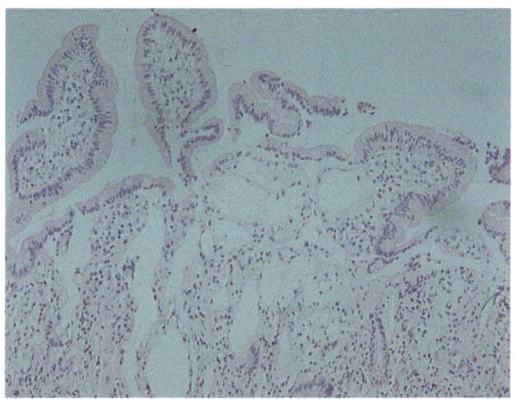

Fig. 1 Pathologic finding of primary intestinal lymphangiectasia: dilated lymphatic duct containing proteinaceous fluid

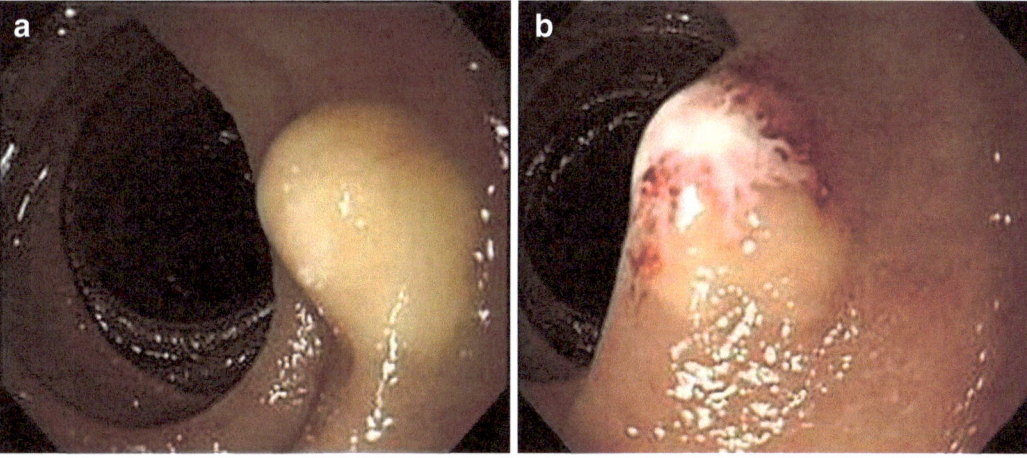

Fig. 2 Enteroscopic findings of primary intestinal lymphangiectasia: (**a**) bulging lesion with white spots; (**b**) lymphatic fluid after biopsy

Table 2 Comparison of primary and secondary intestinal lymphangiectasia

	Primary intestinal lymphangiectasia	Secondary intestinal lymphangiectasia
Cause	Congenital anomaly	Underlying diseases that increase lymphatic occlusion or pressure in the lymphatic system
Associated disease	Von Recklinghausen syndrome	Heart failure due to right-heart dysfunction
	Turnner syndrome	Chemotherapy
	Noonan syndrome	Retroperitoneal lymph node enlargement due to infection
	Klippel-Trenaunay syndrome	Liver cirrhosis
	Hennekam syndrome	Portal hypertension
		Hepatic venous drainage disorders due to high pressure in lymph drainage
		Mesenteric tuberculosis
		Neoplasms involving the mesenteric lymphatic vessels
		Mesenteric sarcoma
		Chronic pancreatitis with pseudocysts
		Crohn's disease
		Whipple's disease

and consistent attention to diet therapy are important for nutrition and growth, especially in children [2]. Octreotide has been reported to be useful in the drug therapy of primary intestinal lymphangiectasia and continuous administration is necessary because discontinuation of octreotide worsens the symptoms [9]. Although the use of antiplasmin therapy, which improves plasma fibrinolysis and increases lymphatic fluid permeability, has been reported, subsequent studies reported contrasting findings [3]. If there is no response to the drug, surgical treatment may be considered. Surgical treatments, such as partial enterectomy, have also been reported [10].

Conclusion

Primary intestinal lymphangiectasia is a rare disease characterized by an enlarged intestinal lymphatic system, which causes lymphatic fluid leakage into the small-intestinal lumen and leads to protein-losing enteropathy. Because lymphatic fluids contain many proteins, fats, and lympho-cytes, lymphatic leaks lead to hypoproteinemia, hypoalbuminemia, hypogammaglobulinemia, and lymphocytopenia. The most common symptoms of primary intestinal lymphangiectasia are intermittent diarrhea, nausea, and vomiting. Lymphoscintigraphy, capsule endoscopy, and enteroscopy are useful for diagnosing primary intestinal lymphangiectasia. Primary intestinal lymphangiectasia is confirmed on the basis of pathologic findings obtained by endoscopic biopsy or surgery. The pathologic findings include enlargement of the lymphatic vessels of the mucosal and submucosal layers, including proteinaceous fluid. The primary treatment is a low-fat, high-protein, medium-chain-triglyceride diet, and octreotide has been reported to be useful as drug therapy. If there is no evidence of proteinuria, hepatic dysfunction, or malnutrition in patients with edema and hypoalbuminemia, intestinal lymphadenopathy can be suspected. Owing to the small number of cases of primary intestinal lymphangiectasia, there are limitations in pathophysiologic knowledge and treatment. Future studies are needed to elucidate these issues.

Fig. 3 Lymphangiography: normal lymphangiography findings without lymphatic fluid leakage or obstruction

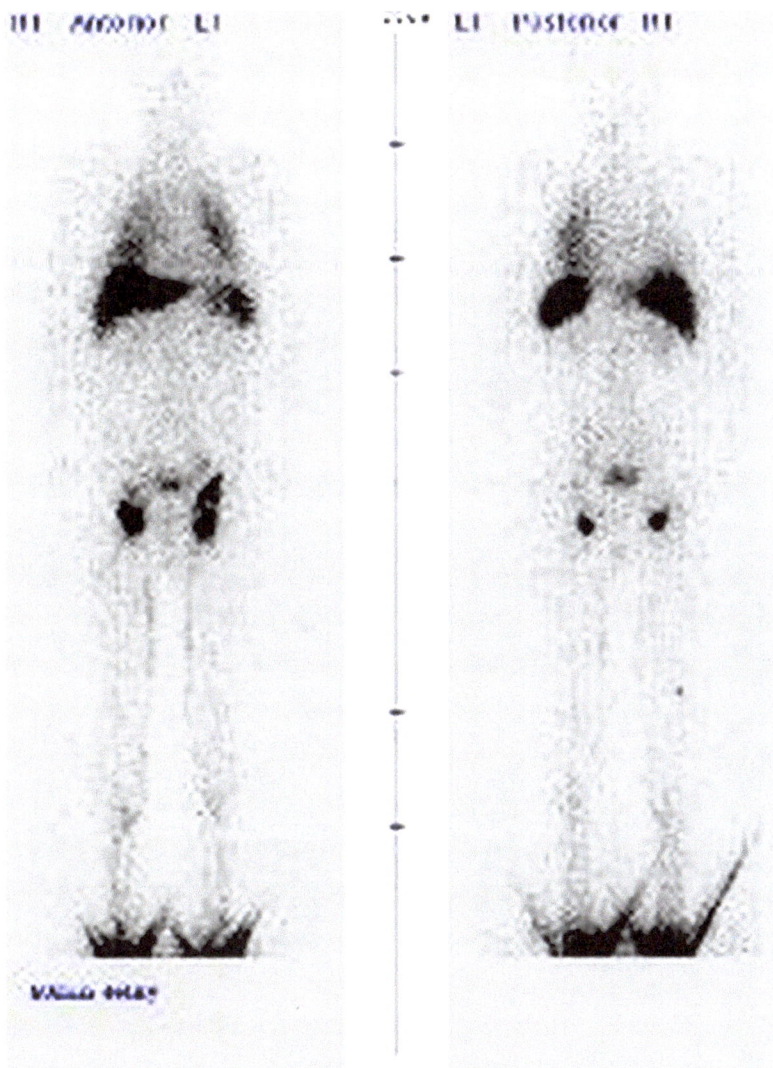

References

1. Waldmann TA, Steinfeld JL, Dutcher TF, et al. The role of the gastrointestinal system in "idiopathic hypoproteinemia". Gastroenterology. 1961;41:197–207.
2. Wen J, Tang Q, Wu J, et al. Primary intestinal lymphangiectasia: four case reports and a review of the literature. Dig Dis Sci. 2010;55:3466–72.
3. Vignes S, Bellanger J. Primary intestinal lymphangiectasia (Waldmann's disease). Orphanet J Rare Dis. 2008;3:5.
4. Oh TG, Chung JW, Kim HM, et al. Primary intestinal lymphangiectasia diagnosed by capsule endoscopy and double balloon enteroscopy. World J Gastrointest Endosc. 2011;3:235–40.
5. Kang HR, Cho YK, Jo YJ, et al. Primary intestinal lymphangiectasia diagnosed by chylous ascites. Korean J Gastroenterol. 2008;87:116–8.
6. Fernandez-Urien I, Carretero C, Division DD, et al. Intestinal lymphangiectasia presenting as abdominal mass. Gastrointest Endosc. 2006;65:522–3.
7. Maamer AB, Baazaoui J, Zaafouri H, et al. A primary intestinal lymphangiectasia or Waldmann's disease: a rare cause of lower gastrointestinal bleeding. Arab J Gastroenterol. 2012;13:97–8.
8. Asakura H, Miura S, Morishita T, et al. Endoscopic and histopathological study on primary and secondary intestinal lymphangiectasia. Dig Dis Sci. 1981;26:312–20.
9. Filik L, Oguz P, Koksal A, et al. A case with intestinal lymphangiectasia successfully treated with slow release octreotide. Dig Liver Dis. 2004;36:687–90.
10. Zhu LH, Cai XJ, Mou YP, et al. Partial enterectomy: treatment for primary intestinal lymphangiectasia in four cases. Chin Med J. 2010;123:760–4.

Index

© Springer Nature Singapore Pte Ltd. 2022
H. J. Chun et al. (eds.), *Small Intestine Disease*, https://doi.org/10.1007/978-981-16-7239-2